"*Outrageous Practices.* And that is not even the sl
—Oprah Winfrey, *The Oprah Winfrey Show,* Oc...

"A valuable resource for anyone concerned with women's health issues . . . An illuminating and compelling call for a new sort of women-friendly health movement."
— *The Washington Post*

"The medical industry gets the microscopic treatment in a scathing new book certain to enrage—and educate—women and their caregivers. Medical journalists Leslie Laurence and Beth Weinhouse expertly chronicle a murky medical underworld of rampant gender bias, systematized discrimination, and pervasive neglect in women's health care in *Outrageous Practices,* an eye-opening look at medicine's treatment of women during the past two centuries."
— *San Francisco Examiner-Chronicle*

"This book is a 'must read' for all women who want documentation of the beliefs they harbor about gender bias. The details are well organized and clearly written. If every medical student and physician who treats women would read this book, we'd see a dramatic improvement in the quality of care we receive."
—National Council on Women's Health

"A comprehensive, meticulously detailed exposé that is destined to mobilize female health-care consumers and prove beyond a doubt that sexist medicine is bad science."
— *Connecticut Post*

"This book will make you mad, but far more important, it will make you aware of what you can do to protect your own health in a biased world."
— *Women's Sports and Fitness*

"*Outrageous Practices* provides ammunition for a vigorous movement by women to demand equal health care." —Barbara Reynolds, *USA Today*

"Self-care is ultimately the best care, and the basis of self-care is following some simple and basic fitness rules: eat healthy, exercise regularly, release stress on a daily basis and find a doctor who has read *Outrageous Practices.*"
— *Houston Chronicle*

"What could, in less-skilled hands, have been a shrill attack is in fact an admirably restrained and thorough examination of how the medical establishment has treated women as patients, as research subjects, and as health care providers . . . Comprehensive analysis, well presented and well documented."
— *Kirkus*

"An up-to-date, comprehensive report on the state of women's health care in the U.S."
— *Publishers Weekly*

OUTRAGEOUS PRACTICES

How Gender Bias
Threatens Women's Health

Leslie Laurence and

Beth Weinhouse

Rutgers University Press
New Brunswick, New Jersey, and London

Library of Congress Cataloging-in-Publication Data

Laurence, Leslie.
   Outrageous practices : how gender bias threatens women's health /
Leslie Laurence, Beth Weinhouse.
     p.   cm.
   Previous ed. published in 1994 with subtitle: The alarming truth
about how medicine mistreats women.
   Includes bibliographical references and index.
   ISBN 0-8135-2448-2 (alk. paper)
   1. Sex discrimination in medicine. I. Weinhouse, Beth.
II. Title.
R692.L38 1997
362.1'082—dc21   97-12096
                                 CIP

British Cataloging-in-Publication information available

First published in paperback in the United States by Rutgers University Press, 1997
First published in cloth in the United States by Ballantine Books, a division of Random House, Inc.,
New York, and simultaneously in Canada by Random House of Canada Limited, Toronto, 1994

Grateful acknowledgment is made to the following for permission to reprint previously published material:

Katherine Fong: Excerpts from "Government Ignores Women's Breasts," *SF Weekly*, March 3, 1991.

Grove/Atlantic, Inc.: Excerpts from *Women and Doctors* by John M. Smith, M.D.
Copyright © 1992 by John M. Smith, M.D. Reprinted by permission of Grove/Atlantic, Inc.

Journal of the American Medical Association: Excerpts from "A Few Words of Advice from a Woman
of Letters—Ann Landers," by Dennis L. Breo, *Journal of the American Medical Association*, 268.14
(1992): 1930–31. Copyright © 1992 American Medical Association.

Ms. Magazine: Excerpt from "Breast Cancer Prevention: Diet vs. Drugs," by Susan Rennie, *Ms.*, May/
June 1993. Excerpt from "What Menopause, Again?" by Margaret Morganroth Gullette, *Ms.*, July/
August 1993. Reprinted by permission of *Ms. Magazine*, © 1993.

Donna Stewart: Excerpts from "Environmental Hypersenstivity Disorder, Total Allergy and 20th
Century Disease: A Critical Review," by Donna Stewart, *Canadian Family Physician*, V. 33, 1987.

Universal Press Syndicate: Excerpts from "Her Health" by Leslie Laurence.

Manufactured in the United States of America

CONTENTS

FOR STEVEN JENKS FORBIS
AND
DAVID GALEF

PREFACE TO THE PAPERBACK
EDITION

In September 1996, five years after women's health muscled its way onto the national agenda, and almost two years after the hardcover publication of *Outrageous Practices*, the federal Office of Research on Women's Health (ORWH) held a little-publicized meeting in Philadelphia to assess the state of women's health research and chart a course for the twenty-first century. That ORWH director Vivian Pinn, M.D., was able to bring together more than 150 top M.D. and Ph.D. researchers and public health officials for the two-day conclave was testament to the continued strength of women's health as a medical and political issue. But while women's health hasn't retreated, the sobering conclusion of the meeting was that it hasn't sufficiently advanced either. When it comes to medical research and care, women are still receiving short shrift.

Heart disease remains the classic example. "We've come almost nowhere in developing diagnostic criteria for women," said Suzanne Haynes, Ph.D., assistant director for science at the U.S. Public Health Service's Office on Women's Health, during one of the breaks. "The whole issue of why women die more frequently than men within the first month after a heart attack . . . , the answer's still not there."

At a session on reproductive health, Ruth Merkatz, Ph.D., of the Food and Drug Administration's Office of Women's Health, told colleagues, "We still don't understand the concept of childbirth."

"We've made progress in preventing neonatal death but we haven't made progress in preventing preterm delivery," said Roberta Ness, M.D., of the University of Pittsburgh's School of Public Health.

"We don't have a good screening method for ovarian cancer," noted Edward Trimble, M.D., of the National Cancer Institute's Division of Cancer Treatment and Diagnosis. "And we don't know enough about assisted reproductive technology and the risk of ovarian cancer."

Experts were dismayed that there were few alternatives to hysterectomy for women with benign uterine conditions such as fibroids. And they lamented the fact that fifteen years into the AIDS epidemic women were still without a vaginal microbicide, a tasteless, odorless compound they could use without their partners' knowledge to protect themselves against sexually transmitted diseases, including HIV. Indeed, in session after session, one message came through loud and clear; you could drive a gurney through the knowledge gaps in women's health.

Emil Skobeloff, M.D., of Philadelphia's Allegheny University of the Health Sciences, argued that it was unrealistic to have expected answers to all these questions in just five years, and suggested that the study of women's health be considered a one-hundred-year project. But women don't necessarily have the luxury of time. The Year of the Woman, 1992, has long since passed, and with researchers competing for less federal funding, women's health issues are in danger of being relegated to the back burner once more.

Since the publication of *Outrageous Practices* in 1994, a new backlash has been threatening women's hard-won gains. At a November 1995 meeting with the Food and Drug Administration, drug company executives balked at the idea of including women in very early clinical trials, the stages at which a drug's basic safety and initial effectiveness are determined, despite two FDA guidelines calling for data on women.

Some pharmaceutical companies are taking a particularly insidious tack: pressuring researchers into conducting gender-biased studies. Investigators at the Philadelphia meeting said they were aware of drug companies that were intentionally designing studies to discourage women from enrolling—for instance, by requiring reproductive-age women to be sterilized or use two forms of birth control. The response to any medical center audacious enough to protest such restrictive policies was swift and severe. The drug firm said it would take its grant money elsewhere. "With federal funds dwindling, there's a lot of pressure on academic medical centers to do these studies," said an unhappy FDA source who asked not to be identified.

The FDA hasn't been able to stop this practice because its drug development guidelines have no legislative teeth: they merely lay out the agency's *expectation* that pharmaceutical companies include women in studies of new drugs. In the near future, however, the guidelines may have the force of law. In 1996, the FDA proposed a rule that would allow it to prevent companies from bringing new drugs to market if they didn't have safety and effectiveness data analyzed by gender. But the fact that the pharmaceutical industry still resists these changes, braying that additional analyses will increase the cost of conducting research, shows how far women have to go to achieve equity in health care, even with legislative efforts in place. Until women's responses to drugs are adequately studied, women's health will continue to suffer.

Medical education is also experiencing a backlash against women, as evidenced by the recent attempt to integrate women's health into the standard curricula. At a meeting of the Council on Graduate Medical Education—an independent body to advise Congress and the Department of Health and Human Services about requirements for physicians—some male medical school deans greeted the attempt to discuss implementing women's health into their curricula by asking, "But what about *men's* health?" as if medical education was somehow biased against them. And that attitude trickles down to the students. Where women's health has been added to the curriculum, it is not unheard of for students to protest the additional course requirements.

Attempts to point out gender bias in medical textbooks have also been met with outrage. In a 1994 study in the *Journal of the American Medical Association* (*JAMA*), five women researchers noted that in physical diagnosis textbooks, females were portrayed in nearly three-quarters of the illustrations relating to reproduction, but only 9 percent of nonreproductive depictions. This reinforces the idea of women as vessels of reproduction and conveys the message that the male body is the norm, the female body an anomaly.

Anyone familiar with the practice of medicine in this country would hardly consider this statement a revelation. But after the study's publication, *JAMA* was deluged with venomous, patronizing letters addressed to the authors. For example:

• "I really wonder why you are getting so steamed up over the gender of illustrations in textbooks. . . . Go away! Get a life!"

• "I can't believe that five women can't find something better to do with their time than writing an article like this. How about shopping?"

• "To take something as simple and honest as an anatomy text and turn it into a fight over gender is ridiculous. . . . May I suggest that your time would be better spent reading or listening to Rush Limbaugh?"

These letters were written by male physicians, outraged by the suggestion of bias in their profession, yet confirming its existence with their protests. The reaction to the article has been so toxic that one of the authors has decided not to include the publication on her resumé, for fear it will hinder a future job search. For most medical researchers, publication in as prestigious a journal as *JAMA* would ensure employment, not jeopardize it. But publicly stating views on women's health can have serious career implications.

Perhaps the most obvious and public example of the backlash has been in Congress, where the battle over reproductive rights continues. In spite of a pro-choice, Democratic president, women's access to abortion is being whittled down thanks to a Republican-controlled legislature with a virulently anti-choice platform. The 1996 Appropriations Bill, by withholding funding, restricted access to abortion for federal workers, military personnel, Peace Corps workers, and women in federal prisons. Just as alarming, the 1996 Congress voted, for the first time ever, to criminalize a specific abortion procedure. The procedure, called intact dilation and extraction (or sometimes partial birth abortion), is a relatively uncommon method used in late-term abortions, often when the fetus is severely deformed or the mother's life is in jeopardy. Although President Clinton vetoed the ban, anti-choice activists have stated their intention to continue targeting late-term abortions and specific abortion techniques. The results of the most recent elections make certain that a Democratic president and Republican Congress will continue their battles over reproductive choice and federal funding in the coming years.

While much about the condition of women's health care in this country remains discouraging, some important changes have been made in the few years since *Outrageous Practices* was first published. New studies are helping to fill in the knowledge gaps in women's health, and new drugs are improving the treatment of some common women's concerns. Some of the most promising developments:

• Postmenopausal women contemplating hormone replacement therapy have received reassuring news on several fronts. Results from the Postmenopausal Estrogen and Progestin Interventions (PEPI) trial found that the combination of both hormones can help prevent uterine cancer while not significantly reducing the cardiovascular benefits associated with using estrogen alone. Data from the Harvard-based Nurses' Health Study confirms this finding. New studies were also published suggesting that estrogen may protect against osteoarthritis and Alzheimer's disease.

• Reproductive-age women concerned about oral contraceptives also received reassurance. An analysis of fifty-four epidemiological studies involving over fifty thousand women with breast cancer and over one hundred thousand healthy women found no long-term increase in breast cancer risk among oral contraceptive users. The study, which included about 90 percent of the worldwide data on breast cancer risk and birth control pills, should allay women's biggest fears about the Pill.

• Continuing genetic research has identified two genes—BRCA1 and BRCA2—associated with the development of breast and (in the case of BRCA1) ovarian cancer. Testing for these genes will enable women who have a family history of the disease to recognize their increased risk and make informed decisions about more frequent screening, preventive medication, or even, in rare cases, prophylactic surgery.

• The FDA has approved Fosamax (alendronate) as an osteoporosis treatment. The medication, a bisphosphonate which prevents bone resorption, also seems to work as a preventative. The drug is a much-needed alternative for women who are at risk of bone loss but prefer not to take estrogen.

• High-tech, automated machinery—Papnet and AutoPap are two examples—has been developed to help analyze cervical cell samples from Pap smears. The new technology should help reduce the number of false-negative results, minimizing deadly delays in treatment for women with cervical cancer.

• Nonsurgical approaches to abortion are inching closer to general use. Experts believe that greater availability of medical (rather than surgical) abortions will not increase the number of abortions, but will decrease the amount of unnecessary surgery performed on women. The abortifacient drug RU-486 (mifepristone) has received conditional approval from the FDA and may be available imminently. And dozens of Planned Parenthood affiliates are participating in tests of a drug combination to induce abortion. The two drugs—methotrexate and misoprostol—are already approved by the FDA for other uses, and are technically available to the public now.

Women have also benefited from action in the legislative and educational arenas.

• Like the National Institutes of Health before them, both the Department of Health and Human Services and the Centers for Disease Control and Prevention have opened offices of women's health to coordinate programs relating to women's health care issues.

• The Accreditation Council for Graduate Medical Education (ACGME) now requires that prospective obstetricians be trained in how to perform abortions. Programs that refuse to include the training may be stripped of their accreditation. (Congress, however, weakened the power of ACGME's new requirement by voting to allow medical facilities that lose their accreditation solely because they refuse to provide training for abortion procedures to retain their federal funding.)

• The medical community, spurred by the American College of Obstetricians and Gynecologists and the American Medical Association, is being encouraged to consider domestic violence as a medical as well as a social issue, and to recognize and treat signs of abuse. Also targeting domestic violence is Congress, which passed the Violence Against Women Act in 1994. This act allocates federal funds for programs aimed at reducing domestic violence, and allows women who are victims of gender-based crimes to sue the perpetrators in federal court.

As these examples illustrate, some legislators and medical professionals *are* making a concerted effort to redress the inequities in health care. Ironically, the next threat to women may come, not from the research community, but from health care administrators. The growth of managed care, which has helped employers slash medical costs by restricting access to services, has tremendous implications for women's health—both negative and positive.

Managed care has the potential to offer women what they have long desired: comprehensive, coordinated care and an emphasis on preventive services. Studies, for instance, show that women who are HMO members are more likely than women with traditional insurance to receive Pap smears and mammograms. Some HMOs have gone so far as to document that they're improving the health of their female members.

Aware that women both use more medical services than men and make the majority of health care decisions for their families, a growing number of managed care companies are targeting services to their women members. Kaiser Permanente in northern California has a program to identify women at high risk for breast cancer and has contributed to studies of the relationship between hormone replacement therapy and breast cancer. Two of its centers are participating in the Women's Health Initiative, the $625 million study of postmenopausal women's health. U.S. Healthcare is taking part in studies of bone marrow transplants for advanced breast cancer. A handful of plans, including Group Health Cooperative of Puget Sound and Harvard Pilgrim Health Care, are teaching their doctors how to screen women for domestic violence. And Oxford Health Plans is covering a wide range of alternative therapies, an area of special interest to women, and intends to introduce a women's health program this year.

While these are all praiseworthy initiatives, other less frequently discussed managed care practices are making it harder for women to get needed services. For example, though nearly 90 percent of managed care plans pay for oral contraceptives (versus about one-third of traditional insurance plans), only 39 percent cover all five major methods of birth control—the Pill, IUD, Norplant, Depo-Provera, and the diaphragm—according to a study by the Alan Guttmacher Institute.

And though three-quarters of plans allow women to see their obstetrician-gynecologists without a referral, about half limit them to a single "well-woman" visit a year. If, during a routine exam, a woman brings up a medical complaint, many HMOs won't let her ob-gyn treat her. She has to see her primary care doctor for a referral and then make another appointment with her ob-gyn. This is more than a nuisance. It can—and sometimes does—delay crucial care.

Perhaps it's no surprise that women in managed care say they're less satisfied with their access to medical services, choice of doctors, and waiting time for routine appointments compared with women who have traditional insurance, according to a survey by the Commonwealth Fund, a New York City philanthropy. Women in managed care are also more likely to say that their doctors don't spend enough time with them.

The reliance on generalists can be especially problematic for women. These days, internists and family physicians are expected to take care of an unprecedented number of problems, from unusual gynecological symptoms to neurological and psychiatric disorders, areas in which they often have no formal training.

In the case of mental health services, which are used more often by women than men, this often results in misdiagnosis and undertreatment. While generalists write at least 70 percent of the prescriptions for antidepressants, studies suggest that they're more likely than psychiatrists to prescribe these drugs at suboptimal doses. They're also more likely than mental health specialists to rely on medication alone—and the wrong medication, in many cases. "I've heard of generalists prescribing tranquilizers for women with depression, which may exacerbate rather than alleviate the condition," says Russ Newman, Ph.D., executive director for professional practice at the American Psychological Association. As a result, women with depression who are denied therapy and pushed to use inappropriate drugs won't get the relief they need.

These practices raise a legitimate question: is managed care's reliance on generalists good for women's health? There are strong hints that the answer may be no. A study of almost 150 internal medicine and family practice residents conducted by researchers at Chicago's Cook County Hospital found that more than 40 percent would not think to provide a healthy woman with information on family planning or German measles immunization, crucial for preventing birth defects should she unexpectedly become pregnant. Generalists were also remiss at counseling women about sexually transmitted diseases, safer sex, and preconception care.

This shocking finding is buttressed by a 1996 Institute of Medicine report that concluded that family practitioners and internists were missing some of the key skills necessary to function the way they are expected to in managed care. Internal medicine residents, for instance, lacked experience in such areas as gynecology and preventive medicine, the supposed bedrock of managed care.

Managed care's policy of getting people out of the hospital as quickly as possible also disproportionately affects women, who receive 50 percent more surgical procedures than men. One hotly debated area involves early maternal discharge: ordering mothers and their newborns out of the·hospital twenty-four hours after a normal delivery and forty-eight hours after a cesarean section (versus 3.9 and 7.8 days respectively in 1970). Perhaps not coincidentally, as hospital stays decreased, the number of infants re-hospitalized with jaundice and dehydration increased. In 1996, President Clinton signed federal legislation designed to halt this practice—although the law won't take effect until January 1, 1998.

"Drive-through deliveries," however, are not the only draconian discharge policies affecting women's health. Doctors are being pressured to send women home so soon after surgery for reproductive tract cancers that they sometimes still have their catheters in place. Some managed care companies have insisted that mastectomies be performed on an outpatient basis. Women can have a breast surgically removed in the morning and be home in time to cook dinner that evening.

It's no wonder women aren't convinced by managed care's feminist rhetoric—that it's protecting them by limiting access to overdone surgeries such as cesarean sections and hysterectomies. What these companies don't say is that while unnecessary or unproven surgeries are being reduced, so are necessary ones. Some managed care companies, for instance, define reconstructive surgery after mastectomy as cosmetic rather than medically necessary and refuse to cover it. Or they pay for the first part of the procedure—the operation to re-create the breast mound—but not subsequent procedures, such as the nipple reconstruction or surgery to adjust the opposite breast so it matches the new one. Even more galling, the same managed care companies that deny breast reconstruction sometimes cover penile implant surgery. "This is outrageously sexist," says Christine Horner-Taylor, M.D., a plastic and reconstructive surgeon in the Midwest. She helped draft legislation, passed in about a dozen states, requiring insurers to cover reconstruction after mastectomy. While managed care has the potential to improve women's health, its restrictive policies and hidden biases will continue to hit women hardest. Unfortunately, the dizzying changes in the health care system—which will become even more pronounced as large numbers of Medicaid and Medicare recipients switch to managed care—combined with the conservative Republican majority in Congress mean that women will have to fight even harder to have their health care needs taken seriously.

ACKNOWLEDGMENTS

It would be impossible to acknowledge each of the nearly four hundred people we interviewed for this book—people who shared their medical expertise, their opinions, or their own medical histories—and the hundreds more who conducted research and wrote scientific reports we relied on for information. All of these individuals are much appreciated.

That said, we would like to single out for recognition a few individuals who were exceptionally generous with their time and knowledge. Our sincere thanks to: Elaine Borins, William Castelli, Frances Conley, Joseph Gambone, Diane Goetz, William Harlan, Florence Haseltine, Janet Henrich, Sherrie Kaplan, Susan Love, Mary Ann Malloy, Kenneth Mayer, Howard Minkoff, Lynn Paltrow, Karen Rothenberg, Ruby Senie, and Jane Sherwood. (And our apologies if we've left anyone out.)

In addition, Sheila Blume, James Goldberg, Maureen Henderson, Margaret Jensvold, Myrna Lewis, Billie Mackey, and Donna Stewart were all gracious enough to take time out of their busy schedules to read portions of our manuscript. Their valuable input helped bring accuracy and clarity to this book.

Our thanks also to the staffs of the following organizations for their help in supplying documents, statistics, and various sorts of information in response to our frequent and varied requests: The Alan Guttmacher Institute, the American College of Obstetricians and Gynecologists, the American Fertility Society, the American Heart Association, the American Medical Association, the American Medical Women's Association, the American Psychiatric Association, the American Psychological Association, the Centers for Disease Control and Prevention, the Center for Reproductive Law and Policy, the Congressional Caucus for Women's Issues, the National Cancer Institute, the National Institute for Allergy and Infectious Diseases, the National Institute of Child Health and Human Development, the National Institute of Mental Health, the National Institute on Aging, the National Women's Health Network, the Office of Research on Women's Health, the Society for the Advancement of Women's Health Research, and the Society for Menstrual Cycle Research. Some of these groups kindly let us sit in on meetings otherwise closed to the press.

Tom Garrigus also helped with much-needed research, and Linda Rattner and Julie Tate were dauntless fact checkers. Pat Volin's efficient, professional fact-checking and research on the completed manuscript certainly helped improve the final product.

Our gratitude also goes to our agent, Suzanne Gluck, who immediately recognized the importance of this project and worked tirelessly to make it a reality; our editor, Joanne Wyckoff, who guided us through the publishing process with calm reassurance; and Andrea Schulz, who kept everything running smoothly throughout.

■ PERSONAL ACKNOWLEDGMENTS

Beth Weinhouse:

My love and thanks to my sister, Amy Weinhouse, for her invaluable legal research and equally valuable emotional support. No one else could have translated abstruse court transcripts and legal articles with such skill and good humor. I am also grateful to my friend, Deborah Schimberg, for her time and research expertise; her hours in the library helped make this a better book.

Much love and thanks go also to my father, Melvin Weinhouse, and my brother, Jerry Weinhouse, physicians in the best healing tradition who care about all their patients, male and female. They have shown me what medicine should strive toward. And much love to my mother, Eleanor Weinhouse, who brought me up to believe that gender is never limiting. Although she wanted a female physician in the family, she has proudly accepted a medical writer instead.

I have also finished this book in better emotional shape than I might have thanks to Jan Goodwin and Linden Gross, long-distance friends who were involved with their own book projects. Our long, commiserating phone conversations helped keep my spirits up during the dark days of approaching deadlines.

Finally, but most important, I want to thank my husband, David Galef, who married me soon after I signed this book contract, and celebrated our second anniversary with me right after the book was finished. In between, he offered the perfect combination of love, encouragement, copy editing, back rubs, professional advice, home-cooked meals, and medicinal hugs. Without him the deadlines would have been much tougher to bear.

Leslie Laurence:
I am particularly indebted to Gail Poulton and Leslie Vreeland, two seasoned journalists whose reporting brought clarity and depth to this project. Words will never be able to sufficiently thank them for their friendship, their endless support, and their professionalism.

A special thanks to Stacey Okun, Jim Brosseau, Daniel Young, John Enright, Harold Goldberg, Clay Terry, John Rittgers, Robin Micheli, Conan Putnam, and Kathleen Harris Maida for their support and for not taking it personally when the final phase of the book took me out of circulation for months at a time.

Eloise Waite offered stimulating conversation and her special brand of hospitality on several of my reporting forays into Washington, D.C. And John and Margaret England and Stu and Cathy Gannes graciously took me into their homes on a reporting trip to San Francisco.

Thanks to Harriet Choice of Universal Press Syndicate for encouraging me to take on the "Her Health" column under the correct theory that it would dovetail perfectly with the book, and to Universal's Lisa Tarry and Alan McDermott for their patience when I pushed deadlines to the limit. I owe a lot to Richard Bussard, my former editor at the *Jacksonville Journal,* who took the time to turn an English major into a reporter.

I'm also grateful for my family's love and support, in particular my mother, Renee Laurence; my sister, Kim Laurence; and my wonderful nonagenarian grandparents, Rose and Joseph Rosner. My brother, Robert Feldman, a caring and compassionate physician, shared his insights about the gender gap in medicine. William Forbis, a top-rate author and journalist, is like a father to me. His unwavering faith in my abilities means more to me than he probably knows.

My heartfelt love and appreciation go to my husband, Steven Forbis, who spent countless hours reading first, second, and third drafts of the manuscript, offering constructive criticism and encouragement. He was a source of solace during an intensely stressful time.

An in memory of Bunny, and to Gorgeous, who showed me the joys of living in the moment.

OUTRAGEOUS
PRACTICES

INTRODUCTION

As health and medical reporters, we have long been aware that women are not always treated with proper respect by their (usually male) physicians. And we know from women physician friends and acquaintances that women in medicine face a great deal of discrimination and harassment. But what we *didn't* know until recently is that women have been excluded from much important medical research. There is a shocking gap between what is known about men's health and what is known about women's. Says Elaine Borins, M.D., a psychiatrist at the University of Toronto, who organized a conference on Gender Science and Medicine in 1990, "A woman who gets a pain and goes to the emergency room is not treated the same as a man. There isn't as much known about what to do for her." Medicine is only as good as the knowledge it's based on, and the best doctor in the world can't compensate for faulty research.

Consider these three outrageous practices:

• In the early 1980s, when the National Institutes of Health set aside money for clinical research on endometriosis, a debilitating condition in which uterine tissue grows inside the abdominal cavity, not a single researcher filed a proposal to utilize those funds. Although endometriosis is not a rare disease—some five million women are affected—most doctors assumed women's excruciating pelvic pain was all in their heads. Why should physicians have devoted precious research time to studying a condition that didn't even exist?

• In 1984, in a required course on human sexuality at the Georgetown University School of Medicine, one of the professors, a male psychiatrist,

3

said that aggression was normal in sexual relations between men and women, and that inhibition of aggression in men could lead to impotence. Another instructor, the head of urology at Georgetown, said that when couples came to him for sex counseling because the woman could not have an orgasm, he reassured them that this was quite normal. According to one of his students, Adriane Fugh-Berman, M.D., now a medical adviser to the National Women's Health Network, "Misinformation about sexuality and women's health peppered almost every course." But how will doctors who bring the misinformation and demeaning attitudes toward women into their clinical practices be able to care for their female patients properly?

• In 1988 a study was published showing that small doses of aspirin could help prevent heart attacks. The research was based on information collected from 22,000 volunteers—all men. When women very sensibly asked if taking aspirin might help them prevent heart attacks, too, their physicians were stymied. There simply were no data to help them make a decision. Yet heart disease has been the leading cause of death in women for most of this century.

In an era of supposed medical enlightenment, the neglect of women's health is only now coming to light. Embarrassed scientists acknowledge the gaping hole in information, but claim that the knowledge gap was a result of inadvertent, benign neglect. But can such neglect be truly termed *benign* when women may die as a result of scientific ignorance?

Researchers claim that it is much more difficult to study women than men. It becomes a challenge to assemble a homogeneous group of women when their hormonal profiles can be so different: they may be premenstrual, taking oral contraceptives, pregnant, menopausal, or taking hormone replacement therapy. The hormones may affect drug dosage, metabolism, and side effects. A pregnancy can make participating in research dangerous. Larger numbers of women are needed in order to obtain meaningful results. Experiments become more expensive. But rather than find a way around these problems to ensure that women are included, scientists have simply taken the easy way out and studied men.

By excluding women from research, scientists seem to be confirming that women's bodies are different and more difficult to study. But then by simply extending their male-drawn conclusions to women, they are implying that—with a few obvious exceptions—women's bodies are the same as men's. In this book we demonstrate why it is so important to look beyond the paradigm of the 70-kilogram (154-pound) male, currently the basis of most medical research and treatment.

Almost no one believes there is a grand, evil, male conspiracy behind the current state of women's health. Says Florence Haseltine, M.D., one of the relatively few ob-gyns at the National Institutes of Health, "I don't think it was malicious or intentional. You want doctors to study what they're interested in, so you have male doctors in their fifties studying other male doctors in their fifties for heart attacks. It was like everything else in our society. Women are second-class citizens, so they are thought of second."

Some of the neglect came out of a misplaced sense of paternalism or protectionism. Since the horrors of the drug thalidomide, which left thousands of children deformed when their pregnant mothers took it in the 1950s to relieve nausea, researchers have avoided exposing women of reproductive age to experimental drugs out of fear of harming a "potential fetus." Yet that means that many new drugs are inadequately studied in women. For instance, when the Food and Drug Administration approved the AIDS drug AZT in 1987, not one of the sixty-three federally sponsored studies had evaluated its effects on women. It should have come as no surprise to clinicians that women were having toxic side effects at the high doses deemed safe and efficacious in men. "The elegant studies on men provide guideposts, but men are different from women," says Howard Minkoff, M.D., professor of obstetrics and gynecology at the State University of New York Health Science Center at Brooklyn. "We can't assume that what we've learned from them is valid for women."

The medical bias extends beyond research; it pervades medicine, beginning with medical-school admissions and education, encompassing research facilities and medical journals, and culminating in how women are treated as patients in clinics, hospitals, and physicians' offices across the country.

Consider these realities about women's health care:

As of this writing, on the eve of health care reform, twelve million American women have no health insurance and millions more have inadequate coverage. Over a twelve-month period more than one-third of 2,500 women in one national survey had not had a Pap smear, pelvic exam, clinical breast exam, or a complete physical, according to the Commonwealth Fund, a private philanthropy.

Women are twice as likely as men to be talked down to by their physicians and told a medical condition is all in their heads. A stunning capper came in 1993 with a study showing that women were less likely to get necessary cancer-screening tests when a physician was male, and particularly if he was an internist or family practitioner. In the Commonwealth study, 41 percent of women—but only 27 percent of men—said they had changed physicians because they were dissatisfied with their care.

So fragmented and inconsistent is women's health care that some advocates are suggesting that women specifically seek out female physicians. Some women have gone even further. Tired of being ignored or humiliated by their male doctors, they are abandoning physicians altogether and seeking health services from nurse practitioners, who teach them how to be caretakers of their own bodies and who view patients as partners, not chattel.

Rhoda Kupferberg, a thirty-four-year-old psychologist, had always been terrified of pelvic exams. Ever since she could remember, she'd been unable to relax when her gynecologist inserted the cold metal speculum. "Sometimes he would yell at me to loosen my muscles," she says. "I felt like crying. I was so tense, I'd bleed for days afterward." Her doctor could have attempted to uncover the source of her discomfort, but he didn't bother. He simply wrote her off as a "difficult" patient.

Then Kupferberg switched to a practice run by nurses. They were the first medical professionals to ask if she had ever been sexually abused. She had. As it turned out, Kupferberg was an incest and rape survivor. Now her terror at having a hard metal object thrust into her vagina made sense. So instead of rushing to perform a pelvic, the nurse practitioner had Kupferberg sit on the examining table in a gown for her first few visits, eventually working her up to the exam. "For the first time in my life I could be examined without pain," says Kupferberg.

We decided to write this book because as health and medical reporters we found ourselves outraged over stories such as Kupferberg's—stories of gender bias, neglect, or discrimination. Our idea was to present these accumulated outrages in a forum where their collective impact could be properly assessed. In this book we've asked—and tried to answer—such questions as:

Why are so many unnecessary surgeries performed on women?

Why is heart disease, the number-one killer of men and women in this country, so under-studied in women?

Why isn't breast cancer a bigger research priority?

Why is most research on women with AIDS designed to protect their unborn children rather than treat the women themselves?

Why has so little research been done on the health issues of postmenopausal and older women?

Why is so little known about the effects of the sex hormones in oral contraceptives and postmenopausal hormone replacement therapy?

Why are women's health concerns more likely to be dismissed as psychosomatic?

Why, in the 1990s, are so many women so dissatisfied with their medical care?

Though it may seem as if there is a glut of women's health books on the market, all of them so far equate women's health with *reproductive* health—contraception, menstruation, pregnancy, menopause, and so on. This is the same mentality responsible for leaving women out of all but reproductive research. But women have bodies beyond those that gynecologists care for. Women's health isn't just PMS, contraception, pregnancy, and menopause. Women have heart attacks, develop colon and lung cancer, get the flu, break their legs. They utilize the health care system more than men and, because they also coordinate the health care for their families, are perfect candidates for preventive health services. But as noted above, even here the medical system fails them. We want to emphasize the vast majority of women's health concerns that are the same as men's but all too often aren't taken as seriously, treated as appropriately, or understood as well.

Until the end of the last century medical science believed that all female health woes stemmed from problems with the reproductive organs. Today, although such theories are relegated to history, modern medicine still seems structured around this belief. Although women have hearts, livers, and lungs in addition to ovaries, fallopian tubes, and uteruses, more than half of all woman see an obstetrician-gynecologist as their primary or even sole health care provider. Just how ludicrous this is becomes obvious if the genders are switched. Who ever heard of a man relying on a urologist or proctologist for all of his health care? Women may have won the right to be seen as more than wives and mothers in society, but in medicine the old beliefs seem to persist.

Specialists tend to look for problems in their area of speciality, so a woman complaining to her ob-gyn of abdominal pain may be tested for reproductive problems when the illness is related to the gastrointestinal tract. Worse, rather than referring women to other specialists, some gynecologists take it upon themselves to treat high cholesterol, prescribe antidepressants, and assess chest pain. Yet when it comes to a service that gynecologists *should* be providing—abortion—even women with private doctors have to

go elsewhere. Most gynecologists are not trained in the procedure, and
even those who are often won't perform it. Gynecology may be the only
medical specialty that allows its residents to choose whether or not to learn
a specific procedure. Could a gastroenterologist decide he doesn't want to
learn how to perform a colonoscopy? Could a radiologist refuse training in
CAT scans?

Also, ob-gyn is a *surgical* subspecialty, which means that surgical remedies for problems are always foremost on doctors' minds. Hysterectomies
and cesarean sections, two controversial and often overdone surgeries, fall
squarely in an ob-gyn's province. Clearly, a training-induced inclination toward surgery, coupled with financial and legal considerations, mean that
these physicians are not always acting in women's best interests. Consider
that approximately one-third of reproductive-age women have uterine fibroids, usually a benign condition, for which the treatment is often hysterectomy. "What benign condition of the adult male genitalia would be
treated with surgical removal?" asks Karen Johnson, M.D., a psychiatrist
who is lobbying for the creation of a new primary care specialty in women's
health.

We also decided to investigate women's health because it seemed like
more than coincidence that every recent health "scandal" has involved
women's health: toxic shock syndrome and tampons, DES, thalidomide, the
Dalkon Shield, breast implants.

It's no wonder that in spite of repeated reassurances by physicians that
certain tests and treatments are safe, women remain skeptical—about the
radiation exposure in mammograms, the cancer risks from oral contraceptives and hormone replacement therapy, the safety of common medications, the necessity of many operations. At a birth control conference in
Virginia, some physicians pooh-poohed women's fears of contraceptive side
effects, but Felicia Stewart, M.D., director of research at the Sutter Medical
Foundation in Sacramento, respected them. Referring to some of these past
health scandals, she said, "We [ob-gyns] do not have a very good history;
our patients remember the procedures and devices we believed were safe,
that turned out later to be harmful."

In the 1970s the feminist movement attacked the medical profession,
advocating that women shun traditional male doctors. The feminists favored special well-woman clinics and "know your body" courses that
taught genital self-exam (using plastic speculums) and even menstrual extraction, which can be used as a form of early abortion. The feminists
urged women to take as much responsibility as possible for their own
health, because by abdicating control of their bodies to physicians, they

thwarted their struggle for equality. Wrote Barbara Ehrenreich and Deirdre English in *Complaints and Disorders*,

> The medical system is strategic for women's liberation. It is the guardian of reproductive technology—birth control, abortion, and the means of safe childbirth. It holds the promise of freedom from hundreds of unspoken fears and complaints that have handicapped women throughout history. When we demand control over our own bodies we are making that demand above all to the medical system. It is the keeper of the keys.
>
> But the medical system is also strategic to women's oppression. Medical science has been one of the most powerful sources of sexist ideology in our culture. Justifications for sexual discrimination—in education, in jobs, in public life—must ultimately rest on the one thing that differentiates women from men: their bodies. Theories of male superiority ultimately rest on biology.

While many of the criticisms the feminists heaped on the medical establishment were valid, in at least one way the feminist movement itself was guilty of what it accused physicians of doing—genitalizing women's health. The feminists focused on contraception, reproductive freedom, and access to safe abortion. They were so focused on the wrongs done in the name of reproductive health, they missed the other big part of the story: They, too, ignored women's bodies from the waist up. It took women *within* the system—people like National Institutes of Health director Bernadine Healy and ob-gyn Florence Haseltine—to blow the whistle and agitate for change.

In the few years since gender bias in medical research has been recognized, a variety of steps have been taken to remedy the inequity. Many new studies have begun, including the enormous Women's Health Initiative, the largest study yet to examine the effects of diet and hormone replacement therapy on cancer, heart disease, and osteoporosis. But a great danger now is the yearning for a "quick fix." Women should resist putting too much pressure on the scientific community for an instant solution. Instead women should demand the same rigorous scientific investigation that has been applied to collecting data on men's health. Studies on women's health should be properly designed and well validated. Otherwise the research is of no value to women.

This book, which starts and ends with the woman *patient*, is divided into three parts. Part I, "Diagnosis: Gender Bias," begins in the 1800s, when women patients were subjected to extraordinary horrors in the name of medical healing, and women who wanted to become physicians faced formidable obstacles. In chapter 2 we chronicle the hardships and sexism that women physicians still face today. Chapter 3 shows how discrimination against women in medicine extends to research, where women's health issues are given short shrift.

Part II, "Second-Class Patients," examines specific medical conditions, such as heart disease, breast cancer, and AIDS, and shows how the male model of medicine jeopardizes women's health care. We discuss how women's reproductive health needs have been marginalized and how such natural life events as childbirth, menopause, and aging have been medicalized. Finally we end the section with a discussion of women's mental health, which is all too often misunderstood and mistreated.

In part III, "Healing the System," we look at outside forces, such as drug marketing and court rulings, that influence women's health care choices. We then examine the interaction between physicians and their female patients and close with our prescription for the future of women's health.

We believe that the time is right for a new women's health care movement. Just as equal work and equal pay galvanized women in the sixties and seventies, and issues of child care and reproductive freedom consumed women in the eighties, health care is promising to become *the* women's issue of the nineties, the "next wave" of feminism. The health care movement of the seventies never went quite far enough. Women can be informed medical consumers only up to a point: they can choose the best physicians and know what questions to ask, but ultimately they and their doctors are limited by what has been studied and what is known. Women should demand that their bodies, their illnesses, and all of their health care needs receive equal funding, equal attention, and equal study.

1

DIAGNOSIS: GENDER BIAS

1

A BRIEF HISTORY OF
MEDICINE
A Legacy of Ignorance

Despite the physicians' maxim to "first do no harm," the history of medicine contains some rather gruesome "treatments" inflicted in the name of healing. Bleedings, purgings, and massive doses of toxic substances were given to both men and women in an attempt to cure what ailed them. Until well into the last century the "cure" was often worse than the disease. But the history of *women's* health care—particularly gynecological and obstetric care—is especially shameful. There were unique horrors visited on women because they were "the other," because few women were included in research and medical practice (except for the midwives, whose reign ended over one hundred years ago), and because there were few voices with the authority to protest effectively.

The roots of gender bias in modern medicine can be most clearly traced to the early 1800s. That was the century when physicians largely replaced midwives in caring for pregnant women, the century when many types of gynecological surgery were developed . . . and then overused, the century when women began to protest the inequities in their care. Unfortunately many of the wrongs they inveighed against persist. To get a full picture of the history of women's health, it is necessary to look at women in their different roles—as patients, research subjects, and health care providers.

■ WOMEN AS PATIENTS

For a good idea of how physicians viewed their female patients during the nineteenth century, consider these quotations from medical writings of the time:

"She [Woman] has a head almost too small for intellect but just big enough for love."

"[It was] as if the Almighty, in creating the female sex, *had taken the uterus and built up a woman around it.*"

"The Uterus, it must be remembered, is the *controlling* organ in the female body, being the most excitable of all, and so intimately connected, by the ramifications of its numerous nerves, with every other part."

"Thus, women are treated for diseases of the stomach, liver, kidneys, heart, lungs, etc.; yet, in most instances, these diseases will be found on due investigation, to be, in reality, no diseases at all, but merely the sympathetic reactions or the symptoms of one disease, namely, a disease of the womb."

"We cannot too emphatically urge the importance of regarding these monthly returns as periods of ill health, as days when the ordinary occupations are to be suspended or modified. . . . Long walks, dancing, shopping, riding and parties should be avoided at this time of month invariably and under all circumstances. . . . Another reason why every woman should look upon herself as an invalid once a month, is that the monthly flow aggravates any existing affection of the womb and readily rekindles the expiring flames of disease."

"[We must recognize] the gigantic power and influence of the ovaries over the whole animal economy of women—that they are the most powerful agents of all the commotions of her system; that on them rest her intellectual standing in society, her physical perfection."

As these passages show, many physicians seemed to see their female patients as collections of reproductive organs, with everything else quite incidental. Scientists believed that individuals had a fixed amount of energy, and that men should direct it toward their work and women toward reproduction. Any other activities that women engaged in, whether intellectual, sexual, or athletic, would jeopardize their reproductive capabilities.

Some physicians believed the uterus was the female body's controlling organ, while others gave that authority to the ovaries. But for all, almost nothing could go wrong in the body without the reproductive organs being blamed. Physicians who attended the forty-fourth annual meeting of the American Medical Association in 1893 heard a lecture listing the five principal causes of the diseases of women: (1) imperfect development of the sexual organs, (2) gonorrhea, (3) septic inflammation following childbirth, (4) lacerations due to childbirth, and (5) miscellaneous causes including constipation, erroneous habits of life, and errors of dress.

Women's psyches, too, were seen merely as an extension of their reproductive capabilities. Doctors at that same conference also heard a lecture about "lactational insanity," a madness that affected nursing mothers.

To cope with the fact that women's maladies had different causes than men's, doctors developed a double repertoire of remedies. Men with a sore throat or headache received treatments aimed at the appropriate body part, while women with these complaints and others—indigestion, curvature of the spine, fatigue, and depression—had therapies aimed at the ovaries or uterus. Possible cures included leeches applied to the vulva (to treat amenorrhea), strong chemicals injected into the uterus, even white-hot iron instruments inserted into the vagina to cauterize the cervix.

Menstruation, pregnancy, and menopause—the most normal of life events for women—were also seen as illnesses. Women were advised to stay in bed every month during their periods to preserve their health. Uppermiddle- and upper-class women were told that the slightest exertion could be risky. (Working-class women, on the other hand, were never advised to take days off from factory jobs or other unskilled labor.) When physicians noticed that women with tuberculosis were not menstruating, they concluded that TB was the result of menstrual problems, rather than the other way around.

Even singing while menstruating could be hazardous. Just over one hundred years ago in the *Journal of the American Medical Association*, then as now a preeminent medical journal, there was an article entitled "Impairment of the Voice, in Female Singers, Due to Diseased Sexual Organs." It stated, "When we consider the intimate connection of the uterus with the great sympathetic nervous system, and the frequent deleterious impression of the stomach, heart and head reflexly therefrom by way of this nervous connection, it is but carrying the same reflex process but one step farther when we assert its reflex influence over the organs of the voice." The author went on to note that if good singers have noticed that their periods adversely affected their singing and tried as much as possible to abstain from singing each month, "then it stands to reason that an inflamed or conjusted [sic] uterus will, at other times, also prejudiciously affect the organs of voice and song. . . ."

This is the part of health history that is most distasteful: the use of the medical, biological, and anatomical sciences to keep women in their place. For instance, in the late 1800s, when science finally came up with the germ theory of disease—blaming illness on poor hygiene and bacteria—it was used as a rationale to urge women to greater heights of cleanliness and good housekeeping. The president of the British Medical Association said that every time he made a house call, he evaluated the cleanliness of the home, because stopping diseases from spreading depended "on the character of the presiding genius of the home, or the woman who rules over that domain."

Perhaps in order to avoid these draconian cleaning standards, affluent women of the late nineteenth century seemed to suffer from one of two then-trendy complaints: hysteria or invalidism. Not surprisingly, since the uterus was one of the body's controlling organs, hysteria became a widespread, almost fashionable disease. The word *hysteria* has the same root as *hysterectomy*, from the Greek word for "uterus." Limited almost exclusively to upper- and upper-middle-class women ages fifteen to forty-five, hysteria caused frenzies of laughing, crying, coughing, sneezing, screaming or fainting. There was no discernible cause and no available treatment. It was Sigmund Freud in this century who finally took "hysteria" away from the uterus and placed the blame squarely on the brain. Yet while Freud's theories removed personality from the reproductive organs, they still tended to blame female problems on the genitals—the absence of the penis. So even into this century women's personalities were still seen to be arising from the gonads, whether their own or the lack of another's.

While some affluent women were agitated and hysterical, others subscribed to the cult of invalidism, which seemed to equate illness with femininity. Women became languid hypochondriacs spending days in bed with headaches, "nerves," or other mysterious complaints. While most of the symptoms were vague, mild, or simply feigned, Barbara Ehrenreich and Deirdre English remind their readers that in many ways women in those days *were* sicker. Tight lacing of corsets, arsenic nipping, maternal mortality, repeated pregnancies and gynecological complications at delivery (such as prolapsed uterus and irreparable pelvic tears) contributed to poor health. And for many women, the real or imagined illness of invalidism was a legitimate excuse for avoiding sex, childbearing, and housekeeping.

Because the victims tended to be affluent, a host of medical "specialists" sprang up overnight to deal with these mysterious—and lucrative—disorders. The cause, of course, was always the reproductive organs.

Once it became fairly well accepted that women's physical and psychological ills arose from their reproductive organs, it was perfectly logical to begin performing gynecological surgery to treat these ills. In the 1860s some physicians even began removing women's clitorises to treat nymphomania and masturbation. Women may have been seen as bodies wrapped around sex organs, but they were definitely *not* supposed to be sexual beings.

In the second half of the nineteenth century, doctors began removing ovaries to "cure" personality disorders and other ills. Dr. Robert Battey of Rome, Georgia, spoke about "normal ovariotomies"—removal of normal ovaries for nonovarian conditions. Writes G. J. Barker-Benfield, "Among the indications were a troublesomeness, eating like a ploughman, masturbation, attempted suicide, erotic tendencies, persecution mania, simple 'cussedness,' and dysmenorrhea. Most apparent in the enormous variety of symptoms doctors took to indicate castration was a strong current of sexual appetitiveness on the part of women." How ironic that less than a century later women's interest in sex would be considered healthy, and doctors would attempt to treat women for "frigidity." How ironic and sad, too, that a hearty appetite for food was considered pathological, as was a loss of appetite. Social constraints dictated a narrow margin of acceptability in women's behavior.

Not all women accepted these explanations of their symptoms and behavior. Mary Livermore, a women's suffrage worker, spoke against "the monstrous assumption that woman is a natural invalid," and denounced "the unclean army of 'gynecologists' who seem desirous to convince women that they possess but one set of organs—and that these are always diseased."

Many women agreed with Mary Livermore and rebelled against the misogynistic practices of traditional medicine. A popular health movement arose in the mid-1800s similar to the feminist health movement of the 1970s. For instance, nineteenth-century women organized "Ladies Physiological Societies," where groups of women met to receive instruction in anatomy and personal hygiene, with an emphasis on preventive care.

The reaction against the painful and mutilating treatments of the "regular" (also called allopathic, as opposed to homeopathic) doctors included alternative therapies practiced by "irregular" doctors. These alternative therapies included the water-cure movement (also called hydropathy or hydrotherapy), homeopathy, and Thomsonianism (a movement based on herbal cures and common sense). Both men and women were adherents of these popular health movements, but women—perhaps because of the prevailing mood in mainstream medicine—were especially enthusiastic. These philosophies did not see female anatomy as pathological, but natural. And rather than "cure" with mutilation, the irregulars proposed gentle therapies to deal with problems. The regular physicians were scathing in their criticism of these treatments, but as Mary Roth Walsh writes in *"Doctors Wanted: No Women Need Apply,"* "Historians have too often dismissed the irregulars as simply quacks and dogmatists. But in an age when there were few medically valid theories available, no one had a monopoly on medical truth."

Samuel Thomson, who began the movement called Thomsonianism in the 1820s, was a poor New Hampshire farmer who, after watching his wife and mother mistreated by regular doctors, became interested in popularizing the folk medicine he had learned as a child. He felt that these natural remedies could often help, or at least do no harm, whereas the "heroic" measures that regular doctors were using—bloodletting, purging, and large doses of toxic drugs—made both men and women suffer. As an alternative he recommended herbs and cold baths, whole-grain cereals, loose clothing (as opposed to the tight-laced corsets women wore), and exercise.

Water-cure enthusiasts built establishments in the countryside where sick people could stay for days to months, eating wholesome food, breathing fresh air, exercising, taking daily baths, and having regular massages and wet-sheet wraps. These were similar to present-day spas, and then, as now, harried wives and mothers saw these resorts as sanctuaries where they could take a break from responsibilities and put their own needs first.

Also as an alternative to the regular doctors' treatments, Lydia Pinkham's Vegetable Compound, introduced in 1875, won a loyal following. The blend of alcohol and herbs (including Jamaican dogwood, pleurisy root, and dandelion root) advertised itself as stimulating the appetite, quieting quivering nerves, and inducing restful sleep. The tonic was supposed to ease menstrual cramps, pregnancy problems, and menopausal symptoms. With the slogan "Only a woman can understand a woman's ills," the product went on to surpass all other patent remedies in its popularity. In 1883, the year Lydia Pinkham died, sales reached $300,000. Lydia Pinkham's tonic is still being sold in drugstores across America, now primarily as over-the-counter relief for hot flashes and other menopausal symptoms. According to the manufacturer, Numark Laboratories, Inc. in Edison, New Jersey, the formula remains essentially the same, with the addition of vitamins C and E.

The idea of women taking care of women, which Lydia Pinkham exploited, is an ancient one. When it comes to childbirth, female midwives have helped women give birth in almost every culture throughout history—until the last century. The virtual extinction of the midwives at the hands of nineteenth-century male physicians is considered a devastating turning point in the history of women's health.

When midwives attended pregnant women, their approach was to interfere as little as possible. They had relatively few means of dealing with extremely complicated births, but for the healthy majority they provided care and comfort—without harm. Yet late in the last century, as medical organizations grew, physicians began to feel threatened by midwives and jealous of their monopoly over the care of pregnant women.

The physicians began their campaign by convincing middle- and upper-class women, who could afford the services of a physician, that their health would be in jeopardy if they allowed midwives to attend them at birth. The doctors pointed to new knowledge and improvements in obstetric care—for instance, the development of forceps—that were withheld from midwives. Finally, the physicians, with their economic clout and political connections, were able to get licensing laws passed to exclude midwives from practicing. All this, they said, was to protect the health of America's women.

Puerperal infection, also called childbed fever, was the leading cause of maternal death. Although the physicians blamed midwives for the high incidence of these deaths, there is no evidence that the doctors' patients did any better. Doctors attended deliveries dressed in street clothes and worked with unwashed hands, unwashed instruments, and barely rinsed sponges. The hospitals they practiced in were breeding grounds for all kinds of bacteria, and the lack of hygiene meant that germs spread quickly from one patient to the next. The midwives' hygiene may not have been any better, but their patients usually gave birth at home, away from the hospital's quagmire of pathogens.

In the 1800s it was common for doctors to graduate from medical school having never seen a birth, let alone attended one. Nonetheless, physicians gradually drove the midwives out of business, in part by their campaign to influence public opinion, but also by imposing formal training and licensing requirements for practicing medicine.

The physicians' dislike for the midwives had more to do with financial matters than concerns for women's health. They simply did not want to share the relatively easy and potentially lucrative business of delivering babies. If women's health were truly the doctors' main concern, it would have been easy enough for them to share their medical knowledge with the midwives—instructing them, for example, in how to use medicated eyedrops to prevent infant blindness from gonorrhea. Instead, the doctors closed ranks and gradually gained a monopoly on delivering babies.

By the turn of the century, just half of all babies born in this country were being delivered by midwives, and most of these mothers were poor and uneducated, often recent immigrants. Middle- and upper-class women accepted the social pressure to switch to physicians. By 1930 midwives had practically disappeared in the United States, having been outlawed in many states. Today just 4 percent of all births are attended by midwives, although modern nurse-midwives are exceptionally well educated and licensed.

With the midwives' disappearance, women lost more than just female birthing attendants. Midwives in the nineteenth century also taught women about contraception and even, when necessary, provided abortions. As they disappeared—and before women physicians were more than a rarity—women lost control over their own bodies. Feminist health writers Barbara Ehrenreich and Deirdre English wrote in 1978, "With the elimination of midwifery, all women—not just those of the upper class—fell under the biological hegemony of the medical profession."

A lot of the objections that women today have with routine obstetric care—most having to do with the fact that they are treated as if they are ill rather than going through a normal, natural process—developed as a result of midwives being forced out of practice by physicians who convinced the government and the public that "medicalizing" pregnancy was beneficial to women and children. Physicians developed obstetrical tools, such as forceps, to ease difficult deliveries. They began using chloroform and ether as anesthesia during childbirth, a development that women initially hailed (although some physicians refused to use it, since they believed that suffering during childbirth was women's punishment from God). Yet the switch from mostly female midwives to mostly male physicians was hardly an unqualified boon for women's health.

Even the verbs used to describe childbirth illustrate the difference. In the eighteenth century and earlier, midwives used to "catch" babies, implying that the mother was responsible for the birth and that the attendant was merely there to help. Doctors, on the other hand, "deliver" babies, as if without their presence the baby would never arrive.

With the shift from midwife- to physician-attended births, women in this country were conditioned to see themselves as ill every time they carried a child. Medical school teaches doctors to view childbirth as a medical condition that requires "managing." It teaches them to deliver fluids through intravenous lines rather than glasses of water, to attach electronic fetal monitors, and to do routine episiotomies (an incision between the vagina and perineum performed to hasten deliveries, though studies show it is of little benefit). Midwives, on the other hand, see childbirth for the natural process it is. They do not look for problems, but recognize them when they occur and know when referral to another specialist is necessary.

When it came to protecting women's reproductive health, many of the most striking advances were not proposed by physicians but by nurses. Concerned with the mother-and-child death rates, a group of Boston nurses originated the concept of prenatal care in 1901. Until that time pregnant women were not given any medical attention until they went into labor. They ate and drank what they pleased, and if they were poor, they often worked long hours in sweatshops right up until delivery and returned to work soon afterward. If they were wealthy, they were confined to their houses for the last several months of pregnancy, because it wasn't considered proper for a pregnant woman to be seen in public.

The Boston nurses, reacting to the growing body of knowledge on the importance of health care during pregnancy, began visiting some of the women enrolled in the home-delivery service of the Boston Lying-In Hospital. By 1912 these nurses were visiting women an average of three times before delivery, performing physical exams, checking blood pressure, taking urine samples. The idea caught on in other parts of the country, and in areas with these first prenatal programs maternal and infant mortality rates began to decrease. Largely as the result of a similar program in Maryland, for example, maternal mortality declined from sixty deaths per ten thousand live births in 1933 to ten in 1948.

And it was another nurse (and midwife), Margaret Sanger, who spearheaded the campaign for access to contraception in the years before the first World War until the 1930s. She coined the term *birth control* and passed contraceptive information on to as many women as she could, in spite of persecution and prosecution. In 1917 she helped found the National Birth Control League, which eventually became the Planned Parenthood Federation of America.

Most physicians at the time were firmly opposed to the idea of contraception. Dr. Augustus Gardner, professor of clinical midwifery at the New York Medical College, referred to contraception as "detestable practices" and said in 1905 that "all the methods employed to prevent pregnancy are physically injurious" and could lead to degeneration of the womb, "moral degradation, physical disability, premature exhaustion and decrepitude." (The American Medical Association did not mention birth control in its service guidelines until 1970.) Sanger's call for motherhood "based on dignity and choice, not ignorance and chance" could be a rallying cry for women today.

■ WOMEN AS RESEARCH SUBJECTS

Common sense dictates that unless women are included in medical research, they will receive second-class medical care, since physicians will know less about female bodies than male. Recognizing this reality, women today are lobbying to be *included* in medical research. But not too long ago research was thought of as something women needed to be protected from.

A look at the past explains why researchers late into this century adopted protectionist policies and why women now are wary about participating even as they recognize the importance of being included in medical research.

One of the most egregious examples of experimental abuse of women was perpetrated by one of the founders of modern gynecology, Dr. J. Marion Sims. Sims shared the prevailing notion that women's psychology was governed by their sex organs; he performed both clitoridectomies and ovariotomies. But Dr. Sims made his reputation by developing a surgical cure for vesicovaginal fistula, a tear from bladder to vagina that can cause urinary incontinence and considerable discomfort. The tear was a common ailment of nineteenth-century woman, and was usually the result of a complicated delivery. While the women who benefited from Dr. Sims's surgical skills were undoubtedly grateful, those who were his research subjects could not have been. For the four years (1845–1849) Dr. Sims worked on developing his method of surgical repair, he operated on Alabama black slave women who never gave permission for the surgery.

Slave owners brought female slaves who had fistulas to Dr. Sims, because the women in such condition were unable to work. It was the *masters* who gave permission for the operations, not the women themselves. Dr. Sims operated on seven women in this way, some repeatedly. The first woman, named Lucy, was operated on without anesthesia (although anesthesia had been developed, Sims was not aware of it). In excruciating pain, she nearly died afterward of blood poisoning—and the operation was not successful. After each of the operations the stitches became infected and the fistulas remained open. Another woman, Anarcha, endured thirty operations, all without anesthesia, until finally the fistula was repaired when Dr. Sims used silver sutures, which resisted infection.

After word of Dr. Sims's success was circulated, white women came to him for the operation. None of them could endure the surgery because of the pain. Dr. Sims relocated to New York, where he continued his work on indigent Irish women in the wards of New York Women's Hospital. (One of these women, Mary Smith, endured, like Anarcha, thirty operations between 1856 and 1859.) While there's no denying that Dr. Sims's work eventually benefited women with vesicovaginal fistulas, there's also no excuse for experimenting on women without their consent, as if they were guinea pigs rather than people.

Sims also coined the term *vaginismus* to describe an involuntary muscle spasm in the vagina that prevented women from having intercourse. One of his treatments for this condition was to go to his patient's house and etherize her so that her husband could have sex with her unconscious body.

Women, of course, are not the only wronged research subjects in the history of medicine. In this century, researchers battle the legacy of Tuskegee, the notorious U.S. Army study in which black men with syphilis were told they were receiving treatment for the disease but were really given placebos and observed until death.

Less well known in this century is an ethically questionable San Antonio study on contraception. In *The Hidden Malpractice* Gena Corea describes the "research." "Dr. Joseph Goldzieher of the Southwest Foundation for Research and Education . . . wanted to see if the nausea, headaches and depression [contraceptive] Pill-users often experienced were real or 'psychological.' So, in 1971, he experimented with 398 Chicano women in San Antonio, Texas. Of these women, seventy-six who thought they were getting contraceptives were given placebos instead. Ten became pregnant within months.

"The contempt Dr. Goldzieher had for these women revealed itself in a statement he made in defense of his experiment. 'If you think you can explain a placebo test to women like these, you never met Mrs. Gomez from the West Side,' he told *New York Post* reporter Barbara Yuncker." Goldzieher's disdain for the women he studied didn't seem to perturb the scientific community. In a footnote Corea goes on to note that the NIH Center for Population Research continued to fund Dr. Goldzieher's work until 1974.

Even more recently, in 1989, *The Nation* reported a study of prostitutes in the Philippines. These women were servicing U.S. military men stationed at Subic Bay Naval Base. Not surprisingly, given their line of work, many developed AIDS. After diagnosis most of the women were given basic information about the disease, although no counseling or medication. However, one group of eight HIV-positive women was singled out for special observation. These women were told nothing about what their diagnosis meant. Instead they were employed by the city government as clerks, given job-training classes, and encouraged to plan for the future. They were then watched to see the value of positive thinking on the course of the disease.

It's no coincidence that all of these horrifying studies were done on women (and men) of color. Physicians report that today minority men and women are especially reluctant to participate in medical research. Suspicions run so high that at a recent NIH-sponsored conference on recruiting and retaining women for clinical trials, one doctor reported that African-American men and women involved in a study at his clinic sometimes refused to partake the free refreshments because they did not believe they were safe to eat. Given the history of medical research, who can blame them?

■ WOMEN AS DOCTORS/HEALERS

Today most people take women doctors for granted, but as recently as 1970 less than 8 percent of all U.S. physicians were women (only South Vietnam, Madagascar, and Spain had a lower percentage of female M.D.s).

Modern women are not the first, however, to enter careers in medicine. In the Victorian era, when delicate sensibilities prevailed, many women preferred their physicians to be female. In 1896, 33 percent of the students at Johns Hopkins Medical School were women (although across the country only 5 percent of physicians were women at the turn of the century).

In spite of Victorian attitudes women had to fight for their admittance to the profession. Books such as *Sex in Education; or, a Fair Chance for the Girls*, by Dr. Edward H. Clarke, argued that women could not be educated along with men because working during their menstrual periods would jeopardize their fertility and general health. Girls, he said, needed to "concentrate" on developing their reproductive organs between the ages of fourteen and eighteen, and then for several days a month afterward. "There have been instances, and I have seen such, of females in whom the special mechanism we are speaking of remained germinal—undeveloped. It seemed to have been aborted. They graduated from school or college excellent scholars, but with undeveloped ovaries. Later they married, and were sterile."

He advocated a separate education for boys and girls, although he did not address the problem of how girls' schools could ever function given that, to preserve their health, girls were not to attend classes or work during their periods. Since girls don't menstruate on the same schedule, it's difficult to imagine how any teaching or learning could take place, with different girls missing different weeks each month. Dr. Clarke also didn't speculate on how women could ever become medical professionals if they had to be unavailable to their patients while menstruating each month.

According to Dr. Clarke, overeducated women not only lost reproductive function, they even failed to grow breasts. He describes one studious young female patient as being so flat-chested because of her education that "the milliner had supplied the organs Nature should have grown." This young woman was lucky, however; at least she didn't die. According to Dr. Clarke, too much studying could even lead to a young woman's death.

Not withstanding Dr. Clarke's dire warnings, there were plenty of women who were called to the medical profession. Some men's objections didn't have to do with concerns over intellectual prowess—even a hundred years ago they knew better—or physical health, but with feminine sensibilities. Men were horrified that women physicians would have to witness disease, surgery, and death (although these sights seemed to be perfectly acceptable when the woman was a nurse). It was the development of anesthesia—ether and chloroform—that helped make the idea of women in medicine more palatable, since doctors would no longer have to hold down their patients and inflict great pain.

Although before the era of medical licensing many women practiced as healers, the title of first female doctor in America belongs to Elizabeth Blackwell, who received her medical degree in 1849. Becoming a doctor was her mission after watching a good friend die of a painful disease (now thought to be uterine cancer) "the delicate nature of which made the methods of treatment a constant suffering to her. She once said to me: '. . . If I could have been treated by a lady doctor, my worst sufferings would have been spared me.' "

Blackwell was refused admittance to twenty-nine medical schools before her final acceptance in 1847 at Geneva Medical College, a small school in upstate New York. The faculty had read the students a letter from a physician urging Blackwell's acceptance and had put the decision to a vote. The students seemed to think the letter was a joke. Yelling "Aye" and throwing their hats in the air, they convinced a stunned faculty—which had assumed the rough country boys would reject the idea of a female classmate—to admit Elizabeth Blackwell.

Once in school, Blackwell met with prejudice and hostility only slightly more overt than what women in medicine deal with today (see chapter 2). Her classmates gave her such a hard time that Blackwell even tried starving herself on the mistaken theory it would prevent her from blushing and embarrassing herself during lectures on the reproductive organs.

Even after Elizabeth Blackwell, admission of women to medical schools was slow. Johns Hopkins Medical School opened in 1893 and agreed to admit women only after several prominent female educators and a network of committed feminists contributed half a million dollars to the institution. Apparently when women loosened their purse strings, men would loosen their admissions policies.

As more women earned their medical degrees, this first generation of female physicians gravitated toward the care of women and children, the fields that would become gynecology, obstetrics, and pediatrics. They were also interested in public health and disease prevention, two big concerns in health care today. "We should give to man cheerfully the curative department, and women the preventative," announced Dr. Harriet Hunt in 1852.

Dr. Amanda C. Price wrote in her 1871 senior thesis at the Women's Medical College of Pennsylvania, "How many men do we find teaching the laws of health . . . ? It seems to be their ambition to cure disease, and very seldom do any of them think it worth their while to teach their patients how to prevent a return of their maladies."

Although small in number, women physicians also served as a tempering influence—they were not enthusiastic about the craze for pelvic and gynecological surgery in the nineteenth century. Mary Walsh quotes a woman physician of the time as saying, "The profession went mad in the direction of gynecological tinkering, womb prodding, and probing, and woman was rarely permitted to have an ache or pain referable to any other part of her anatomy." And in 1894 a disgusted doctor, Mary A. Spink, wrote in the *Woman's Medical Journal,*

> As for the removal of the ovaries the fact is, that women physicians object to the wholesale onslaught upon those innocent organs, which originated with so-called reputable physicians and has been continued by men mountebanks to the degree that nearly every city in the land has several "private homes" or "sanitarioms" [sic] for the purpose of removing those organs, removing them for nervousness produced by a thousand outside causes, removing them because the husbands request it, removing them for everything but disease.

Women in medicine were also attracted to the study of topics that benefited women. In 1876 Mary Putnam Jacobi was the first woman to win the prestigious Boylston Prize from Harvard for the best essay in medicine. Her paper, entitled "The Question of Rest for Women During Menstruation," made a convincing case that rest each month during menses was medically unnecessary. Judging for the competition was blind, and the judges who awarded the prize did not realize the paper had been written by a woman.

Other women physicians set out to prove that women were not physically incapacitated each month, and that there was no reason women couldn't handle the practice of medicine. In 1881 three female physicians on the staff of New England Hospital published a study on 430 women physicians who had graduated from medical school since 1870. They found that only 13 of them complained of poor health, and only 4 of those ascribed their illness to the pressures of medical practice. And only 34 of 307 women who answered a question about menstruation reported that they were incapacitated each month. "We do not think it would be easy to find a better record of health among an equal number of women, taken at random from all over the country," declared the authors.

Other early female physicians who devoted themselves to improving the care of women included Dr. Eliza Taylor Ransom, a Boston physician, best known for her pioneering work early in the century on the "twilight sleep" method of anesthesia for childbirth (scopolamine and morphine).

After a brief heyday in the late 1800s, however, the number of women in medicine declined. One reason was the fading of Victorian delicacy, which meant that fewer women patients insisted on seeing female physicians. Male doctors no longer saw the need to give up half their potential patients to women—and they definitely weren't thrilled with the idea of women physicians caring for men. In the early days of Johns Hopkins Medical School, female doctors were reportedly allowed to examine male patients only from the neck up, even though women in hospital charity wards endured their pelvic exams in full sight of male interns and students.

There was also an institutional backlash. In the face of medical reform and state licensing requirements, many of the all-women's medical colleges that had opened after Elizabeth Blackwell received her degree were closed. By 1903 women's medical colleges had virtually disappeared. And many formerly coed colleges began shutting their doors to women once more. Women professors lost their jobs because the coed schools did not hire them. With their loss, there were no role models for female medical students.

Those medical schools that remained nominally coeducational during the period from the late nineteenth century to the 1920s admitted far fewer women. At Johns Hopkins the percentage of women students dropped from 33 percent in 1896 to 10 percent in 1916. At the University of Michigan the decline was from 25 percent in 1890 to 3.1 percent in 1910. And those women who were fortunate enough to be admitted to medical school still faced enormous obstacles to practicing. Many hospital internship and residency programs refused to admit women to finish their training, even though the states were starting to make hospital training a requirement for licensing.

World War I was a small "break" for women doctors. The war created a demand for physicians, but also cut the supply of young men as many entered the military. Some medical schools began admitting women for the first time. Women physicians also served in World War I, some establishing hospitals in Europe, others working as contract surgeons, although they were not granted military status or benefits. (Some American women physicians volunteered for the French army, which not only accepted them but awarded them the Croix de Guerre for meritorious service under fire.)

At the same time, women already practicing medicine were beginning to chafe at changes in their profession. Medicine was becoming less human and more technological, they charged. In 1930 M. Esther Harding, a psychiatrist, wrote to Bertha Van Hoosen, a prominent female surgeon and founder of the American Medical Women's Association (AMWA), "I have been struck recently more than once at the meetings of a Psychotherapeutic Society. Usually the men lead off with scientifically arranged data, followed by statistics and rather abstract theory. Then presently a woman speaks up and nearly always her voice is raised to remind the group that after all the patient is a human being and not merely the subject of certain symptoms or mechanisms. And this I think is characteristic."

World War II was another break—Rosie the Riveter wasn't the only woman to benefit from the conflict. Thanks to lobbying by the American Medical Women's Association, women physicians were finally allowed to serve in the military. Dr. Emily Barringer, chair of the AMWA committee to secure military commissions, attended the congressional hearings on the Celler and Sparkman bills in support of women serving in the army's and navy's medical corps. She charged that the military was not making the best use of American doctors. Medical historian Mary Roth Walsh writes, "Noting that the army had taken some of the most skillful male obstetricians abroad and left at home some of the best female plastic surgeons, Barringer dryly added that if there was one type of operation that soldiers did not need, it was a cesarean section. Finally, on April 16, 1943, President Roosevelt signed into law the Sparkman-Johnson Bill enabling women to enter the Army and Navy Medical Corps."

The immediate result of this victory was that the percentage of women medical students rose from 4.5 percent of the 1942 entering class to 14.4 percent in 1945. Even Harvard finally broke down and voted to admit women to the 1945 freshman class. Yet there was another backlash after the war as women physicians lost their jobs to make way for returning men.

It wasn't until 1970 that aspiring women physicians had their next big break. In 1970 Congress' Special Subcommittee on Education, Discrimination Against Women, cited a survey in which admissions officers in nineteen of twenty-five northeastern medical schools admitted that they accepted men in preference to women unless the women applicants were demonstrably superior. In October of that year the Women's Equity Action League (WEAL) filed a class-action suit against every medical school in the country. The result was a sharp and immediate increase in the number of women medical students. Between 1970 and 1975 the number of female medical students tripled, and today 40 percent of medical students and 18 percent of practicing physicians are women.

While the 1970 suit was a victory for women, it did not mean instant enlightenment for men. Women physicians still had to contend with the same Victorian sensibilities that worried about reconciling women's "feminine" nature with the harsh world of medicine. In 1974 the *New England Journal of Medicine* published excerpts from letters recommending women to the intern selection committee at a California hospital. They included the following: "Patty is an attractive, mature, personable young lady who is a pleasure to have around and who has no 'hang-ups' sometimes associated with female physicians." "Nancy proved to be a very pleasant and friendly individual who is delightfully feminine at all times." "Ms. ———— is intelligent, mature, pleasant, and dependable—she is also an excellent cook." Old stereotypes die hard.

Certainly there have been gains in the last two decades for women in medicine. Some of that has to do with a changing medical profession. As physicians become more regulated and less independent, as they lose some of their prestige and godlike status, as health reformers attempt to cap their pay, the way is opened for women. But the path still isn't easy. As women physicians gain in numbers, they suffer a backlash of sexual harassment and discrimination on the job (see chapter 2) not much different from that reported by Elizabeth Blackwell over a hundred years ago.

■ GENDER BIAS PAST AND PRESENT

There is unfortunately a clear path from the ignorant attitudes about women's bodies prevalent in the last century to the ignorant attitudes that exist today. A century ago physicians removed women's ovaries to treat a variety of unrelated complaints. They believed women's reproductive organs were responsible for almost everything that can and did go wrong with the human body. How much has changed? Recent medical students say that, during anatomy lectures on the female reproductive system, lecturers take pains to describe the female reproductive system as inefficient, badly designed, and prone to problems. Since doctors are supposed to fix body problems, how much of a leap is it to the case of Dr. James C. Burt, of Dayton, Ohio, who took it upon himself to redesign women's anatomy with surgery? For twenty-two years, until he relinquished his medical license in 1989, Dr. Burt operated on more than four thousand women, many without permission. He rearranged their sexual organs because he believed that women's bodies were "functionally inadequate" for sexual intercourse and that his "love surgery" would cure them. Instead he left women mutilated, in pain, and sexually impaired. Although no longer practicing medicine, Dr. Burt still faces dozens of malpractice suits.

We may be horrified by the "ovariotomies" and "clitoridectomies" of the nineteenth century, but what of the hundreds of thousands of unnecessary hysterectomies being performed today (not to mention the clitoridectomies performed on young girls in some Muslim countries)? Nearly 550,000 hysterectomies are performed in the United States each year, making hysterectomy one of the most common operations of all. Yet the vast majority of these operations are elective, not lifesaving. When the American College of Obstetricians and Gynecologists recently announced its wish for ob-gyns to become the primary-care physicians for postmenopausal women, one woman doctor retorted, "If they want to do that, they're going to have to leave some organs in first."

How far have we really come from the days when women were told their psychological symptoms were due to physical problems and their reproductive organs were removed as a cure? Today women are frequently told that their very real physical symptoms—chest pains, menstrual problems, endometriosis, gastrointestinal pain—are psychological, and are handed a prescription for antidepressants or tranquilizers.

The medical textbooks of the 1800s may seem laughably ignorant today, but as recently as the 1970s physicians were being taught that morning sickness was caused by a woman's resentment at being a mother, PMS was also a psychological disorder, and menopause represented the end of a woman's usefulness in life. And the doctors who were trained with those textbooks are still practicing medicine.

Instead of putting today's inequities in perspective, the examples of past abuses of women serve only to show that we haven't come as far as we thought.

It's also important to remember that medical advances and practices are closely tied to social factors. For instance, when obstetrical anesthesia (ether and chloroform) was introduced in the 1800s and then improved in this century ("twilight sleep" and then spinal or epidural anesthesia), women hailed the developments. Yet by the 1960s and 1970s many women were spurning anesthesia in favor of natural childbirth.

Safe cesarean sections were also an important factor in reducing maternal and fetal death rates. For most of the 1800s women whose deliveries were difficult or whose babies were too large had no choice but to sacrifice the child—physicians had to deliver the child piecemeal to save the mother's life. Now cesareans are considered so safe that almost one-quarter of the babies born in this country are not delivered vaginally, far more than can be explained by the rate of complications. And women are making known their displeasure with the overuse of this medical advance, too.

The same issues that course through the history of medicine with regard to women are still unresolved, the same general sexism and "genitalization" of women occurs, the same prejudice against women doctors and scientists, the same callousness with regard to gynecological surgery. Sadly, the women who participated in the popular health movement of the nineteenth century, and the women who fought to be admitted to medical school, would not be surprised by the inequities in women's health today. In over one hundred years women have still not received the medical educations or the medical care they deserve.

2

SCIENCE AND MEDICINE
Where Are the Women Now?

After a distinguished three-decade career as a neuroscientist, Susan Leeman achieved one of the highest honors in her field. On April 30, 1991, she was among five women and fifty-eight men elected to the prestigious National Academy of Sciences, the private nonprofit agency that advises the U.S. government. Although this award recognized Leeman's important contributions to science, her career nonetheless has been fraught with difficulties.

At Brandeis University in the 1960s, Leeman was never appointed to a full faculty position, despite being honored with a career-development award. After nine years at Harvard Medical School, it became clear that she would not be promoted to tenure there either. Perhaps most telling was the fact that she wasn't turned down for tenure—no one had put her up for it in the first place.

In 1980 Leeman was finally awarded tenure at the University of Massachusetts, but the small slights continued. For instance, the month after being elected to the Academy, the dean of the medical center called her to the library's rare books room where a meeting of an accreditation committee was being held. "I was totally surprised," she remembers. "People seldom asked me my opinion on university matters." But when Leeman arrived, the meeting was over. "They hadn't intended for me to be at the meeting," she later realized. "I was there because I was the first person from the university to be elected to the National Academy of Sciences. If you were a man and had just been elected to the National Academy, you'd expect to have been asked there to comment on a scientific matter, not merely to be an exhibit."

Recently, Leeman was asked to chair a study section for the National

Institute of Mental Health. Normally these scientific panels, which conduct peer reviews of NIH research projects, have a single chairperson, so Leeman was surprised to learn she had a male cochair. "He let me call the first meeting to order and then he quickly took over and actually began running the meeting. He called on the first person, the next person, and the next person. I sat there and thought, 'If I protest I'll look ridiculous, but if I don't do something to regain control, the administrative committee will think I'm a wimp.' So I decided to act as if I had delegated the trivial aspect of running the meeting to him and I would handle the scientific part."

Leeman, now sixty-four, managed to save face. But why, long after having proven herself a stellar scientist, is she still faced with these small competitive putdowns? And why, after all these years, does it still matter to her? "If you were to tell this to a man," she says with a sigh, "he would say you're just being supersensitive. I would hope that I'm in a generation where that kind of behavior is over and younger women have it easier."

If only that were so. A generation later, Kym Chandler, who at thirty-four is young enough to be Leeman's daughter, has fought similar battles. At a Canadian medical school in the late 1980s, one of Chandler's male supervisors tried to fire her from her neurosurgery residency when she refused to put her name on scientific papers in which he had falsified data. With the support of other faculty members, Chandler managed to hang onto her position, but the supervisor made her life hell. She was disproportionately assigned such menial tasks as conducting physicals and taking medical histories, and had difficulty getting into the operating room with the supervisor, who attempted to keep her from participating in his cases. "I tried to bring up this differential treatment," she says, "but nobody wanted to hear about it. There's no question the men got better training."

Chandler, who is African-American, knows only too well what it means to constantly have to overcompensate just to remain at par with her colleagues. "It's something women and minorities have to go through," she says, somewhat resigned to the realities of her profession.

A generation ago, when Susan Leeman was cutting her teeth on neurochemistry, a female medical student wouldn't consider blowing the whistle on an abusive boss. But today women doctors—from Columbia to Stanford—are speaking out against the sexism and gender bias that run rampant in their profession. In a male-dominated profession that makes a show of welcoming women but turns around and places obstacle after obstacle in their way, women undergo training that bears a striking resemblance to a fraternity hazing.

Sexual harassment—demeaning comments and sexual come-ons—sends a strong message that women physicians are not valued members of the team. Sexual discrimination—which can manifest itself as salary inequities; forcing women into lower-paying, less-prestigious jobs; excluding them from the informal networks crucial for career advancement; and insensitivity to their needs as working mothers—makes it almost impossible for them to rise to the top of their fields.

These inequities follow women from medical school all the way through their careers as faculty members, researchers, practicing physicians, and even scientists working for the federal government. That women are abused at this country's most respected teaching institutions is at odds with what academic medicine is supposed to be all about. We want to believe that medical training is a meritocracy, a civilized, politically correct culture where the keepers of the Hippocratic oath embody justice and shun prejudice.

Likewise the federal government is supposed to be the guarantor of civil liberties. When it tolerates—some would say, even promotes—sexist behavior in its research community, our faith in the very essence of our public health system is shattered. Perhaps it's no surprise that the National Institutes of Health, the same governmental body that had its hands rapped for not enforcing its policy of including women in clinical trials, would also be blind to the mistreatment of women scientists who work both at its sprawling Bethesda campus and in the research institutions whose studies it funds.

It's not difficult to have empathy for the plight of women physicians. After all, these women are our sisters and daughters, mothers and friends. Their anguish matters to us. As a nation that prides itself on advances in treatment and biomedical research, we also have a responsibility to care. For when female physicians are abused and prevented from fulfilling their professional potential, we all suffer.

The obstruction of women's careers puts a chokehold on their research. And when that research happens to focus on women's health, it means a delay in answers to the kinds of questions we've all been asking—for instance, how do drugs affect women differently than they do men? Does the progestin in hormone replacement therapy negate the heart-healthy effects of estrogen?

Women who are treated by doctors who verbally abuse and impede the careers of their female colleagues also suffer the fallout. "Any woman patient coming into the care of an arrogant, superior physician isn't going to get the type of sensitive health care she may want. She certainly will not have somebody who will sit down and explain things to her," says Frances Conley, M.D., the Stanford neurosurgeon who resigned in 1991 charging then-acting department chair Gerald Silverberg with gender insensitivity.

■ A HOSTILE ENVIRONMENT

But just how forbidding is the climate in which women physicians work? And what can be done about it? In 1992 the federal Office of Research on Women's Health held a major national conference to find out. Later that same year the nonprofit Society for the Advancement of Women's Health Research kicked off its own series of workshops on the subject. For many of the women in attendance these meetings provided the first opportunity to publicly discuss the horrendous conditions under which they were required to function. For the men—most of whom were deans or department chairs—the dialogue was like a jolt from the blue. How amazed they were to learn that the women at their institutions were having the life slowly kicked out of them by an oppressive sexist system. That the realities of women's work lives caused these men to have a collective epiphany speaks volumes about what is wrong with our medical institutions. Like a steamroller that couldn't be stopped, women physicians around the country began enumerating the barriers that held them back:

• *A lack of mentors and role models.* Mentors provide guidance and offer access to information that is critical to the success of a medical career. However, men are often reluctant to mentor women. With a dearth of women in leadership positions, female medical students are presented with few positive role models. Without adequate mentoring, they lack access to the informal networks in which they learn basic survival skills, such as salary negotiation and promotion strategies.

Women who do find male sponsors say the mentoring relationship is easily misunderstood and often results in their being victimized by the person on whom their future success depends. "We've all had mentors and we've all had bad relationships with our mentors," says an ob-gyn at the New York Hospital–Cornell Medical Center. "The setup of the older man mentoring the younger woman in this Pygmalion relationship is a setup for romantic overtures to be made. I had one traumatic experience. He was among the most influential people in my career."

Although she was married, this ob-gyn says her supervisor tried to convince her to sleep with him. "On the one hand there's a hint of a peer relationship. Part of being equal is that he touches you." As long as she went along with the fantasy and let everyone believe she was the man's mistress, she could be center stage with one of the most important doctors in her field. "He was very distinguished, very well known. He told me, 'I'll make your career,' sort of like George Balanchine. He opened doors. I met people I never would have met without him." But on a business trip, the ob-gyn told him the sexual advances had to stop. "Our relationship was never the same after that. He punished me by excluding me from projects and no longer promoting my career. Since that experience all my important professional relationships have been with women."

Willa Drummond, forty-eight, a tenured professor of pediatrics and physiology at the University of Florida Medical School, had a similar experience. At age thirty, and recently separated from her husband, her mentor—a world-renowned pediatric cardiologist—tried to seduce her at a medical conference. Over the years Drummond has fended off unwanted advances from other male mentors. "If they're successful, mentor relationships are always emotional relationships," she says. But when they cross the line, a junior woman has little recourse. She can't speak out because, "you need them not to be mad at you. You need them to write you recommendations."

It's a sad comment on the state of medicine when Drummond—echoing scores of other female physicians—says, "What this guy gave me was more than he took away." For in the end, he took away a lot. Partially as a result of her unpleasant experience, Drummond dropped out of pediatric cardiology, a field of only two hundred people nationwide, a field she feared was too small for the two of them.

• *An atmosphere of exclusion.* While women are not overtly kept out of informal networks, they're not likely to attend "meetings" at the golf course, racquetball court, or local watering hole. As Nadine Bruce, M.D., the American College of Physicians' former governor for Hawaii, says, "As a woman I think twice before I ask a colleague out for a drink. His wife may not understand it and he may not understand it."

But what message does it send when a professor offhandedly tells faculty members that some of his best networking takes place at the men's urinal? Or when a group of male physicians goes to talk shop at the "Chili Bordello," where the beers are cold, the barmaids hot? The message, of course, is that women are outsiders, they do not belong.

As a result women become isolated and invisible. Out of the loop and apart from the day-to-day functioning of their departments, they're less apt to be considered as candidates for awards, honors, and leadership positions.

As students they even miss out on important training. Adriane Fugh-Berman, a general practitioner in Washington, D.C., will never forget the first day of her emergency medicine rotation at the Georgetown University School of Medicine. When an instructor asked who had had experience placing a central intravenous line, almost all the male students raised their hands. None of the women did. "For me it was graphic proof of inequity in teaching," says Fugh-Berman. "The men had had the procedure taught to them. The women had not. Teaching rounds were often, for women, a spectator sport."

- *Diversion into less-prestigious specialties.* While women are no longer barred from high-status specialties, subtle messages often discourage them from entering the more lucrative, demanding fields. One study found that medical school faculty still pigeonhole women into traditional fields. For instance, only 8 percent of women in that study identified pediatrics as their chosen specialty, but one-third later entered pediatrics residencies. Likewise only 14 percent of surgery residents are currently women.

If this trend continues, medicine will become a two-tiered system, with women in the moderately remunerated areas of family medicine and primary care, and men in the richly rewarding surgical subspecialties.

- *Their interests exploited and used against them.* Women are more likely than men to be placed in a position in which they can't do the necessary work to get promoted. For instance, a radiologist was told by her department head that he was not happy with her publication record. "No one had told her what the expectation was, yet most of the men knew you were supposed to publish two peer-reviewed articles per year," says Sharyn Lenhart, M.D., chair of the American Medical Women's Association's Gender Equity Committee. When the woman took a closer look at her schedule, she realized she had been assigned twice as much clinic time as the other people at her level, mainly because she loved patient care. The department, however, was exploiting her interest in clinical work in such a way that it was impossible for her to publish enough to advance professionally.

- *Being pushed into clinical medicine.* Common wisdom holds that women are "good with patients," so female physicians are being shunted into clinical medicine, while men dominate the more prestigious and lucrative world of research. Women who attempt to do both clinical practice and research "have difficulty getting protected research time," says Lynn

Gerber of the Clinical Center of NIH. "Women are usually delegated to second-string clinical research, and then they're often not acknowledged for their work."

• *Difficulty getting grant support.* Women receive only 21.5 percent of all research project funds, and their grant awards are, on average, $30,000 less than those of their male counterparts. "Women are less apt to be in control of million-dollar grants," says Bernadine Healy. "They get the $100,000 grants."

• *Difficulty getting first authorship on papers.* When she was at the University of Washington, a female physician wrote a grant proposal and filled out all the data-collection forms for a project to study the prevention of high-risk behaviors in adolescents. But when the research was completed and it came time to submit an abstract to the international AIDS meeting, her male supervisor listed her as fifth author and a junior man—who had attended only two of the weekly study meetings during the year—as first author. She says almost every woman physician she knows can relate a similar experience. But the University of Washington doctor refused to take it in stride. She took her case to independent arbitration—and won. Still, she says, "it knocks everything out of you to go through this. It takes time away from important research you should be doing."

• *Fights for lab space.* When Phyllis Gardner, M.D., was hired as an assistant professor of medicine and pharmacology at Stanford in 1984, she was promised a 450-square-foot lab. But when she arrived, her lab was a mere 150 feet. It took years to up that space to her current 650 square feet. "I've had to battle for each extra increment," she says, pointing to a big pile of memos she's written on the subject over the years.

• *A lack of secretarial help.* Gardner says her chairman was upset with her for encouraging three junior women in her division to fight for better positions and salaries. As punishment he failed to post a secretarial position for her, which resulted in a long delay in her getting office support. "It's hard to differentiate one single act as gender-based, but if you take the cumulative effect, you begin to wonder why you seem to be fighting more for your space and secretarial support than other people," says Gardner. "I publish regularly in the right places, such as *Nature* and *Science*. It's not that I'm not doing what I'm supposed to do.

"A lot of these incidents don't happen to men. It's very demoralizing, unless you're a reasonably strong person. And if you're a reasonably strong person, you have to object, and that takes a lot of energy, and your productivity goes down."

• *Biases in the tenure process.* Trying to balance career and family responsibilities and garner enough publications before the tenure clock runs out is particularly problematic for women: the years in which they must "publish or perish" often coincide with their peak childbearing years. The fact that the majority of medical schools still adhere to the seven-year tenure track established in 1913 underscores just how unresponsive the promotion process is to the realities of women's lives. Sharyn Lenhart describes it as the "seventy kilogram career track."

Aware of the shortcomings, a handful of establishments have started to reform the tenure process. The Yale University School of Medicine, which in 1991 started an Office for Women in Medicine, allows women taking maternity leave to extend by six months the probationary period between their initial appointment and the tenure decision. Some schools have increased the probationary period by one to three years. Others now limit the number of publications needed for promotion or place more weight on teaching in the promotion process.

"Tenure is an anachronism for females as well as males," says David Brown, M.D., dean of the University of Minnesota School of Medicine. "To think you can achieve a strong record and publish in that period of time is ludicrous. To attempt to accomplish, people play it safe and abandon striking out in new areas. It works against scholarship and originality." And particularly against women.

• *Difficulties juggling medicine and motherhood.* In a study reported in the *Journal of the American Medical Women's Association (JAMWA)* in July–August 1992, 81 percent of the women physicians questioned said they experienced conflicts between their personal and professional responsibilities. So far only about a quarter of residency programs have maternity policies. In some programs women who become pregnant are shunted onto the "mommy track" against their wishes, or experience outright hostility from their male colleagues, who resent having to cover for them. It doesn't matter that these same men have no qualms about taking extensive sick leave when necessary. As one second-year house officer said, "When I needed to limit my on-call hours during the last month of my pregnancy, I was told I wasn't fulfilling my obligations. However, when John hurt his knee skiing and needed the time off for physical therapy, it was treated as perfectly acceptable."

Unlike male doctors, who often have wives to handle domestic chores, women tend to bear the brunt of child-rearing and housekeeping duties. On-site child care is a rarity. "The lack of adequate maternity-leave policies, available part-time work arrangements, child care, and more flexible promotion policies accommodating the multiple responsibilities of young faculty members with families are all perceived by women faculty as significant barriers," noted the *JAMWA* report. One study found that 78 percent of women holding faculty positions felt that their careers had been held back by childbearing. "For women the presumption is sometimes made that family responsibilities will automatically interfere with professional activities; for men the assumption is often that marriage and children will make for greater stability and professional success," writes Bernice Sandler in *The Campus Climate Revisited: Chilly for Women Faculty, Administrators, and Graduate Students*.

Some women, fearful of being knocked off the tenure track, delay motherhood indefinitely. "Medicine is very conducive to young women postponing children until it's too late," says Willa Drummond knowingly. Preoccupied with her career, she let motherhood pass her by. "I will always have that regret."

• *Pay disparity.* In 1988 female physicians made only 62.8 cents for every dollar earned by their male colleagues. In family practice female physicians make 27 percent less than men, in internal medicine 29 percent, and in pediatrics 34 percent. According to the American Medical Association, the average net income of male doctors was $152,000 versus $96,000 for female physicians.

Because women are excluded from informal networks, they often have no idea how salary decisions are made, nor are they aware of where they stand in relation to their peers. An associate professor at one academic center accidentally learned that she was earning $16,000 less than a junior colleague. "She had had mentors," says Sharyn Lenhart. "She was a real leader at her medical center."

When she went to her department head and asked him about the pay disparity, he said, "Well, you haven't published as much." The woman checked and found that she had published a little more than her junior colleague. When she went back to her department head, he told her, "Don't make waves. We know your family has always come first." Her husband, who was also a department chair at the institution, told her she should be appreciative of how much her bosses respected her and had helped her career.

• *Racial discrimination.* All the barriers to women's full participation in academic medicine are even more pronounced for women of color. In 1992, black women accounted for less than one-tenth of all female medical school graduates and only 3 percent of the graduating class. As one physician says, "For many minority women, to be in a position where a glass ceiling comes into effect would be a significant improvement."

• *Discrimination by search committees.* When a department-chair slot becomes available, a medical school dean appoints a dozen or so people to search out the best potential candidates. Occasionally there are women among the top ten applicants, but rarely do they make it to the top three, and when they do, they're often knocked out of the running for vague reasons. "The criteria seem to change for women," says Susan Blumenthal, M.D., deputy assistant secretary for women's health at the Department of Health and Human Services. "If she has strong organizational skills, then she needs more clinical skills. If she's interpersonally difficult, she's too aggressive." Michelle Harrison, M.D., director of the Women's Health Fellowship Program at the Robert Wood Johnson Medical School, concludes facetiously, "It must be biological, since men don't have difficult personalities that prevent appointments."

Most women physicians are tired of being the token female on the recruitment list, the person the search committee can point to just to say they considered a woman. A search committee's top candidate, Carol Nadelson, M.D., the first female president of the American Psychiatric Association, recently interviewed with a medical school dean but lost the job to a man who had no administrative experience and fewer publications than she. Another time Nadelson lost a job because her curriculum vitae was too long. "If you're looking for an excuse not to hire a woman," she says ruefully, "you'll find one."

As a result of search-committee biases, women are not represented in sufficient numbers to change the workplace culture. Although women comprise almost half of all entering medical school classes, in many specialties they account for less than a quarter of all residents. In some of the highest-paying fields, their showing is downright dismal: a mere 14 percent in general surgery, 7 percent in neurosurgery, and 5 percent in urology.

• *Underrepresentation in leadership positions.* Women are conspicuously absent from leadership positions in all areas of medicine. Of the more than two thousand chairs of academic departments, ninety are women. Only four of the 126 medical school deans are women. In fact the majority of women are clustered at the lower-paying levels of assistant and associate professor, wallowing in what former NIH director Bernadine Healy has described as "academic ghettos." In pediatrics, for example, in which more than half of all residents are women, 50 to 60 percent of men but only 30 percent of women are at the associate-professor or professor level. Of 126 academic pediatrics departments in the United States, only six are chaired by women.

The record is equally grim in professional medical and scientific societies. Consider:

- The American College of Obstetricians and Gynecologists, whose mandate is to provide reproductive health care to women, has not had more than four women on its seventeen-member executive board at any one time in its forty-three-year history. Only once has a woman been president.
- The American Medical Association, the largest organization of physicians in the world, has never had a woman president in its 147-year history. Of the twenty doctors who sit on the AMA's board of trustees, four are women.
- Of the 2,028 members of the National Academy of Sciences, seventy-six are women. Most of them do not have voting privileges.
- Although the National Institutes of Health recently had its first woman director, Bernadine Healy, M.D., until recently only two of its seventeen institutes—the National Institute of Nursing Research and the National Institute of General Medical Sciences—were headed by women. (Former General Medical Sciences head Ruth Kirschstein, M.D., is now deputy director of NIH.) Women make up 17 percent of the section chiefs and only 4 percent of the lab chiefs of NIH.

■ SEXUAL HARASSMENT

Women's exclusion from the boys' club that is medicine is partially the result of perceptual biases that guide the way men and women both view each other and themselves. In medicine as in the larger society women are stereotyped as dependent, weak, incompetent, subordinate, emotional, fragile, and fickle, whereas men are viewed as independent, powerful, competent, dominating, logical, and decisive, as leaders and protectors. Every time these biases are brought into medical school classrooms, academic departments, and research centers, women can't help but lose. "When women demonstrate traits that are predominantly attributed to men—even if they're appropriate in the workplace they're in—those traits are received in a negative fashion," says Sharyn Lenhart. Women who don't remain in their places are easy targets for sexually-harassing men. These women learn that the sex bias they encountered in medical school will stay with them way beyond their training.

No one knows the true prevalence of sexual harassment in medicine, but recent studies suggest it is ubiquitous. In a 1992 report in the *Journal of the American Medical Women's Association*, 30 percent of the 229 women doctors surveyed said sexist behavior was common in the workplace. Another survey, of 133 internal medicine residents at the University of California, San Francisco, found that 73 percent of the women but only 22 percent of the men said they had been sexually harassed at least once during their training.

One of the female residents in the San Francisco survey said she had been asked out by two different attending physicians before they had completed their evaluations or letters of recommendation. A third-year medical student said she was meeting privately with her attending physician to discuss her evaluation when he suddenly asked, "Have you ever seen the movie *Deep Throat?*" When she shook her head no, he leaned across his desk, opened his mouth and ran his tongue slowly around his lips. During a surgical rotation the senior resident, a man, told a female resident to stand next to him in the operating room, where he proceeded to rub his groin against her during surgery.

Frances Conley, the Stanford neurosurgeon, knows firsthand how damaging harassment can be. Her bold move in 1991—bringing the ongoing sexism in her medical school department to the media and consequently into people's living rooms—made harassment in medicine a national issue. Before Conley came forward, stories were shared behind closed doors, if at all. Now it's impossible to attend a conference or seminar on gender discrimination in medicine without hearing her name invoked. Sharyn Lenhart makes a habit of kicking off her workshops and talks on the subject with pictures of both Anita Hill and Conley. "I owe them a debt of gratitude," she says. "Without the publicity they generated for this issue, people like myself who have been interested in doing research in this area probably would not be asked to speak."

Like many transformations, the radicalization of Frances Conley came in fits and starts. Unbeknownst to her, the Stanford Faculty Senate meeting she attended shortly before she resigned in 1991 was to be a turning point. Usually limited to faculty representatives from various academic departments, this meeting was open to anyone who wanted to discuss issues of sexism at Stanford. Dozens of aggrieved women students showed up and gave Conley and others an earful. One student reported that during a lecture on pulmonary physiology a male professor showed a slide of an inflatable sex doll and said, "Meet Angel, your new companion." Another student described an incident in an ob-gyn course, in which a male instructor discussed uterine contractions by saying, "Well, none of you are ever going to experience this. Your wives may." He didn't notice that more than one-third of his class was female. Still a third student talked of a professor who discouraged a young woman from going into surgery because, he said, she didn't have "male genes."

Conley was floored at the student accounts. Nothing had changed, she felt, since she began medical school in 1961. She knew she could no longer remain silent, and decided to resign in protest.

An op-ed piece she wrote about her resignation for the *San Francisco Chronicle* became headline news. Conley appeared on *Good Morning America* and *Today* and was featured on the cover of *People*. She testified before Congress about sexism in medicine, and the invitations to speak came pouring in. Conley, a surgeon who had devoted the previous twenty-five years of her life to studying nervous system disorders, had become the unofficial spokesperson for a generation—really several generations—of oppressed women doctors.

Conley had had the chutzpah to say what most of them only dreamed of saying. She had tenure and had nothing to lose—or so she thought—when she told the dean of her medical school, Dr. David Korn, that Gerald Silverberg was a "sexist pig" who was not fit to lead her department. For years, she says, she'd shrugged off his sexual advances and the demeaning way he addressed her as "honey" in front of her peers. She'd watched with embarrassment as he hugged nurses.

For Conley it had become second nature to look the other way. A lone woman in a sea of often-hostile men, she had learned to be one of the boys. As long as the inappropriate comments and lewd behavior didn't affect her ability to do her job, she could laugh them off.

But when Silverberg became acting chair, the equation changed. Conley says her name was removed from department stationery, she was excluded from important meetings, and was prohibited from interviewing the residents with whom she'd be working. "I had a staff that felt they had to do what he wanted, and what he wanted was to belittle me. Silverberg and I had a clinic together. My patients would sit for two hours before they were put in an examining room. I'd see them at seven-thirty at night because his always got priority. That impacts patient care, and it's not right. That's when it's time to draw the line."

The bottom line for Conley was the fact that, if promoted, Silverberg would become a role model for the next generation of doctors. "As soon as you put somebody into an executive leadership position, their behavior is validated. All of a sudden that becomes appropriate behavior," she says, her voice rising in pitch and intensity. "We've seen this in our residents. They copy him. And *they* go handle nurses incorrectly, pinching them on the butt, doing egregious things that should not happen to any woman in a professional environment. It was wrong, not so much for what happened to me but for what was happening to the junior women who couldn't speak up. I thought, 'I can live *with* him. I cannot live working *for* him.' "

As a result of her charges Gerald Silverberg lost the neurosurgery chairmanship and Conley eventually rescinded her resignation. But Conley lost a lot too. The woman who used a 1985 sabbatical to earn a master's degree in business so that she would be prepared for an administrative position in academic medicine—perhaps someday a chairmanship or deanship—knows she can kiss that dream good-bye.

"Look, you have certain things that are realistic and certain things that are not," she says, dressed in her signature slacks and running shoes. "What I did was to just get into the field. When I entered neurosurgery, there were only three other woman who had boards. I'm the only one who's spent ten years as a full professor. If I had gone any farther, it would have been a big frog's leap into a dean type of situation. That's not going to happen now. I'm out of the loop. I'm a nothing. I *do not* exist."

Margaret Billingham, a professor of pathology who's had her own share of problems at Stanford, says Conley is not exaggerating. "Fran realizes she is a beacon. Most women admire her tremendously for what she did. But we fear for her. She's been hurt badly."

Some might argue that Conley has not been hurt. After all, she's succeeded, even flourished, in a male-dominated specialty. As neurosurgeon Kym Chandler says, the field is such a boy's club, "you can practically smell the testosterone." But women who know Conley say the slights and slurs have taken their toll. Her trip from the cloistered world of neurosurgery to the rough-and-tumble arena of feminism has left her isolated, a doctor in Siberia.

Taken individually, each demeaning comment—for instance when a male colleague told Conley he could see the outline of her breasts through her lab coat—is easy to shrug off. But as the comments accumulate, like so many drops in a bucket, they overflow and affect the work environment. Mary Rowe, a labor ombudsman at the Massachusetts Institute of Technology, says these microinequities serve to exclude women—even women as strong as Frances Conley—undermining their self-confidence and making them less productive. Female physicians describe it as being hit by a ton of feathers.

Sometimes the slights are deliberate and send a clear message that women are not welcome. Other times no one is out to consciously hurt the woman physician, but she's excluded from networks and her work is devalued compared with that of her male counterpart. As Lenhart explains, "Perceptions are held about her commitment to her work or her capacity for work without much discussion with her." But whether unintentional or malicious, the slights and harassing behavior adversely affect a woman's career. "They're tough," says Lenhart, "because you don't always notice them and because you can't complain about this stuff every time it happens. On the other hand, to say nothing about some of these things, particularly if they're having an impact, is also a mistake."

Both quid pro quo harassment—when a sexual relationship with a supervisor is made a condition of employment—and harassment that creates a hostile work environment—such as verbal advances or offensive body language—are punishing to women professionally and emotionally.

Mary Rowe documents the numerous ways these microinequities hurt women's careers. At one extreme are the women who lose their jobs, never finish their degrees, or abandon their careers entirely. But even the women who hang onto their jobs feel the pressure. When women are treated as though they can't perform well, they come to believe it themselves. When they're loaded down with trivial tasks, they have little time to do more important creative work. And of course microinequities create barriers between men and women, making it difficult for them to work cooperatively and collaboratively.

Equally troubling, when sexist behavior is pervasive, it's difficult to know where to begin to respond. Reacting to every incident would be emotionally draining and probably get a woman branded as hypersensitive or hysterical.

Some women do what they've been trained to do: deny and repress, internalize blame. They feel guilt and shame, but they don't dare talk about it. They may begin to suffer from anxiety, poor concentration, headaches, sleep disturbances, and depression. Some experience post-traumatic stress reactions: periods of numbness and dissociation alternating with periods of intense emotions, nightmares, and flashbacks of the original harassing experience. And the feathers continue to pile up.

Some women isolate themselves. Many live in a state of chronic ambivalence, waffling between feelings of anger and insecurity. The University of Florida's Willa Drummond coped by developing what she calls "a defensive persona of standoffishness." It has cost her promotion after promotion. One fellow faculty member told her, "You're perceived as being angry. If that perception wasn't there, you'd find doors opening up for you." But the perception is there because she *is* angry, and justifiably so. Yet her anger is one more strike against her. Proof that she's not to be trusted, she's not a member of the club.

"Most women grieve and mourn when they become fully aware of the impact of these losses," writes psychiatrist Sharyn Lenhart. "These include loss of income, job, opportunities for career development, important mentor or teaching relationships, [and] opportunities for specialized training and education."

■ MEDICINE'S GLASS CEILING

If sexual harassment can erode a woman's confidence in her professional abilities and perhaps change the course of her career, gender discrimination can fully destroy that career. A woman who has become nationally renowned and has her research in prestigious publications expects her achievements to be rewarded just like her male counterparts. Instead, on the verge of being promoted into a senior position, she experiences an unexpected setback that she attributes to circumstance. But after another unexpected inequity, she realizes she has cracked her head on the glass ceiling. Another brilliant career is on the skids.

The stories women tell are remarkably similar, but the case of Heidi S. Weissmann illustrates the dangers in being a whistleblower. From early childhood, Weissmann wanted to become a doctor and, after skipping three grades, she entered the Mount Sinai School of Medicine at the age of nineteen. After completing a radiology residency at New York City's Albert Einstein College of Medicine–Montefiore Medical Center, and a fellowship in ultrasonography and computed tomography (CAT scan) at New York Hospital–Cornell University Medical Center, Weissmann joined the Montefiore radiology department as an instructor. By twenty-eight she was world-renowned for her research and teaching and had made significant contributions to her field, including the development of a safer and more efficacious method of diagnosing acute gallbladder disease that today remains the gold standard.

In recommending that Weissmann be promoted early to associate professor, her department chairman M. Donald Blaufox, M.D., wrote to then-acting dean Ernst Jaffe, that Weissmann "has repeatedly presented at peer reviewed national meetings and receives invitations on an almost daily basis to discuss the role of Nuclear Medicine in her area of interest throughout the country and indeed throughout the world. . . ." He went on to note that "Weissmann's contributions to the scientific literature have clearly achieved national and, indeed, international recognition."

Weissmann was only thirty-three when she got the promotion. Then she hit rough waters. Her trouble started when she was asked to serve a four-year term on an NIH study section, a position that would bring prestige to her medical center and make an important contribution to the national research agenda. Several days before her first critiques were due, Weissmann realized that her three-page handwritten documents had been sitting on the department secretary's desk for weeks. When Weissmann went to Leonard Freeman, M.D., the chief of her division, to discuss the situation, he offered no support. Finally, she paid the secretary out of her own pocket to have the papers typed.

When she discussed her problems getting secretarial help with Dr. Blaufox, he leaned back in his chair and said, "That's the way it should be. You're a junior woman. I haven't been asked to serve for a four-year term on an NIH study section." He told her that she wasn't getting the message and that she should resign. "At that point," she says, "I got the message. I had to be hit over the head."

Discouraged and without institutional support, Weissmann resigned from the study section after serving for only a year. Subsequently, Blaufox recommended a male associate professor to take her place.

Weissmann says that, unlike her male colleagues, she was discouraged from participating in professional activities that would have advanced her career, was denied a promotion to division chief (a junior male faculty member was subsequently hired for the job), and earned less than her male counterparts.

When Weissmann complained, an associate dean told her, "It's clear there's discrimination going on here, but I don't believe in anyone becoming a martyr. Your CV is incredible, and I think you could get a job anywhere you wanted, so my best advice to you is to just bide your time and move on when an opportunity presents itself."

Weissmann thought about it. Then she decided, "It wasn't my career goal to become a martyr." So instead of filing a complaint, she requested a six-month sabbatical at full pay to write a book—a request previously granted at her institution. What she got was a one-year sabbatical at half pay because, she was told, hers was a second income and she could afford the salary cut. She was surprised to learn that the sabbatical was approved not to write a book, but to write a grant proposal. A book, Freeman argued, would only benefit Heidi Weissmann. A grant, he said, would bring money into the department.

Though not the terms she'd hoped for, Weissmann took the leave. But three-and-a-half months into her sabbatical she received a letter saying she would be reappointed on a probationary basis. One colleague told her, "Freeman wants to shake you up and put you in your place." (Weissmann later learned that there was no such thing as probationary reappointment for someone in her position.)

In 1988 she filed a sex-discrimination suit against her employers. Now, she says, "It's amazing how effectively I've been shut out." Weissmann, who previously won a copyright-infringement lawsuit against Leonard Freeman for plagiarism of her work, cites a litany of discriminatory actions that includes retaliation. For instance, the day after filing her copyright-infringement lawsuit against Freeman, Weissmann was stopped by security guards, locked out of her office, and searched. By the end of the day, the entire contents of her office had been packed. Six weeks later, Blaufox notified Weissmann that he considered that she had resigned because she hadn't reported to work. Between her copyright-infringement case and this suit, she's devoted the last seven years of her life to fighting her former medical institution. While Freeman's legal fees have been paid by Montefiore, Weissmann is footing her own bills, which are over half a million dollars. Not only has Freeman been promoted to vice chairman of the department of nuclear medicine at Albert Einstein, he has received honorary membership in the national medical honor society. Weissmann, forty-three, has been unable to find work in her field. "I'm trying to give as much meaning as possible to the derailment of a career I loved," she says. "I have a thirteen-year-old daughter. I'm fighting for her—and for the next Heidi Weissmann."

Walter Stewart, Ph.D., an NIH employee who developed a software program to root out scientific misconduct and plagiarism, knows that unless harassers are held accountable for their indiscretions, there will continue to be more Heidi Weissmanns. "It's incredibly depressing watching these brave, persistent women get the life slowly crushed out of them by this enormously heavy system. First the man attempts to steal a woman's work. Then it turns out he's stolen other people's work. But there's no question all these episodes originate from the abuse of power. This thing is institutionalized. It's perfectly clear the system functions as an abuser of women. And women have more that the system can steal now."

Weissmann realizes how far women have come. If she'd lived at the turn of the century, she wouldn't even have gotten into medical school. Today women are no longer denied internships and residencies, nor are they openly barred from appointments at good hospitals, from membership in group medical practices, or from directorships at laboratories. But, as in other professions, women who aspire to the top tier in medicine hit invisible barriers. Judith Lorber, Ph.D., a professor of sociology at the City University of New York, explains that women are kept from top positions through a subtle process, a kind of "colleague boycott"—not keeping women out entirely "but not including them in ways that allow them" to reach the top of their professions.

"The reason men are so reluctant to allow women into their inner circles is their fear that if too many women become leaders, the profession will 'tip' and become women's work, and men will lose prestige, income, and authority," she says. "To move up, a young person's worth has to be recognized and encouraged. Promising young men are still groomed by senior management. Promising young women are left to fend for themselves."

Lorber describes this process as the "Salieri phenomenon—a combination of faint praise and acceptable denigration of their abilities to lead that delegitimates women physicians' bids to compete for positions of great authority." (In the play *Amadeus* the court composer Salieri blocked Mozart's career by offering not direct opposition but lukewarm support.)

This colleague boycott occurs because women frequently work in what are called "skewed" groups; that is, workplaces that have less than 20 percent women. Women physicians who work in such a setting encounter problems independent of their personalities and, often, independent of the personalities of the men with whom they're working. "If you do well, it's perceived quickly by everyone," says Lenhart. "If you do poorly or just have an average number of mistakes, the whole world sees it. These are group phenomena and are largely unconscious, but they're very, very powerful."

In a "tilted" group, women constitute about 30 percent of the workforce, equivalent to the proportion of women in medical schools right now. "Individuals are still not seen well as individuals," says Lenhart. "There's a fair amount of misperception and bias. But they do have enough clout to form a constituency and to begin to voice their concerns. That's what women physicians are starting to do now. It's why people like myself are being asked to talk. But we don't have leadership positions yet, and that's typical of a tilted group."

When the percentages reach fifty-fifty or even sixty-forty, women physicians will be part of a "balanced" group. As Lenhart describes it, "You're evaluated for who you are, and stereotyping based on gender is not as predominant because the group mixes better. People are used to seeing women as people, as workers, not just as sex objects, wives, or mothers. If they're in the workplace to that degree, a lot will happen just based on the numbers."

Unfortunately the American Medical Association does not project a balanced workplace until well into the twenty-first century. Other researchers say the minority group—in this case women—has to make a complete turnaround and constitute closer to 75 percent of the workforce in order to effect change in deeply ingrained behaviors. If this turns out to be true, gender equity in medicine is a very long way off.

■ NIH: THE NATIONAL INSTITUTES OF HARASSMENT

If women are abused in academic medicine—the home of the skewed group—some would say it's no surprise. But women doctors and researchers might expect to be treated better by the federal government. Not so. Margaret Jensvold, a thirty-seven-year-old Washington, D.C. psychiatrist, expected to have a successful research career at the National Institute of Mental Health. Little did she know when she began her fellowship there in 1987 that no female physician had ever received tenure by advancement through NIMH's fellow program. This, despite the fact that the doctors accepted into the program are among this country's best and brightest.

Jensvold seemed to have been groomed for the job. Women on both sides of her family had been successful in men's fields at least three generations back. Her great-aunt, Jeanette Piccard, had set the high-altitude record and was considered the first woman in space. "I knew my mother's and grandmothers' generations had opened doors my generation would be able to walk through," Jensvold says.

She had every reason to believe she would follow suit. She graduated Phi Beta Kappa from UCLA and was in the top third of her class at Johns Hopkins. Prior to her appointment at NIMH she was named one of the six most promising psychiatry residents in the United States.

At NIMH Jensvold was eager to begin biological psychiatric research on premenstrual syndrome and depression in women. But within two months of entering the fellowship program, she knew something was seriously amiss. In a suit filed in December 1990, Jensvold says her boss, David Rubinow, M.D., chief of the Section on Behavioral Endocrinology within NIMH's Biological Psychiatry Branch, created a "sexually hostile work environment" by making sexist comments about her, her female colleagues, and women patients, that she was assigned to research projects and then abruptly removed, and that she was prevented from completing her projects. "The men co-authored," she says. "I didn't. They wrote review papers. I was forbidden to write review papers."

In addition, she says, Rubinow used a computer screen-saver image of model Cheryl Tiegs in a low-cut swimsuit and, long after the holidays, displayed a Christmas card showing a male colleague in a military uniform holding a large phallic-looking syringe. A miniskirted nurse knelt before him with her face in his crotch, simulating oral sex.

When Jensvold asked to do work comparable to what the men were doing, Rubinow told her she was narcissistic and not sufficiently dependent upon him. What's more, he replied, people didn't want to work with her in the laboratory because she was "attractive and competent." As a condition of employment, Rubinow told Jensvold she would have to enter psychotherapy and gave her the names of three male psychiatrists. When Jensvold asked for a female therapist, Rubinow told her there were no good ones in Washington. "It was a very powerful message that I had to do everything he said or my fellowship wouldn't be renewed."

Not only is it unethical for a manager to force a subordinate into therapy, it is forbidden by federal law. But Jensvold wanted to continue her fellowship, so she started therapy. During her third session she was stunned to learn her psychiatrist was employed by NIMH and would not guarantee her confidentiality. She discontinued therapy and, several months later, was told she would not be allowed to continue her training. Rubinow says Jensvold was fired because she failed to "demonstrate excellence" in her work while displaying "considerable distress" over "personal life issues."

Jensvold left without publishing any of her NIMH research. "I'd gone to NIMH with the dream of getting tenure there, or at least having three good years to publish papers and establish a track record," she says. Midway through her fellowship, Jensvold learned that two women who had preceded her in the fellowship program had also complained of discrimination.

One of them, Dr. Jean Hamilton, began a two-year fellowship in NIMH's clinical neuropharmacology branch in 1980. Her plan was to study women and depression, and sex differences in pharmacology. Women, she knew, suffered depression at twice the rate of men and made up the majority of users of psychotropic drugs, but no one had bothered to study whether women responded differently to these medications.

As the only female clinical associate among dozens of men, Hamilton was immediately branded as "other," "different," an "outsider." In an Equal Employment Opportunity Commission (EEOC) complaint she filed in 1983 she said that most fellows were assigned to the wards for a year but that she was required to spend most of her two years on the wards. A superior, Fred Goodwin, M.D., whom she named in the suit along with Rubinow, told her that women were good clinicians because they were "warm" and got "along well with the nursing staff," qualities Hamilton knew would never get a woman tenure.

Unlike her male colleagues, Hamilton says, she had higher clinical loads and was denied the secretarial and technical assistance needed to score and analyze data. This prevented her from conducting further research and writing papers. On one occasion she even had to hire outside help at her own expense. She was repeatedly denied opportunities to collaborate on research projects with other physicians in her branch and was excluded from authorship on papers to which her contribution was equivalent to that made by male physicians, who did receive credit.

Although she was told she would not be retained for a third year, Hamilton managed to stay on—but only because a male colleague decided at the last minute to leave. Near the end of her third year, however, she was not asked back for a fourth. There were no funds to keep her. Funny, there was money in the budget to retain every white male fellow.

Goodwin said Hamilton was let go because she was working in "low-priority" areas. No one seemed to notice that she had the first approved protocol to study PMS at the NIMH, or that when David Rubinow came along with the second PMS study, he was told—and refused—to collaborate with Hamilton. One can only conclude that PMS research is a low priority when studied by a woman but a high priority when conducted by a man.

"I was invisible," Hamilton says. "I was just a high-status nurse while the boys did high-status work, which was science."

In 1986 Hamilton settled out of court. A gag order prevented her from discussing the terms of the settlement. But when Hamilton testified at Margaret Jensvold's sex discrimination trial in 1994, the gag was lifted. Hamilton is now a tenured, full professor at Duke University, where she's happily doing the research that was neglected at NIMH. But she's sad at the lost opportunities, opportunities denied her simply because she was a woman who dared enter the lion's den that is the National Institutes of Health.

Of course NIH isn't just any lion's den. The nation's premier research institution, it has an annual budget of $11 billion and funds 85 percent of the biomedical research conducted in the United States. In short it decides who gets to study what. For young researchers an NIH fellowship is often the ticket to academic stardom—in particular the coveted job of department chair. In fact three-fourths of all academic chairs have done training at NIH. But if that training is rife with sexism, the inappropriate behavior becomes legitimized and is modeled to the next generation of medical students as appropriate. And the circle of sexism continues.

"What goes on internally in the federal government has a big effect on academia," says a female NIH administrator, who has a sex-discrimination suit pending against her division. "If the government starts enforcing the law in its own agencies, other institutions are going to get the message. Right now it's an old boys' network between [NIH] and the medical institutions that receive its grants."

What is often left unsaid is that when sexism occurs in this country's most prestigious medical research institution, it affects all women. It doesn't take a brain surgeon to figure out that discrimination against women leads to discrimination against their research. And when their research focuses on women, that work is at best delayed, at worst stopped dead in its tracks. For instance, Jean Hamilton had to leave NIMH in order to pursue research on gender differences in drug metabolism, despite the clear need for this kind of research. Most of the PMS work Margaret Jensvold started at NIMH has been shelved: she doesn't have the resources to conduct the large clinical trials necessary to provide good scientific data. She's had two small papers published—including one in which she got good results adjusting dosages of antidepressants across the menstrual cycle—albeit several years behind schedule. Another, on the relationship between a past history of sexual abuse and PMS symptoms, has yet to see the light of day.

"People think researchers are altruistic and they're not," says Billie Mackey, an NIH administrator and president of Self Help for Equal Rights (SHER), a women's organization at NIH. "They research the things they're interested in. If most of your researchers are men, you'll find a tremendous amount of research on men's diseases." And little on women's.

Says the NIH administrator, "It's total greed, men wanting all the power, all the money, all the visibility, not willing to share with anybody." Clearly it's holding women back. A report of an NIH task force convened in 1991 to assess the career development of women scientists at NIH found that, as discussed above, women make up only 17 percent of the section chiefs and a paltry 4 percent of the lab chiefs, positions that determine what research gets funded at NIH. Women make up 18 percent of the tenured scientists on campus and 30 percent of the fellows in the postdoctoral training program. At NIMH, as of the early 1990s, a woman physician had not been promoted to the level of section chief in fifteen years.

Perhaps most discouraging to women, whether working in academia or for the federal government, is the extent to which harassers are protected and promoted while the women are excommunicated and blacklisted. Maureen Polsby, M.D., a neurologist with the then National Institute of Neurologic and Communicative Disorders and Stroke, says that when she refused to go to bed with her lab chief, Thomas Chase, M.D., the man who had recruited her for her fellowship, he threw her to the wolves. "I got assigned all the scut work and saw patients no one else wanted to see." A male fellow who started at the same time she did was allowed to do his own research full-time, an opportunity she was denied. When she did manage to do work with promising results, she says Chase took the projects away from her and gave them to a male colleague. The third time it happened, she filed an EEO complaint. And then all hell broke lose.

Polsby says she was not allowed to use her two years as an NIH fellow toward completion of her residency, a privilege routinely granted and one that was promised her at the outset. Without residency training she would not be board eligible.

Billie Mackey says this sort of retaliation is typical. Female whistleblowers frequently lose their lab space and resources, are excluded from departmental meetings, and are prohibited from attending medical conferences, which prevents them from both reporting on their work and learning the latest advances in their fields.

After filing her complaint, Margaret Jensvold says she was prevented from writing up her research. On her last day of employment three administrators physically removed her keys and beeper. She was told that her library and parking privileges would be terminated immediately. Normally they lapse after a month. One female administrator describes the retaliation as "not unlike prisoner-of-war tactics. It's psychological warfare every, every, every day."

Ironically, while the female victims of sexism get revictimized for speaking out, their accusers get raises, bonuses, and awards. Rubinow, for instance, has received a promotion, and in 1992, with Jensvold's sexual discrimination and retaliation suit still pending, was named the Distinguished Clinical Educator at NIH. Jensvold can only say, "It's a sad commentary on what NIH has to offer in terms of mentoring." Before his departure in 1993 Steven Paul, M.D., former scientific director of NIMH and the subject of at least two EEOC complaints, chaired the Committee on the Status of Intramural Women Scientists at NIMH, the purpose of which was to promote the careers of women in the organization. All of which sounds suspiciously like sending the wolf in to mind the sheep. In 1994 Thomas Chase received the prestigious Fred Springer award at the annual meeting of the American Academy of Neurology. And NIMH lab chief Michael Brownstein, M.D., was named acting scientific director of NIMH, despite the three EEOC complaints pending against him.

"These men should not receive raises, they should be penalized," says Mackey. "The message that's sent when nothing happens is that it doesn't matter, the government will send a lawyer out to defend them."

Indeed the minute a woman enters the Byzantine EEOC process, the deck is stacked against her. A complainant has forty-five days from the time of the incident to see an EEOC counselor and document what happened. The counselor then has one hundred eighty days to conduct an investigation and write up a report. But women complain that counselors, all of whom work elsewhere in NIH and devote one-quarter time to EEOC matters, spend all their time interviewing character witnesses for the alleged harassers but fail to interview the people who can corroborate the victims' charges. Although women naively expect an impartial investigation, they learn that in fact "the process is set up to protect the institution at all costs," says a female administrator. "The institution is out to prove it's right and you're wrong. It tests your resilience right down to your toes."

If no resolution is reached after receiving the counselor's report, a woman has fifteen days to file a formal complaint with the Department of Health and Human Services (HHS). But SHER's Mackey says the EEOC often sits on investigations without issuing a report so that women are delayed in proceeding along the formal route. This could explain why in 1992 only thirty-seven formal complaints were filed versus 242 informal ones. NIH has every reason to string the process out. Informal charges remain confidential; formal ones become public.

If a woman hasn't been beaten down early in the process, she has the option of going to court, where the government's big guns continue to bear down on her. As of early 1994, five sex-discrimination cases were pending against NIH, including Margaret Jensvold's. "For women with these cases it's a very alone place to be. It's scary and a very, very risky thing to do unless you're filthy rich," one female administrator says.

Of course it shouldn't be this way. Although former NIH director Bernadine Healy promised to battle sex discrimination at NIH, it took her until the spring of 1993, only months before she was to vacate her post, to admit publicly that there was a problem of sexism at the agency. This was disappointing, as it came one full year after Billie Mackey and seven other SHER members met with Healy to ask that changes be made. Among their requests was that an ombudsman—someone not paid by HHS—be appointed in the Office of Personnel Management, that the number of EEOC counselors be increased from thirty working one-quarter time to ten working full-time. They also asked for a list of accusers who had gotten raises and requested that all pending cases be settled promptly. At the time of Healy's departure in June none of those requests had been met, leading Billie Mackey to conclude that "this was not a top priority" for NIH.

To be fair, Healy did attempt to address the problem. On June 11 and 12, 1992, NIH, along with the Office of Research on Women's Health, held the first national meeting to discuss ways to advance the medical careers of women. At eight that morning the congressional ballroom at the Bethesda Marriott buzzed with electricity as more than three hundred mostly female clinicians and researchers gathered to make their voices heard. Instead of being part of a substantial minority, they were now the majority. It was positively exhilarating.

After two days of deliberations the women recommended, among other things, that NIH develop a model sexual-harassment policy, take steps to increase the number of women reviewers in study sections, and make funding contingent upon an institution's success in promoting women and its having policies on sexual harassment in place.

They also asked that medical centers be encouraged to develop incentives to advance and promote women faculty members, that each institution create a commission on the status of women, that formal mentoring structures be developed, and that studies be conducted on the prevalence of sexual harassment and its effects on the health of those who are harassed.

One message came through loud and clear: It was time for a change. As Jimmie Holland, M.D., a psychiatrist with Memorial Sloan-Kettering

Cancer Center in New York, said at a similar meeting four months later, "We're witnessing an incredibly different time. When I went to medical school in the fifties, there was not even an opportunity to protest. Today young women demand more and expect more."

Not long after the NIH conference there were signs that some of those demands might be met. Bernadine Healy approved a proposal to nominate women scientists to apprise the directors of each NIH institute of the problems and issues specific to women. The Office of Research on Women's Health implemented a recruitment and reentry program awarding grants of $50,000 a year for two years to women whose biomedical careers had been interrupted by such things as childrearing. At the same time scores of medical institutions began developing sexual-harassment policies and made a concerted effort to recruit more women and promote them into senior positions. Some were following the lead of Harvard, which in 1988 started annual career-planning conferences in which senior faculty help junior women—and men—map out their careers. Others, like Stanford, began sensitivity training for men and women alike.

"We're victims, but we need to make sure we don't play the role of victim," says Fran Conley. "If you're a victim, all of a sudden you're not responsible for anything that happened to you. Well, goddammit, I am responsible for what happened to me in that I have succeeded. I have a curriculum vitae that any man in this world would be proud of, and I am responsible for that."

Like most female physicians who have successfully bucked the odds, Conley does not want pity. She doesn't want a pat on the shoulder, doesn't want to hear, "Gee, I'm so sorry for you." "I want people to congratulate me for standing up, to feel empowered by it and to say, 'Look, okay, this is one step. Let's take the next step forward. We don't need to feel sorry for each other. We need to gain from what's happening to us.'"

But Conley, like other women of her generation, believes progress will be hard won. In fact she doesn't expect to see much improvement during her lifetime. As one female physician told a meeting of academic deans and faculty members, Conley included, "Nothing will change until the men of my era retire or die." Many of the male doctors in attendance agreed—as if to emphasize how far women have come and how far they still have to go.

Postscript:

On March 11, 1994, Montefiore Medical Center and the Albert Einstein College of Medicine of Yeshiva University agreed to pay Heidi

Weissmann $900,000 to end her sex-discrimination suit. She refused to accept a gag order, but had to agree not to seek employment at Einstein or any of its twenty-nine affiliated medical centers in the New York area. The federal judge on the case found that Weissmann's filing of EEOC charges appeared to have been "followed closely by discriminatory treatment" and noted the absence of "contemporary written documentation" confirming M. Donald Blaufox's version of events.

Several weeks later, on April 1, a Baltimore jury ruled that David Rubinow had discriminated and retaliated against Margaret Jensvold, resulting in damage to her professional reputation. Experts say that in recognizing discriminatory mentoring as a form of sex discrimination, the case has set a legal precedent. As of this writing, Jensvold was awaiting a decision on damages and possible reinstatement.

Maureen Polsby's case is expected to come to trial in 1994.

3

THE RESEARCH GAP

In June 1990, American women got a rude shock. For all the complaints women leveled against the health care system—most having to do with insensitive male doctors and dissatisfaction with gynecological and obstetric care—the majority of women still assumed that at least they were included in America's state-of-the-art medical research. But they were wrong. For at least the past several decades women in this country had been systematically excluded from the vast majority of research to develop new drugs, medical treatments, and surgical techniques.

It was on June 18, 1990, that the government's General Accounting Office (GAO) released its report of an audit of the National Institutes of Health (NIH). The audit found that although NIH had formulated a policy in 1986 for including women as research subjects, little had been done to implement or monitor that policy. In fact, most researchers applying for NIH grants were not even aware that they were supposed to include women, since the NIH grant-application book contained no mention of the policy. Because the 1986 policy urged rather than required attention to gender bias, most institutes, and most researchers, had simply decided to ignore it altogether or pay it only slight heed: "It used to be enough for a researcher to say, 'Women and minorities will not be excluded from this study,'" explains one woman in NIH's Division of Research Grants. But not excluding women is very different from actively recruiting and including them.

Patricia Schroeder (D-Colo.), one of the congresswomen who had requested the audit, was outraged. "This was nothing but window dressing," she said of NIH's 1986 policy. "The audit found that most of the people there didn't even know they had adopted this so-called criterion." Recognizing the implications of the exclusion, Schroeder stormed, "American women have been put at risk by medical practices that fail to include women in research studies. The health of American women will stay at risk until NIH fully implements its inclusion policy. American women deserve better treatment from the research community."

The GAO found that women were being underrepresented in studies of diseases affecting both men and women. In the fifty applications reviewed, one-fifth made no mention of gender and over one-third said the subjects would include both sexes, but did not give percentages. Some all-male studies gave no rationale for their exclusivity. "The [NIH] may win the Nobel Prize, but I'd like to see them get the *Good Housekeeping* seal of approval," said Congresswoman Barbara Mikulski (D-Md.), voicing her hopes that the behemoth medical institution could be made more woman-friendly.

As if medical research were some kind of exclusive male club, some of the biggest and most important medical studies of recent years had failed to enroll a single woman:

• The Baltimore Longitudinal Study, one of the largest studies to examine the natural process of aging, began in 1958 and included no women for its first twenty years because, according to Gene Cohen, then deputy director of the National Institute on Aging (NIA), the facility in which the study was conducted had only one toilet. The study's 1984 report, entitled "Normal Human Aging," contained no data on women. (Currently 40 percent of the participants in this study are women . . . although 60 percent of the population over age sixty-five is female.)

• The by-now-infamous Physicians' Health Study, which concluded in 1988 that taking an aspirin a day might reduce the risk of heart disease, included 22,000 men and no women.

• The 1982 Multiple Risk Factor Intervention Trial, known as Mr. Fit, a long-term study of lifestyle factors related to cholesterol and heart disease, included 13,000 men and no women. To this day no definitive answer exists on whether dietary change and exercise can benefit women in preventing heart disease.

• A Harvard School of Public Health study investigating the possible link between caffeine consumption and heart disease involved over 45,000 men and no women.

• Perhaps most unbelievably, a pilot project at Rockefeller University to study how obesity affected breast and uterine cancer was conducted solely on men. Said Congresswoman Olympia Snowe (R-Me.) upon hearing of this study, "Somehow, I find it hard to believe that the male-dominated medical community would tolerate a study of prostate cancer that used only women as research subjects."

Once the floodgates had been opened, revelations about gender bias in medical research suddenly came from a variety of sources. The Society for the Advancement of Women's Health Research, which had helped spur Congress to request the audit, revealed that though women spend more money on health care than men do and comprise 51 percent of the population, the money spent to research women's health was woefully inadequate. Only 13.5 percent of the 1987 NIH budget was being spent to study diseases that exclusively, predominantly, or more seriously affect women, or that have different risk factors or treatments in women.

This statistic caused some consternation among women, but male scientists were predictably defensive. William F. Raub, then–deputy director of NIH, calculated that using the same criteria to identify research on men's diseases, NIH devoted only about 5 percent of its 1987 budget to research issues pertaining primarily or exclusively to men.

But Dr. Raub's figures are misleading. Because of women's complex reproductive anatomy and hormonal cycles, far more diseases are exclusive to women. Yet not only were women being left out of research on diseases that affect both sexes, but just 13.5 percent of the total NIH budget was being used to look at breast cancer, all gynecological cancers, infertility, pregnancy, and contraception. Conditions such as fibroid tumors of the uterus, endometriosis, menstrual cramps, and premenstrual syndrome—all of which are quite common—were being virtually ignored. And diseases such as arthritis, Alzheimer's, and osteoporosis—which primarily affect women—were also being shortchanged.

Even the structure and staffing of the National Institutes of Health, which conducts or funds the lion's share of medical research in this country, seemed designed to put women's health second. At the time of the GAO report, NIH had only three gynecologists on staff, but thirty-nine veterinarians. There was, and is, no obstetrics and gynecology program on campus in Bethesda, Maryland. The National Institute of Child Health and Human Development—the only institute that looks at contraception, infertility, and pregnancy—receives only 5 percent of the total NIH budget and spends less than 10 percent of this on departments of ob-gyn. The institute's focus has traditionally been more pediatric than gynecological. Of over three thousand individuals on the NIH advisory committees, only twenty-six were ob-gyns, even though the most common causes for admissions to acute hospitals are for ailments that fall under this jurisdiction. Clearly women's health needs were not a priority at the nation's premier research institution.

NIH's two largest and most generously funded institutes, the National Cancer Institute and the National Heart, Lung and Blood Institute, were also guilty of bias. A study of thirty years' worth of randomized clinical trials of drug therapy for heart attacks (trials sponsored by NHLBI as well as others) found that fewer than 20 percent of the patients were female. And at the National Cancer Institute, a look at 1989 studies of fifteen different malignancies found that women were underrepresented in all but breast, endometrial and ovarian. For example, in studies of colorectal cancer, which kills more women than all gynecological malignancies combined, 44 percent of study subjects were women. Yet 51 percent of colorectal cancers occur in women.

As NIH's bias was revealed, other medical institutions and professional organizations scrambled to examine their own policies, and other reports were released equally critical of the state of women's health research in this country. The Institute of Medicine released a report showing that there was inadequate funding for obstetrical and gynecological research. Although the moral and political maelstrom surrounding contraception and abortion was one reason, another was that without an obstetrics or gynecology program at NIH there was no focal point for reproductive research. "With no women's institute at NIH, it's nearly impossible to get an obstetrical or gynecological grant accepted," said a frustrated maternal-fetal medicine specialist.

Ezra C. Davidson, Jr., M.D., then-president of the American College of Obstetricians and Gynecologists, which had not previously gone on record as being critical of NIH, rushed to jump on the bandwagon: "Women, who are the biggest users of the American health care system, are faced with a national research agenda that has too little research into the health issues that are of most concern to them personally. Research on early detection of ovarian cancer, effective and safe methods of contraception, osteoporosis and menopause are just four of the many areas in women's health that should be but are not high on this nation's research agenda."

The American Medical Association's Council on Ethical and Judicial Affairs released a report in July 1991 outlining gender disparities in patient treatments. "Our concern," said the authors, "is that medical treatments for women are based on a male model, regardless of the fact that women may react differently to treatments than men or that some diseases manifest themselves differently in women than in men. The results of medical research on men are generalized to women without sufficient evidence of applicability to women." One of the report's obvious conclusions: "More medical research on women's health and women's health problems should be pursued."

In January 1992 the National Heart, Lung and Blood Institute, the American Thoracic Society, and the American College of Chest Physicians sponsored a two-day meeting to discuss women's respiratory health and lung disease. After considering the body of information on smoking-induced disease (including lung cancer), asthma, cystic fibrosis, sleep apnea, respiratory infections, and environmental illnesses, the scientists came to an appalling realization: "The overwhelming conclusion of the participants was that relatively little is known about respiratory health and disease in women."

■ BRINGING BIAS TO LIGHT

What brought about the GAO audit that started this domino effect of damning evidence? In 1985, five years before the audit, the Public Health Service had warned that the lack of medical data on women was limiting the understanding of women's health care needs. In 1986 an NIH advisory committee recommended that women always be included in NIH-sponsored clinical trials unless researchers could legitimately justify their exclusion. In spite of these recommendations, however, women were still being ignored. Women within NIH were well aware of the problem, but didn't know how to effectively expose it without irreparably damaging their own careers. In 1990 several prominent women scientists and women's health advocates, along with political lobbyists Joanne Howes and Marie Bass, formed an organization called the Society for the Advancement of Women's Health Research. It was this organization that brought the problem to the attention of the Congressional Caucus for Women's Issues.

Lesley Primmer, director of the congressional women's group, devised a political solution to the research problem. She realized that since NIH was supposed to have a policy mandating the inclusion of women, Congress could legitimately request an audit to see if that policy was being enforced. So Congresswomen Schroeder and Snowe, who chaired the bipartisan caucus, along with Congressman Henry Waxman (D-Calif.), chairman of the House Subcommittee on Health and the Environment, called for the General Accounting Office to scrutinize NIH's inclusion of women. Finally NIH was going to be held accountable to its own policy. "I gave Lesley [Primmer] a crowbar as a gift," says Florence Haseltine, M.D., director of the Center for Population Research at the National Institute of Child Health and Human Development, "in gratitude for figuring out how to use the GAO audit as a wedge."

The reaction to the flood of findings was swift and furious. Congresswoman Snowe charged that "NIH's attitude has been to consider over half the population as some sort of special case." As more and more information on gender bias in medical research came out in the press, the public was treated to such unbelievable and infuriating "trivia" as the fact that even the rats used in medical research were almost exclusively white males. Said Congresswomen Schroeder, "If anyone thinks women are going to keep paying half the cost of health care and have researchers so elitist they won't even use female rats in the research, they're nuts."

But excluding women as subjects is only one aspect of research bias. The real problem is much broader, and women are excluded at nearly every level of scientific research.

"Who decides what ideas are worthy of pursuit?" asks Elaine Borins, M.D., an assistant professor of psychiatry at the University of Toronto who has extensively studied the issue of gender bias in scientific research. "Whose ideas are they? Who funds what? Who decided that heart disease is more important than breast cancer in terms of allocation of resources? Who gets to do the studies? How do they do them? Who gets published? Who gets publicized?"

The answer to these questions, as Dr. Borins well knows, is middle-aged, predominantly white men. Medical journals, textbooks, and libraries are filled with data on this segment of the population, in articles researched, written, edited, and published by demographically similar professionals.

Medical journals have been particularly reluctant to admit to bias. In 1990 Marcia Angell, M.D., executive editor of the *New England Journal of Medicine*, dismissed the idea that excluding women from participating in medical research affected their health, saying, "Gender bias is not serious in a way that distorts research. It doesn't serve women well to see sexism where it doesn't exist." Three years later she seemed less adamant, but still unconvinced. Writing in a July 22, 1993, editorial in the journal—long after all the reports listed above had been released—she said, "Whether diseases in women have been inadequately studied is difficult to say."

But the women scientists who read the journals felt otherwise. "The typical study published in the *New England Journal of Medicine* has twenty-nine men and one woman testing a new drug that has never been tried before the study," says Dr. Borins. "The one woman never actually participates in some of the preliminary exercises that the men do—she never takes the treadmill test. Then the drugs are given. Then this group is compared to a control group of twenty-six men and four women, or no women. Then the results come out that this is a good drug—or not—for everybody. It's really incredible."

Borins and her colleague Karen Williams, M.A., examined articles published in the *New England Journal of Medicine* in 1989, searching for examples of gender bias. They looked at the study topics, the study subjects, the authors, and the methods; they also scrutinized the articles for sexism in the language or underlying ideas of the study. They found that over 80 percent of the published research was flawed with regard to gender.

But when Borins attempted to publish these findings in a medical journal, she was repeatedly stonewalled. The *New England Journal of Medicine* (*NEJM*) sent a cursory rejection note, without explanation, and without even sending the study out for peer review. "People think of *NEJM* as the ultimate journal, state-of-the-art," she says. "That's what's so sad. That 80 percent of the studies are wrong." Other medical journals were similarly reluctant to publish a study that pointed an accusing finger at their industry.

Because Dr. Borins's study was not quickly published, other women researchers, unaware that the work had been done, completed similar studies, showing over and over again, with scrupulous statistical analysis that few would ever read, how the studies were biased.

At Albert Einstein College of Medicine in New York, Pamela Charney, M.D., and Carole Morgan, Ph.D., did a survey of the 1990 medical literature. They looked at the three highest-subscribed-to U.S.-based medical journals—the *New England Journal of Medicine*, the *Journal of the American Medical Association*, and the *Annals of Internal Medicine*. They considered every article that involved an intervention or treatment, and categorized diseases as gender specific, potentially gender-associated, or unaffected by gender. One hundred and twenty-two studies met their entry criteria, involving 67,000 subjects. But only 13,000 of these subjects were women. In studies of cardiovascular disease, of 42,000 patients studied, only a bit over two thousand—or 5 percent—were women. Of the seventy-seven studies that did include men and women, only 14 percent reported any gender analysis at all, and only 5 percent bothered to analyze the data specifically to interpret gender findings. "People thought that when researchers started including women, there would be a greater understanding about gender and health, but that hasn't happened yet," says Dr. Charney.

In Washington, D.C., at Georgetown University, similar research was being done. Jean M. Mitchell, Ph.D., and Christine M. Cushman, M.P.P., examined 366 clinical trials published in the *New England Journal of Medicine* and the *Journal of the American Medical Association* between January 1986 and October 1992 to determine whether the studies adequately included women. They counted a total of 216,118 men included in these studies, and only 90,717 women. In other words these clinical trials studied more than twice as many men as women. Thirty percent of the studies included 20 percent or fewer female subjects.

As of mid-1994 only Dr. Borins's study had been published—in the September–October 1993 issue of the *Journal of the American Medical Women's Association*. Unfortunately, publishing in *JAMWA*, which is read almost exclusively by women physicians, is like preaching to the converted. Or like publishing an article about women's rights in *Ms.*, whose readers already believe in them, instead of in a magazine where opinions might be swayed.

■ FIGHTING FOR A FAIR SHARE

As with women's rights in general, the controversy over women in medical research is a complex issue with its origins in social and governmental bias against women. After all, the National Institutes of Health is a government institution funded by tax dollars, and women have always had to fight for their fair share of money and power. "How we spend our research dollars has to do with whatever pressure is out there from interest groups," explains Irma L. Mebane-Sims, Ph.D., an epidemiologist at the National Heart, Lung and Blood Institute. "Groups focusing on women's health issues are now able to exert some pressure." In other words, the feminist fight over medical research is just beginning.

Under pressure from congressional women and the American public, the government and the scientific community began to take steps to open medical studies to women and allocate more money for women's health. Within months of the GAO report, in September 1990, NIH established the Office of Research on Women's Health (ORWH). Led by acting director Ruth L. Kirschstein, M.D., the office was set up to address the inequities in women's health and serve as a focal point for women's health research at NIH. The office exists to strengthen research into women's diseases and health conditions, to ensure that women are appropriately represented in research studies, and to help further the careers of women in biomedical research. Says current ORWH director Vivian W. Pinn, M.D., "Women cannot gain from new advances in therapy and interventions if they are not included in the clinical trials that assess safety and efficacy."

The office does not fund studies directly, but supplements ongoing grants or co-funds new initiatives in collaboration with other NIH institutes and centers. The awards are intended to encourage researchers to include more women in a study population or to fill a gap in knowledge regarding women's health. One of the first special research initiatives was co-funded with the National Institute of Child Health and Human Development to study endometriosis and uterine fibroids.

Federal legislation supporting these efforts was slower in coming, in part because of the Bush administration's apparent disdain for women's health issues, which it seemed to group together with abortion rights and fetal-tissue research as moral affronts. It was abortion politics that killed early versions of legislation—the NIH Revitalization Amendments of 1991—that would have put federal law behind the inclusion of women and minorities in clinical trials, and would have ensured the continued existence of the Office of Research on Women's Health. The amendments would also have provided increased support for studies on breast and ovarian cancers, contraception, infertility, and osteoporosis. But because of a clause providing for fetal-tissue research, the Senate voted against one version, and President Bush vetoed another, apparently fearing that women would be so selfless and altruistic that they would get pregnant in droves simply for the chance to have an abortion and donate the fetal tissue to science. (Because of President Bush's—and President Reagan's—aversion to fetal-tissue research, United States doctors have had to import fetal tissue from the former Soviet Union in order to treat Parkinson's patients.)

It wasn't until June 10, 1993—almost three years to the day after the infamous GAO audit—that the revised bill, now called the NIH Revitalization Act of 1993, was signed by President Clinton. Finally there was federal muscle to mandate that NIH enforce its own policies. The NIH Revitalization Act ensures the continued existence of the Office of Research on Women's Health and specifies that studies must not only include women (and minorities) but be carried out in such a way that gender and racial differences can be analyzed. The analysis is crucial. Too many researchers were simply including women in their studies to obey the letter of the law, but omitting the important step of breaking down the results by gender to see if there are differences in the way men and women react (to a drug, a treatment, a diet). Now their omission wouldn't just be lazy; it would be illegal.

Even before it had congressional legislation behind it, the Office of Research on Women's Health had begun to develop an agenda and target the areas of women's health that needed attention. The list, outlined in a report titled, "Opportunities for Research on Women's Health," was vast, beginning with heart disease, cancer, and stroke, the leading killers of both men and women. The report stated that "the startling realization is that most of the biomedical knowledge about the causes, expression, and treatment of these diseases derives from studies of men and is applied to women with the supposition that there are no differences." Diseases that affect disproportionate numbers of women were listed, such as Alzheimer's disease, depression and other mental disorders, osteoporosis, sexually transmitted diseases, immunologic diseases (such as rheumatoid arthritis and systemic lupus erythematosis), diabetes, multiple sclerosis, lung cancer, and respiratory illnesses.

Other areas were more specific to women: breast and gynecological cancers, pre- and post-natal care, uterine fibroids, endometriosis, pelvic inflammatory disease, contraception, infertility, gynecological disorders, menopause, menstruation. The report cited the "pervasive sense in the research community that many of the health issues of women are of secondary importance, especially those that occur solely in women and those that occur in men and women but have already been studied chiefly in men." Obviously there was, and still is, a vast amount of work to be done.

WHY WOMEN WERE LEFT OUT

Even nonscientists know that women's bodies are different from men's, and it's not a great leap to recognize that both sexes must be studied for medical research to be valid. The scientific community did not so much have a blind spot as a willful disregard for women's health. But researchers have a number of excuses for why they proceeded as they did. They claim that including women as research subjects complicates their work for a variety of reasons:

* *Study populations would be less homogenous and therefore harder to analyze.*
  But who decided the 70-kilogram (154 pound) man is the measure of all research? In fact, a smaller female body represents more of the population and would be more of a true scientific standard. Also, since women's average life expectancy is seven years longer than men's, women suffer more

of the diseases of aging, and are better suited to long-term studies. If research is to single out one gender, that gender should logically be female. Since no one is suggesting that men be left out of research, scientists will simply have to learn to factor in and analyze one more variable in their studies.

Leaving women out of studies, or not analyzing studies for gender, can lead to erroneous conclusions. For example, a recent study comparing surgery-plus-chemotherapy versus surgery alone for rectal cancer found a survival advantage for the combined treatment. But when the data were broken down by sex, it turns out that the benefits of chemotherapy are restricted to men.

- *Studies would be more expensive because they would require more subjects.*
  Though studies may become more expensive with larger study populations and more variables to analyze, women's health is worth the expense. While old NIH policy accepted cost as an excuse for not including women in research, the newly passed NIH Revitalization Act expressly forbids financial considerations as justification for leaving women out.

- *Women are harder to recruit into studies.*
  That all depends on where researchers are looking. Many scientists have relied on easily identifiable groups of men—army recruits, veterans, physicians—as participants. Now they'll have to identify comparable groups of women. For example there is currently a Nurses' Health Study, a large observational study of 120,000 female nurses, that examines how lifestyle (diet, exercise, smoking) affects women's health. Recruitment tactics may have to be modified to attract women. Targeting publications and community groups with special appeal to women will give researchers access to the large numbers of women they need. They may also have to consider special requirements such as transportation and child care, in order to ensure participation by a cross-section of women and not just those with the time and/or money to participate. But the success of several recently launched women's studies, such as the Women's Health Initiative, in recruiting thousands of volunteers proves that plenty of women are both willing and able to be a part of medical research.

One African-American woman who had participated in a breast cancer trial in 1989 found the experience so positive that she now volunteers her time as a speaker, encouraging other women to sign up for studies. "I felt really special while participating in the trial," says Barbara S. Brown, of

Richmond, Virginia. "I felt that I was making a contribution to other women and their health and well-being."

- *Women's various hormonal states and cycles—menstrual cycles, pregnancy hormones, oral contraceptives, menopause, hormone replacement therapy— might confuse research results.*

Using women's hormones as an excuse to exclude them is a puzzling defense, since hormonal differences are one of the most important reasons why women must be included. It defies logic for researchers to acknowledge gender difference by claiming that women's hormones can affect study results—for instance, by affecting drug metabolism—but then to ignore those differences, study only men, and extrapolate the results to women.

Important information on drug dosage and timing is being missed by not including women. Some scientists feel that drugs may have to be studied twice in women—before and after ovulation—in order to assess how women metabolize the medication. According to the Office of Research on Women's Health, "If a drug is eliminated from a woman's body more slowly than from a man's, the woman might have a greater risk of side effects or might need a lower dosage. Furthermore, hormonal changes during the menstrual cycle may alter the effects of drugs in women, as noted in the use of antidepressant drugs." Evidence is now emerging that the effects of certain antidepressants vary over the course of the menstrual cycle. Premenstrual women taking a constant dose of these drugs may be getting too much during some parts of the month, too little during others.

Not taking hormonal factors into account means that eventually women's hormones are going to confound treatments that were developed without regard to them. For instance, recent studies suggest that surgery for breast cancer is most successful in the second half of a woman's monthly cycle rather than during the menstrual flow. The same might be true for other types of surgery. But no one will ever know unless women are included in the studies.

- *Women report more drug side effects.*

That women report more drug side effects than men is precisely why they *should* be a mandatory part of research. Drug manufacturers have been shirking their responsibility to women by obtaining drug approvals with male data and ignoring the possibility of side effects in women. Once the drugs are approved, they can be prescribed to both men and women, even if women were not included in the research.

Another reason women may suffer more drug side effects is that drug dosages are geared to the 154-pound man. Not only does the average woman weigh less than the average man, but she has a greater proportion of body fat, which can increase the amount of medication that is absorbed and retained. The current recommended doses of many drugs may be *over-doses* for women, and too much of any medication can lead to unwanted side effects.

PROTECTION OR PATERNALISM?

The objection to women's participation in health research that is most difficult to counter is the concern over exposing a fetus to a drug or treatment that might be dangerous, or at least has not been proven safe. Recent history makes it impossible to dismiss these fears. In the 1950s the drug thalidomide, given to European women to combat nausea during pregnancy, caused thousands of children to be born with severe deformities. In this country the drug diethylstilbestrol (DES) was widely prescribed to pregnant women during the 1940s and 1950s to prevent miscarriage, but has led to gynecological cancers and other medical problems in the offspring of the women who took it.

But in their effort to expose the fetus to "zero risk," scientists have shied away from including not just pregnant women in their studies, but any woman who could potentially become pregnant.

Translated into research practice, that meant that no woman between the ages of fifteen and fifty could participate in the earliest stages of new drug research unless she had been surgically sterilized or had a hysterectomy. (And since many studies have an upper age limit of sixty-five, that leaves a narrow window of opportunity for women to participate.) Exceptions were made only in the case of extremely severe or life-threatening illnesses.

While policies to protect unborn children seem to make sense on first reading, upon closer examination they represent protectionism run amok. An increasing number of studies are showing that exposure to chemicals and environmental toxins can affect *sperm*, yet no one is suggesting that men be excluded from research in order to protect their unborn children. When Proscar, a drug used to treat enlarged prostate glands, was found to cause birth defects in the offspring of male animals given the drug, men in the drug trials simply had to sign a consent form saying they would use condoms. Women weren't given the option of using contraception during the trial. By grouping together all women between the ages of fifteen and fifty as potentially pregnant, researchers were implying that women have no control over their reproductive lives.

The exclusions approached the absurd. Women who were not sexually active could not participate in early stages of new drug research. Women whose partners had had a vasectomy could not participate. Lesbians who had no intention of becoming pregnant could not participate. Women taking oral contraceptives could not participate. The list went on.

The absurdity was compounded by the fact that many trials last only a few months or less, and it would have been simple enough to require sexually active women to use contraception and take inexpensive pregnancy tests. Any potentially dangerous treatment could be discontinued in the earliest stage of a pregnancy. Most studies would pose little risk even if a woman were to become pregnant. The chances of a fetus being harmed by a test of new eyedrops, for example, are small.

The issue of protecting unborn children involves law as well as ethics. Medical researchers are terrified that if a woman participating in research does become pregnant, and the fetus is harmed, they will be legally and financially liable. Even when women offer to sign an informed-consent form acknowledging that they are not to become pregnant during the course of the trial, and to sign a waiver of responsibility, medical institutions and pharmaceutical manufacturers still worry that they will not be adequately protected if they are sued.

The scientific community bases its fears on the example of medical malpractice law, where enormous sums of money are regularly awarded to people who claim they've been damaged by medical treatment. Any jury seeing a malformed baby whose mother was a volunteer in a medical study, say scientists, would certainly hold the researchers responsible for the tragedy.

But lawyers say that medical malpractice is the wrong model, and that there have been few successful lawsuits by people who were harmed by medical research after signing an informed-consent form. Some lawyers now say that excluding women from research may actually be a more dangerous legal stance. Researchers—pharmaceutical researchers in particular—leave themselves more open to legal lawsuits by *not* including women in their studies. Rather than protecting women, exclusion has actually exposed them to more danger by introducing new drugs and new treatments that are not well understood in women. And pharmaceutical manufacturers could be vulnerable to lawsuits charging that they have exposed women to unknown risks and harm by making drugs available to the public that were not adequately tested on women. Only eleven drugs, for example, have been specifically approved for use during pregnancy, but many more are prescribed without certainty that they are safe.

Women may also have a constitutional right to be included in medical research, provided they give their informed consent. One case often cited as precedent is the 1989 court case against Johnson Controls, a battery-manufacturing company. A group of female employees sued the factory for not allowing them to work the more lucrative assembly-line jobs, because if they were to become pregnant, the lead exposure could harm their unborn children. The women argued, successfully, that they had the right to be informed of the risk and make their own decision about whether they wanted to expose themselves to it.

The Food and Drug Administration's (FDA) policy designed to protect unborn children went on the books in 1977. The policy was supposed to be reevaluated every eighteen to twenty-four months, but was not examined again until 1992, in part at the urging of women's health advocacy groups. The restrictions finally loosened in 1993, after the FDA, like the National Institutes of Health, was confronted with a government audit.

Taking the same approach they had used to expose NIH's exclusion of women, the Congressional Caucus for Women's Issues requested in 1992 that the government's General Accounting Office do an audit of the FDA. As they expected, they found that women were underrepresented in drug trials, especially in the earliest stages of new drug research. The GAO examined the clinical trials of fifty-three new drugs subsequently approved by the agency over the course of three and a half years. They found that while women had been represented in each trial, their numbers had sometimes been too low. In nearly two-thirds of the drug trials, the proportion of women tested was less than the proportion of women with the corresponding disease. Women were particularly underrepresented in trials of new cardiovascular drugs.

And in more than half the trials, the results had not been analyzed to determine whether men and women responded differently, even though in 1988 the FDA had issued guidelines emphasizing the importance of analyzing trial data by gender. For instance, a trial with an equal number of men and women might find that 15 percent of the participants developed a rash as a result of taking an experimental drug. But when the results are broken down by sex, it may be that only 5 percent of men, but 25 percent of women, suffer this side effect. And this would be important prescribing information for physicians. "Practically all drugs on the market should have a warning label that says, 'This drug has never been studied in women, particularly women of childbearing age,'" states Alice Dan, director of the

Center for Research on Women and Gender at the University of Illinois at Chicago. "Women prescribed drugs now are essentially experimental subjects without knowing it, agreeing to it, or wanting it."

As a result of the GAO audit and pressure from congressional women and the public, in July 1993 the FDA announced new guidelines for including women in drug research, loosening many of the restrictions it had imposed on researchers. The 1977 blanket ban on including women of "childbearing potential" was lifted, with the proviso that these women sign informed-consent forms acknowledging the possible risk to a fetus if they become pregnant and stating they will use contraception throughout the trial. The FDA is also recommending that new drug research include studies on drug interactions with male and female hormones. Oral contraceptives can sometimes block the effects of other drugs, and other medications can sometimes prevent contraceptives from being effective.

The GAO report found that only 12 percent of new drug studies included analysis of hormonal or oral-contraceptive interactions in women. This omission is potentially deadly. Women are the main consumers of over-the-counter diet pills, for example, yet phenylpropanolamine (PPA), the main ingredient in these drugs, was never adequately tested in women. A major side effect of this chemical is high blood pressure. Since oral contraceptives can also elevate blood pressure, diet pills may not be safe for women taking birth control pills. Hypertension and even strokes have already been reported in some young women taking PPA.

The new guidelines bring the FDA's policy more in line with the National Institutes of Health's. Research submitted to the FDA is largely privately funded, while NIH's budget comes from taxpayer dollars. Since many researchers receive money from both sources, and all of the policies were binding, the double set of standards was confusing. "Researchers had the NIH telling them they *must* include women and the FDA telling them they *can't*," says Tracy L. Johnson, former program director for the Society for the Advancement of Women's Health Research. "It was a mess."

■ THE FEMALE MODEL OF MEDICINE

Now that including women is a visible policy at both NIH and the FDA, specific groups of women are speaking up to insist on their representation. African-American women, Hispanic women, Asian women, older women, and lesbian women want their medical needs addressed. At a meeting in Bethesda, Maryland, sponsored by the Office of Research on Women's Health to discuss recruitment and retention of women in clinical

trials, these groups and others stood up to demand that their health be researched.

Many scientists are terrified by the idea of breaking down their research populations into smaller and smaller subgroups, each requiring
separate analysis. They argue that studies will become impossibly unwieldy
and that too many subgroups will leave them with numbers so small as to
be statistically insignificant. There is concern, too, that racial and ethnic
breakdowns may be misleading. Many people have a diverse racial makeup,
making them difficult to categorize. Also, basing medical conclusions on
race can lead to erroneous conclusions. Pima Indians, for example, have a
greatly increased risk of developing diabetes, while other Native American
groups do not.

Racial diversity in medical research does not only concern women;
most research in the past has not been conducted on a cross-section of
men, but predominantly on white men. And it's difficult to answer the
question of how much diversity is necessary, since so little is known about
racial and ethnic differences in disease. "How many ways must we slice and
dice in the interest of fairness?" asks Marcia Angell of the *New England
Journal of Medicine*.

The answer, for now, is at least *two*: male and female. Before the pie
can be served, it must first be cut in half.

Recently NIH's requirements have been strengthened with regard to
the inclusion of women and minorities. Now not only must the *people* being studied be a diverse group, but even identifiable *tissue samples* must
conform to the new NIH Guidelines on the Inclusion of Women and Minorities as Subjects in Clinical Research. These tissue samples were often
obtained from soldiers killed in action, or accident victims—mostly men.
The rationale was that for some studies researchers needed tissue from people who were healthy until their death. The gender of samples isn't crucial
for studies where researches simply grind up the tissue and study cell par-
ticles such as mitochondria. "But if you're going to examine heart arteries
after coronary bypass surgery, for example, it would be essential to the
study to include both men and women," explains Judith H. LaRosa,
Ph.D., deputy director of the Office of Research on Women's Health.

In all of the NIH's and FDA's new guidelines, one glaring omission remains. Currently neither NIH nor the FDA has guidelines for including
female *animals* in scientific research. For many of the same reasons that human females have been excluded from studies—their hormones complicate
research and confuse results, studies become costlier (in this case because
female animals are more expensive)—female rats, monkeys, and other an-

imals are generally not used in laboratories. Little is known of the estrous cycle of rats, for example, or how it affects metabolism. "Scientists even use only male rat urine in research," says the University of Toronto's Dr. Borins. "They say female rat urine is too complicated."

Just as women scientists looked at the medical journals to assess the number of women included in clinical trials, Jeri A. Sechzer, M.A., Ph.D., of Pace University examined scientific journals to assess the number of male and female animals that were studied. Her results were disturbingly similar to the human findings. In the journal *Behavioral Neuroscience* in 1991, for instance, eight male animals were used for every female. Yet human studies are often based on earlier findings in animals, so it seems crucial that even at the earliest stages of research female animals be included.

Although there are obviously still gender inequities to be remedied, in the years since the GAO report was released there's been a frantic flurry of activity. Dozens of committees have held meetings, issued reports, and made recommendations. New guidelines have been released, and new studies have been funded.

The centerpiece of all these efforts is the Women's Health Initiative (WHI), a $625-million, fourteen-year study of 160,000 women ages fifty to seventy-nine. The largest clinical trial ever sponsored by the National Institutes of Health, the WHI will attempt to determine whether cardiovascular disease, cancer, and osteoporosis can be prevented or forestalled by dietary, behavioral, and drug interventions.

One arm of the trial is a randomized controlled trial of promising but unproven approaches to prevention: low-fat diet to prevent breast cancer, colon cancer, and heart disease; hormone replacement therapy to prevent heart disease and osteoporosis; and calcium and vitamin D supplements to prevent osteoporosis and colon cancer. The second part is an observational study to identify predictors of disease. And the third part is a trial of community approaches to develop healthful behaviors.

The study's scope and size make it an important milestone in women's health research, though, like any study of this size and cost, it has come under its share of criticism. Some scientists argue that the study should have been split into several smaller studies, because metaphorically putting all the eggs in one basket means that if the study does not reach definite conclusions, the entire, gigantic effort will have been a waste. Yet supporters of the study argue that its size is its strength, and that any conclusions it reaches will carry the weight of an enormous sample population.

Another criticism is that the study will expose women who volunteer for the hormone replacement therapy arm of the trial to hormones that may raise their risk of cancer. For instance, giving estrogen without pro-gesterone to women who still have their wombs has been associated with an increased risk of endometrial cancer. But adding progesterone to ne-gate this cancer risk *may* lower the heart- and bone-protective effects of the hormone. The comprehensive, ten-page informed-consent form women must sign to participate in the trial acknowledges the risk and advises that women on either of these regimes will be carefully moni-tored. Treatment will be discontinued if endometrial changes are de-tected. Increased risk or not, these hormonal regimens are being prescribed to hundreds of thousands of postmenopausal women across the country. A study to determine the risks and benefits seems long over-due. "We've been using Premarin [the most commonly prescribed estro-gen] for forty years; I often say we've been engaging in perhaps the largest mass experiment, uncontrolled, for four decades, and we still don't have the answers," says William Harlan, M.D., who oversees the Women's Health Initiative.

Yet another concern of critics is that the trial may not be long enough to properly assess cancer risks. Cancers may take years or even decades to develop, and will only occur in a small minority of women. The study would do better, some critics say, to focus on the role of diet in preventing heart disease rather than breast cancer. Although there have been no prom-ises, and certainly no guaranteed funding, the scientists hope to follow up the women in the trial for years after it has ended, continuing to compile data on cancer risk and prevention.

Finally, the trial has come under fire for not including enough women scientists. Bernadine Healy, ex-director of NIH, said in 1992 that "I would hope that a lot of the PI's [principal investigators] end up being wom-en. . . . [If] you ask me who's the most effective in recruiting women to a trial, it's going to be women." Yet only three of the first sixteen principal investigators named were women (the remaining twenty-nine had not been named as this book went to press).

Despite all these concerns, WHI is still a step in the right direction. But it is only one step. There is a danger in looking to one study for all the answers. Women may read about WHI and feel reassured that within a few years medical research will have quickly brought knowledge about women's health on a par with men's. But WHI is a beginning, not an end, and it's entirely too soon to be complacent. It will take more than one study to remedy inequities in medical research.

In a sense the Women's Health Initiative is a catch-up study, an at-tempt to bring women's health research up to speed. "It will add some new information, but basically we're trying to get the type of data that we already have on men. We can't go forward on women's research without it," says NIH's Haseltine. "For instance right now we only have estrogen and estrogen-like drugs for contraception and menopause. When there are more contraceptive choices and menopause is treated with a variety of approaches, as hypertension is, then we'll have succeeded."

Although there's an impulse to produce quick answers, scientific catch-up can only mean *starting* the new investigations promptly, not rushing the results. There's a grave danger in looking for a quick fix. Women should resist the impulse for fast answers and instead insist on scientifically valid results, realizing that these may take decades to come.

Another danger in complacency is neglecting the very real problem of enforcement. "We can't make any assumption that women's health research and the larger focus on diversity is guaranteed," says Irma Mebane-Sims, board member of the Society for the Advancement of Women's Health Research. "There are too many issues that can alter it."

Careful monitoring, by the Office of Research on Women's Health and government agencies, must ensure that researchers do not look for loopholes in the new guidelines. Including women and minorities as study variables—meaning they must not only be included but also analyzed separately and accounted for in all findings—means extra work for researchers. Their reaction to the new guidelines has not been uniformly positive. "It's frightening a lot of researchers," says Nancy Reame, R.N., Ph.D., professor at the Center for Nursing Research, University of Michigan. "When an NIH staff member brought this up in a meeting, white male scientists got up and said it was outrageous. Several people even got up to the microphone and said they would lie, would say they're going to analyze gender but then not do it."

Public attention to this issue will go far toward ensuring compliance. And since scientific studies are generally funded for one year at a time, money can and must be awarded with regard to gender inclusion and analysis. "Public pressure has to be maintained, but I think the pressure will be maintained," says Dr. Haseltine.

Other problems with medical research in this country go beyond gender. Medical research will always involve an element of risk for those who volunteer, whether male or female. But because for much of history women have been subjugated to men, there is concern that their risk at the hands of largely male researchers is greater than men's.

This is a valid concern, but slightly outdated. Now that women's economic and political power is rising, and women are among the "establishment" in the medical research community, women's risk from research should be no greater than men's. As long as women are apprised of all study risks, they can make a knowledgeable decision and sign an informed consent as responsibly as a man can.

Women themselves may need a little bit of convincing to volunteer. The legacy of Tuskegee and other shameful incidents in research history lingers. The association of study-volunteers with guinea pigs persists. To combat a poor public image, scientists will have to woo women by impressing upon them the benefits they hope to provide to *all* women. The thousands of women who called about participating in the Women's Health Initiative as soon as it was announced proved that this should not be a problem.

Another concern with much medical research in this country is that it tends to be quantitative rather than qualitative. There are few studies into quality of life, which is something women researchers might be more interested in studying. For instance, if a woman has breast cancer, a doctor can tell her, based on previous studies, what her chances for survival are with each form of therapy available. Obviously that's crucial information. But what a doctor can't tell her is how other women who were faced with similar decisions feel about their choices, whether they would make the same decision again, and what they would recommend to others in the same position.

The same is true of older women who are considering motherhood. There are tables of statistics about the increased risk of having a low-birthweight baby or a child with Down syndrome. But there are almost no studies on whether older mothers feel more tired than younger ones, whether they suffer more or less morning sickness and varicose veins, whether their recovery after pregnancy is slower.

Support groups fill some of this function and help answer some questions, but the information needs to be obtained more rigorously. Women and men should not have to rely on a random sampling of anecdotes to help them make health care decisions. Unfortunately these kinds of qualitative studies don't win tenure or get published in the medical journals.

Medical research has also not grappled well with the difficulty and cost of long-term studies. New drugs may be approved after volunteers have taken them for only a few years. Yet many drugs prescribed preventively or to treat chronic conditions are taken for decades. Oral contraceptives, for example, were first approved for marketing in 1960 after less than five years of study. And on the basis of that scanty evidence, the sexual revolution was launched, possibly at the expense of women's health. Today millions of women may start taking birth control pills in their teens and continue taking them until menopause, when they may switch to hormone replacement therapy. But *no* studies have evaluated the safety of such long-term hormone use.

In the end, the most effective appeal to the scientific community on all of these issues is not to charge sexism or callousness, even if such accusations are valid. Instead it is to point out all the problems in the system and show why ignoring them is not just sexism—a charge that can be too easily shrugged off—but bad science. That's hitting the research community where it hurts. Addressing these inequities is not just good for women, it's good for everybody.

II

SECOND-CLASS
PATIENTS

4

WOMEN'S HEARTS
The Deadly Difference

Kathy O'Brien (not her real name), a forty-two-year-old smoker, had been experiencing chest pains on and off for about a year. Her father and two of her uncles had died of heart attacks when young. She went to a clinic in the rural area of northwest New Jersey where she lived, and there the local doctors told her she probably had gallstones. When the pain got worse, she went back to the clinic, where they told her she'd have to have a sonogram of her gallbladder. She left without having it done. Instead Kathy went home, collapsed from chest pain, and nearly died. She had suffered a massive heart attack and gone into cardiac arrest. Technically dead, she had to be defibrillated with electrical shocks on the way to the hospital. The following day she was transferred to a larger, teaching hospital, where doctors did an angiogram and found a blockage in a major blood vessel. After bypass surgery she recovered well. But why, wondered the cardiologists at the larger hospital, didn't anyone recognize heart disease in a heavy smoker with chest pain and a serious family history of death from heart attack?

Though it has been the leading cause of death in American women since 1908, heart disease is one of the best-kept secrets of women's health. It wasn't until 1964 that the American Heart Association sponsored its first conference on women and heart disease. Held in Portland, and sponsored by the Oregon affiliate of the AHA, the conference was advertised as "for women only" and attracted an audience of ten thousand. So many groups of women traveled to Portland from smaller towns around the state that the police finally had to ask local radio and television announcers to warn motorists of the traffic jam around the coliseum where the conference was being held.

The real topic of this conference wasn't women and heart disease, however. It was how women could take care of their *husbands'* hearts. "Hearts and Husbands: The First Women's Conference on Coronary Heart Disease" explained to women the important role they played in keeping their spouses healthy. "The conference was a symposium on how to take care of your *man*: how to feed him and make sure he didn't get heart disease, and how to take care of him if he did," explains Mary Ann Malloy, M.D., a cardiologist at Loyola University Medical Center in Chicago, and head of the AHA's local Women and Heart Disease committee. The conference organizers prepared an educational pamphlet called "Eight Questions Wives Ask." There was no discussion at all of ways for women to recognize their own symptoms or to prevent the disease that was killing more of them than any other, no mention of how women could look after their own heart health. And no one objected, including women, because, for the medical profession and the public, heart disease was an exclusively male problem.

Both physicians and the public still harbor the misconception that women do not suffer from heart disease. Yet many more women die from cardiovascular disease—478,000 in 1993—than from all forms of cancer combined, which are responsible for 237,000 deaths. Although women seem to fear breast cancer more, only one in eight women will develop it (and not all of them will die of it), while one in two will develop cardiovascular disease. And for those who persist in thinking of heart disease as a male province, in 1992 (the most recent statistics available), more women than men died of cardiovascular disease. Among women, 46 percent of all deaths are due to cardiovascular disease; in men it's 40 percent. Because heart disease tends to be an illness of older, postmenopausal women, the incidence of heart disease, and the number of deaths, have been rising as women's life expectancies have increased. "Women didn't die of heart disease when the median age of death was the fifties or sixties," says Nanette K. Wenger, M.D., professor of medicine (cardiology) at Emory University School of Medicine in Atlanta.

Yet despite these ominous numbers, the vast majority of research into coronary artery disease, the type of heart disease that causes most heart attacks, has been done on middle-aged men. "We're very much in an infancy in terms of understanding heart disease in women," says Irma L. Mebane-Sims, Ph.D., an epidemiologist at the National Heart, Lung and Blood Institute. Compared with men's hearts, women's hearts are still largely a mystery.

Researchers justify their focus on men as an effort to prevent *premature* heart disease. Heart disease often occurs in middle-aged men, but tends to occur in postmenopausal women, as levels of the hormone estrogen (thought to be protective) drop. Researchers talk about a ten- to fifteen-year age gap between women and men who develop heart disease. And many cardiac researchers defend their focus on men by saying it is more important to try to prevent heart attacks in men in their forties or fifties than in women (and men) in their sixties, seventies, and beyond.

Unfortunately the issue is not so simple. It's true that if you look at a group of sixty-year-old men and women, statistically only one in seventeen women will have suffered a heart attack, versus one in five men. But there's another way to look at this group of sixty-year-olds, and that is to ask, How many of these people will have a heart attack in their lifetime? How many will die of heart disease? The answer is that as many of the women as men will eventually succumb to heart attacks and cardiac death. And the risk factors that lead to the eventual heart attack can begin decades earlier.

How is it possible to define a "premature" heart attack, anyway? In an era when a vast number of adults will live productive, healthy lives well into their seventies, eighties, and even nineties, when does a premature heart attack occur? At sixty-five? seventy? seventy-five? Does the fact that a woman's average life expectancy is about seven years longer than a man's mean that a premature attack for her occurs later? These are tough questions to answer, and perhaps recognizing this, the American Heart Association has recently stricken the word *premature* from its statement of purpose.

If coronary disease in postmenopausal women can be dismissed by physicians because the women are often quite elderly, coronary artery disease in younger, premenopausal women is often overlooked entirely. "We were taught in medical school that premenopausal women don't have heart attacks, so we don't look for heart disease in premenopausal women," confesses one middle-aged internist.

Even when a woman suffering chest pain is fortunate enough to see a physician who takes her symptoms seriously, she still faces steep obstacles to proper care and treatment. Many of the tests used to diagnose heart disease, such as the exercise treadmill, have poor accuracy rates in women. The drugs used to dissolve blood clots or treat conditions like high cholesterol, high blood pressure, erratic heart rhythms, or angina have not been properly tested in women.

When women do have heart attacks, they are much more likely than men to die within the first few weeks. Studies show that many of the new, high-tech interventions used for treating severe heart disease—such as angioplasty and bypass surgery—are not recommended for women as often as for men, and are not as successful in women when they are performed. These differences can be shown even when studies are age-adjusted. It's not just women's older age and poor health that are responsible for the outcomes. Their gender is also a factor.

Obviously, then, considering women's poor prognosis once they have a heart attack, preventing attacks from occurring in the first place seems especially important. Unfortunately most studies of risk factors and lifestyle changes have been done on men. While there are efforts being made to redress the gaps in knowledge, many heart experts feel it will be decades before the knowledge on women's hearts equals the knowledge on men's.

In 1989, twenty-five years after the American Heart Association's first conference on heart disease in women, the AHA held another national meeting entitled "Women and Heart Disease." Finally this one dealt with *women's* health. At the opening session a speaker referred ironically to the earlier meeting in announcing the "twenty-fifth anniversary" of the conference.

This more recent, "real" women-and-heart-disease conference came about because Dr. Bernadine Healy—who was then president of the American Heart Association but would soon become the first woman director of the National Institutes of Health—and the AHA communications department recognized that cardiology was largely ignoring women. "The impetus for the meeting really came out of the communications department, not out of a medical committee or epidemiology department," says Dr. Malloy. "The chairman was Anne Golden, a woman who was about to become the chairman of the board at AHA. Until then the issue of women and heart disease was almost a stepchild in the AHA rather than a primary focus."

With the new focus on women came the realization that much of the research on risk factors—cholesterol, blood pressure, stress, and diabetes—came from research done on men. "A fair amount of women have been included in the observational studies, the population studies," says Dr. Mebane-Sims. "But women have tended not to be included in the clinical-trials area. We need to improve the depth of research that has been done."

Much of the information about cholesterol in women comes from the famous Framingham Heart Study, which included women from its start forty-six years ago. "That beats anybody in the history of medicine," says William Castelli, M.D., the director. Framingham is an observational study, meaning that the health of a designated population is monitored over time, but people are not assigned to different groups to try specific treatments such as drugs or surgical procedures.

The Framingham study has found that what's dangerous for a man may not be a problem for a woman. For instance, Framingham has found that in men, high levels of the "bad" LDL cholesterol may be most predictive of future heart trouble. In women, however, low levels of "good" HDL cholesterol may be a bigger risk. Also, high levels of triglycerides do not seem to be a risk factor for men, but may be predictive of heart trouble for women.

What that means is that the public health message to keep total cholesterol levels to 200 mg/dl or lower may not be relevant for women, public health screenings and women's magazine articles to the contrary. Keeping total cholesterol down makes sense for men, because it helps ensure that LDL will be low, too. But a high total cholesterol in women may not be harmful provided the HDL level is high, also. It may be the ratio between the two components that is more important than the total blood cholesterol level. (At menopause, LDL rises and HDL sometimes falls, changing the ratio between the two for the worse.)

The Framingham study found that women with cholesterol over 295 mg/dl had the same or lower risk of heart disease as men with cholesterol of 204 mg/dl. A study in Scotland found similar results: Women with cholesterol levels over 278 mg/dl had a lower risk of coronary heart disease than men with values below 193 mg/dl. And a University of Pittsburgh study found that older women with high total cholesterol were dying at no greater rate than women with normal cholesterol.

While a high total cholesterol may not be dangerous for women, a low total cholesterol isn't necessarily safe either. "Women can have low or normal levels of cholesterol, but have a high triglyceride at 150 or higher, and an HDL under 50," explains Dr. Castelli. "These women pay a terrible price in terms of heart disease—in Framingham they produce twice as many heart attacks as any other lipid disorder we study—but they're missed in American medicine. Most doctors, and even some lipid experts, only pay attention to LDL cholesterol or total cholesterol."

For women, these findings call into question the current guidelines for prescribing cholesterol-lowering drugs and, as will be discussed later, low-fat diets. Framingham and other studies continue to discover gender differences in cholesterol risks, yet the message that physicians and the media continue to circulate is that it's important to get cholesterol levels under 200. Women have the right to ask: Important for whom?

High blood pressure is another major risk factor whose body of knowledge is based almost exclusively on male bodies. Most experts feel that hypertension is as unhealthy for women as men, although there is some doubt. For instance, some scientists feel that young women with high blood pressure may be less at risk because estrogen protects the heart by making blood vessels more flexible.

But when it comes to treating this major risk factor, the lack of information on women is infuriating enough to make anyone's blood pressure soar. "We need information about some very basic issues," says JoAnn Manson, M.D., codirector of women's health at Brigham and Women's Hospital, Harvard Medical School. "We know from one study of hypertension in the elderly that reduction of systolic hypertension is important in both men and women in preventing heart disease and stroke. But there are other studies suggesting that there may be less of a benefit to treating women when the diastolic pressure is only mildly to moderately elevated. It may be a combination of how the high blood pressure affects women, and how the drugs used to treat it affect them."

A study in New York hospitals, done by the Woman's Caucus, Working Group on Women's Health of the Society of General Internal Medicine, found that while hypertension was certainly unhealthy, treating women with the current recommended doses of available drugs could be *more* unhealthy: an analysis of the data revealed an *increase* in mortality for white women who had received drug therapy for hypertension. (Black women in the study did benefit from treatment.)

In reporting these results, the researchers deplored a near total lack of information on the side effects of common antihypertensive drugs in women. There is reason to suspect, they wrote, that these medications may have an adverse effect on blood lipids and cause sexual dysfunction. (The drugs cause impotence in men, but have not been specifically studied for sexual problems in women.)

That's no surprise, considering that studies of cardiac drugs—to lower high blood pressure and cholesterol, treat chest pain, regulate irregular heartbeat, and prevent heart attacks—have largely excluded women. Women of reproductive age have been banned from new drug studies because of potential harm to a potential fetus. But even more important with heart drugs, the upper age limits imposed on many studies—often sixty-five—serve to exclude the very population of women most at risk from this disease. Researchers assume that drugs that work for men work the same way for women, but that's a dangerous assumption.

"You tend to hear about more side effects—dizziness, weakness, tiredness—in women who take these drugs," says Audrey F. von Poelnitz, M.D., a cardiologist at Morristown Memorial Hospital in New Jersey. "There's a gut feeling that women, because they are smaller, need a lesser dose of many cardiac drugs, that you can get the same result with less. But that's just a feeling. Most of the initial drug trials were done on men, and the doses and responses were based on those studies."

Some physicians believe that calcium channel blocker drugs, such as Procardia (nifedipine), Cardizem (diltiazem), and Isoptin (verapamil) used to treat angina, may be more suitable for women than other types of drugs used to treat chest pain. These drugs may be more potent in women because their clearance is slower, meaning that women might need lower or less frequent doses. Also, calcium channel blockers relax the arteries, and since women's arteries may be more prone to spasm than men's, the drug may work better on women than the alternatives. Some of those alternatives are beta-blocking drugs—Inderal (propranolol), Lopressor (metoprolol), Corgard (nadolol)—which are also used for treating high blood pressure. These drugs may be less acceptable for women because of their unpleasant side effects: depression, sluggishness, insomnia, sexual dysfunction, hair loss, and weight gain.

This last side effect, weight gain, may be an independent risk factor for heart disease. But in women new studies are showing that the risk from excess weight may depend more on where it's carried than on how much there is. Fat that clings to the hips and thighs—the classic female "pear" shape—may be less of a heart risk than weight deposited around the stomach and abdomen, creating an "apple" shape in those whose tummies bulge but whose legs and hips are slim. "This central obesity in women is very dangerous," says Dr. Castelli. "It produces the syndrome of high triglyceride, low HDL, increased insulin resistance, and high blood pressure."

The women who curse their ample thighs may bemoan the fact that they can't fit into designer blue jeans, but they may not need to fear heart attacks if their waists are slim. Yet these are the same women who may try to defy nature by continually dieting, and—according to nearly every study on weight loss—continually gaining the weight back. And it's this "yo-yo" dieting that can turn what was a relatively benign amount of excess weight into a heart risk.

While no medical experts believe that excess weight is healthy, the studies are still inconclusive as to whether it is an independent risk factor for heart disease in women, or whether instead it often accompanies other problems that are, such as high blood pressure and diabetes.

Diabetes is a major heart risk factor in women, much more so than in men. "Postmenopausally diabetes may contribute to as many as one in five heart attacks," says Dr. Manson. Women with diabetes don't just have a higher risk than other women; they even have a higher heart disease risk than most men. When a women gets diabetes, she starts to run the same heart attack risk as for diabetic men, which is much higher than normal men.

Lack of the hormone insulin is the cause of diabetes. But lack of the female hormone estrogen, or an excess of androgens (male hormones), is also a heart risk for women. Women tend to have smaller coronary arteries than men, and smaller arteries can be more easily blocked with plaque, making it harder for blood and oxygen to get through. This anatomical difference should mean that women have *more* heart attacks than men, and have them younger. The fact that they don't is mainly due to the protective effect of female hormones. This hormonal risk factor is the only one that is completely different in men and women.

Estrogen's protective effect ends at menopause. "You might think of it as a mistake to let women go through the menopause," says Dr. Castelli, speaking, one hopes, purely as a cardiac researcher. "Once they go through the menopause, they start to fill up their coronary arteries. Women have much smaller coronary arteries than men. Once they start to fill up, it only takes about six to ten years to fill them." Women who have undergone a surgical menopause (removal of the ovaries) also have an increased risk.

In one of the most ironic exclusions of women from clinical research, studies in the late 1960s on the risks and benefits of the female hormone estrogen were done on *men*. Observing that premenopausal women—women whose bodies produced high levels of estrogen—seemed to have a lowered risk of coronary artery disease, researchers decided to put this theory to the test in the group they perceived to be at risk for heart disease. "It seems preposterous now," says Dr. Manson. But apparently it didn't occur to anyone at the time that the idea of testing female hormones on men was ludicrous, and that not including women in the study was even worse.

Researchers were simply acting on the prevailing notion that heart disease was a male problem. "The concern was that men were dying of heart disease; at that time the diversity issue was a nonissue," says Dr. Mebane-Sims. So a group of male volunteers was given estrogen in a dose many times higher than the normal replacement dose for women. Not surprisingly, the men complained of a lot of side effects (including impotence), and they received no heart benefits at all; in fact they died of cardiovascular disease in greater numbers than the controls. Faced with that evidence, physicians began to believe that maybe estrogen was a heart risk for women, too, and it was dropped as therapy. It was nearly two decades later, as results from the Nurses' Health Study emerged, that estrogen's heart-protective benefits were confirmed in women. But how many women were harmed because of the delay caused by testing estrogen in men?

Today women have to decide whether or not to take postmenopausal hormones based on shockingly scanty evidence. Most physicians believe that women who use estrogen supplements after menopause do receive some protection against heart disease. And estrogen seems to help prevent osteoporosis, too. But there's also evidence that taking estrogen alone after menopause leads to an increased risk of endometrial cancer. So physicians add progesterone to the mix and give women with intact uteruses (those who haven't had a hysterectomy) estrogen in combination with progesterone. But it's possible that adding progesterone minimizes or even negates the heart benefits. It's also possible that progesterone accentuates the benefits, or has no effect at all—no one really knows.

Many studies are currently under way to answer the questions about hormone replacement therapy (HRT). The large and ambitious Women's Health Initiative is studying this issue. Another trial, PEPI—Postmenopausal Estrogen/Progestin Interventions—the only randomized clinical trial to date on HRT, is examining the effect of various estrogen/progestin treatments, including pills and patches, on blood lipids, cardiovascular disease, and cancer in women ages forty-five to sixty-four. These results should be released imminently. And HERS—Heart and Estrogen/Progestin Replacement Study—is looking at women who have had heart attacks, angioplasty, and bypass surgery to see if these women do better with or without hormonal replacement. Taking place at fifteen centers throughout the country, it will take six years to get answers.

In the meantime physicians don't really know which postmenopausal women would benefit most from replacement therapy. And they don't yet know the ideal regimen to recommend. As the population of women entering menopause continues to grow in size and economic clout, these women are demanding better answers to some hard questions.

For premenopausal women the hormones in birth control pills have also been implicated in some cardiovascular risks. The old, high-dose oral contraceptives, especially in conjunction with smoking, have been linked with a higher risk of blood clotting, heart attacks and stroke. On their own, these hormones can raise blood pressure and change lipid profiles for the worse by raising LDL, decreasing HDL, and increasing triglycerides. The newest generation of birth control pills contains much smaller doses of hormones. But because they are dominant in progestins—hormones that may be androgenic—many scientists feel the new pills need to be evaluated for their long-term effects on heart disease. So far these studies have not been done.

As if making decisions about contraception or hormone replacement therapy based on paltry information weren't stressful enough, stress itself has been implicated in cardiac disease. The link is still rather tenuous: some studies have found a connection, and others find none. Researchers are still arguing about what the relationship is, but one thing is certain: "Similar to other research, the original research done on personality, stress and heart disease was very male-oriented," says Marianne J. Legato, M.D., associate professor of clinical medicine at Columbia University College of Physicians and Surgeons, and author of *The Female Heart.*

Everyone has heard of the typical Type-A personality, who is supposedly prone to coronaries: impatient, hard-driving, hostile. The description is generally used to describe a middle-aged man. The original Type-A study was done on a group of over three thousand California business*men*, and no women.

The Framingham study found that Type A could be a risk for women too, if their husbands were Type A, that is. Framingham found that Type B, or passive, women married to demanding, Type-A men were at increased risk. And for both men and women, Framingham data indicate that high levels of unexpressed hostility and anger can increase the risk of heart disease. Other studies have shown that high anxiety and fear may be more of a heart risk than hostility for women.

Many social observers commented that when women entered the workforce in large numbers there would be a corresponding rise in heart disease as the stresses in their lives began to match those in men's. In fact, studies have found that women staying at home are more at risk of a heart attack. Women who work outside the home tend to have lower blood pressure and cholesterol, and often weigh less. But the issue is not quite so simple. The woman who works outside the home may be in a physically active job, or she may sit behind a desk all day. The woman at home may run around after toddlers, clean house, garden, jog, and play tennis, or she may sit in front of the television eating candy and smoking. Also, how can someone determine whether an outside job, which may be cushy or pressured, is more stressful than staying home, which may be peaceful or chaotic, depending on the family situation? It's possible that staying home used to be less stressful for women when they were expected to fill traditional roles. Now that women are encouraged to engage in outside work, those women who stay home may feel unhappy and undervalued.

The Framingham study found that different psychosocial factors predicted the incidence of heart attack in women who stayed at home as opposed to those who were employed. Lack of education, tension, financial concerns, and infrequent vacations were heart risks for both working women and homemakers, but the women who stayed at home had a further grab bag of concerns that threatened their hearts: being lonely during the day, having difficulty falling asleep, and believing they were prone to heart disease. The researchers described the homemakers as possibly being in a "coronary-prone situation" where tension is exacerbated by too few vacations and feelings of isolation.

Statistically stay-at-homes have a higher heart risk, but women who work outside the home aren't safe from heart disease, either. The lowest risk seems to be among professional career women—doctors, lawyers, business executives, investment bankers—who have a degree of power and control at work, and feel a sense of reward for what they do. Those whose risk is highest are the women in pink-collar jobs, jobs with little control, such as secretary, waitress, file clerk. These women, especially when they have a double load and must assume responsibility for a family as well, may be at highest risk of heart disease from stress.

"Women in these kinds of jobs may have bosses who have no insight into what they're dealing with at home," explains Jane B. Sherwood, R.N., research nurse coordinator at the Institute for the Prevention of Cardiovascular Disease at Deaconess Hospital, Harvard Medical School. "If the kids give them a hard time in the morning, then they get in trouble for being late for work. The women with the highest heart risk are those who have few supports, incredible amounts of responsibility with family, and little hope of getting out of the situation they're in."

As Susan Faludi pointed out in *Backlash*, the opponents of the women's movement who predicted that increased opportunities for women would lead to a greater incidence of heart attacks got it all wrong. It's the women with opportunities who have the healthiest hearts. Women in dead-end jobs or who stay home unhappily are the ones who are most at risk.

■ SILENT SYMPTOMS, SILENT WOMEN

Although it is the leading cause of death, heart disease inspires no terror in American women. When a woman feels a lump in her breast, her first terrified thought is likely to be breast cancer, even though only one in ten breast lumps turns out to be malignant. But when a woman feels a pain in her chest, chances are she'll think she's got a touch of indigestion, has pulled a muscle, or has been living under too much stress. Heart attack, or any kind of heart disease, might never occur to her. Heart disease still has a macho image, although it's women who often bear the pain more stoically.

"Women are brought up to experience pain and not pay much attention to it," says Jane Sherwood. "Girls learn as teenagers that the world doesn't stop because they have menstrual cramps. And women work throughout their pregnancies, then go home within a day of giving birth and take care of their babies, even if they're in pain from the episiotomy or cesarean." Because women learn from these experiences that pain is not necessarily a sign that something is wrong, says Sherwood, they are more apt to try to ignore even severe pain and just wait for it to go away. "But men see pain as a signal that something is wrong. They stop what they're doing and go to the doctor." Adds Dr. Malloy, "I've had women tell me they didn't really take the pain seriously because they thought heart attack symptoms would be at least as severe as childbirth pain, so they were waiting for it to get worse."

The result is that many women, when they start experiencing the pain of angina or a heart attack, try to ignore it and continue with their usual activities. More than a third of all heart attacks in women go unnoticed or unreported by their victims (versus just over one-quarter in men). "I've been amazed at what women have accomplished after the pain of their heart attack started," says Sherwood. "There was one woman who gave a dinner party for twelve people and didn't come to the hospital until it was over."

According to Dr. Malloy, "A woman will get her male partner to a doctor a lot quicker than she'll get herself there. Women will try to complete certain tasks and get their families in order before going to the hospital." But women are penalized for putting others first, because the delay can be deadly. Certain lifesaving procedures, such as clot-busting drugs, must be administered within a few hours of the onset of a heart attack.

When women do finally see their doctors or show up in the emergency room with their chest pain, they are usually astonished to find out they are having a heart attack. Sherwood tells of women who, in the emergency room in the midst of massive heart attacks, assess their pain on a scale of one to ten as "probably a three." Women may also be surprised by their diagnosis because their symptoms often do not fit the classic "elephant sitting on your chest" description of heart attack pain. They may not have the pain radiating down the left arm that men learn to fear. Women are more likely to suffer from what doctors call atypical symptoms, such as vague abdominal discomfort, nausea and vomiting, fatigue, shortness of breath, arm pain. Of course the term *atypical* is used because "typical" heart attack pain is that experienced by the majority of people who take part in medical studies: middle-aged white men.

Bernadine Healy has coined the term *the Yentl syndrome* to describe the gender bias in recognizing and treating women's heart symptoms. Yentl was the nineteenth-century heroine of Isaac Bashevis Singer's short story, who had to disguise herself as a man in order to study the Talmud. Healy says that physicians tend to ignore symptoms of heart disease in women until the women show they are "just like a man" by having severe coronary disease or a heart attack. Only then are the women offered the same treatment that men would normally receive.

Because women's symptoms may be vague, physicians may not be properly alarmed when a female patient, especially a premenopausal one, comes in complaining of symptoms that might indicate heart disease. Both women and men are likely to experience chest pain for a variety of reasons, only one of which is heart disease. One study found that women ages twenty-five to fifty-four are twice as likely as men the same age to suffer from severe angina (chest pain). Yet women this age are also far less likely to suffer heart attacks. Physicians have to be skilled at determining which chest pains may predict a future heart attack.

Ironically it was one of the few studies to have included women, the famous Framingham Heart Study, that first suggested women's chest pains were not a cause for alarm and that women with chest pain rarely went on to develop heart attacks. "The Framingham study inadvertently misled people for a long time with the idea that angina was a benign illness in women," says Dr. Malloy. "The follow-up had not been long enough. It wasn't until they'd been following up women for a long time that they discovered differently. Hindsight is always twenty-twenty." Unfortunately, in the two-decade interim many physicians read the Framingham findings and interpreted them as justification for ignoring women's chest pain.

According to Dr. Castelli, the initial reports came out before enough women had been studied. Although at its start Framingham actually in-

cluded more women than men, in the early days of the study most of the
women were premenopausal. So there were very few women with chest
pain, and even fewer suffering from heart disease or heart attacks. "The
early report was based on pretty small numbers," admits Castelli. "But
once all the women in the original cohort went through the menopause
and got to the area of life where they developed these diseases, we found
differently. Our most recent data show that when you get good histories of
chest pain in women, they get heart attacks and die at maybe only a
slightly lower rate than men."

Now Dr. Castelli is anxious to spread the word among physicians and
the public that women's chest pain *should* be taken seriously. "One of the
great fallacies is that chest pain in women is in their head and not their
chest, but that's not exactly true," he says. "It is true that most chest pain
in men and women is not caused by a malfunction of the heart. But if
you take a detailed history of that chest pain, you can separate out which
is which. Chest pain that may indicate a heart attack is usually in the
central part of the chest and is brought on by exercise, exertion, excitement, anger, stress. It can radiate to the neck or down the arm or into
the stomach. It usually makes people feel sick to their stomach, break out
in a cold sweat, get short of breath, feel life is about to be over. And the
pain is relieved within four to five minutes of relaxing. It's not a true
pain, but a tightness in the chest, a heaviness. But too often when
women go to the hospital with that chest pain, they're told it's in their
head." Yet in spite of the new findings, chest pain is still underdiagnosed
and undertreated in women.

Sadly it is also often *mis*diagnosed. Dr. von Poelnitz describes a recent
case:

Sarah Johnson (not her real name), a forty-two-year-old woman who
was a heavy smoker, was having some achiness in her chest and some
pain in her left arm. It was summer and everyone was afraid of Lyme disease. So she went to her doctor and told him that's what she must have.
She asked for a Lyme-disease blood test. The test came back negative,
and the doctor never questioned her more about her chest pains, so she
figured it was nothing. Meanwhile she was getting ready for her daughter's wedding. It was on the receiving line at church that Sarah had her
heart attack. She felt suddenly sick and dizzy, had a funny feeling in her
chest, and pain in her shoulder. But she didn't want to ruin
her daughter's wedding, so she didn't tell anyone what she was experiencing. An hour later she ran to the bathroom and vomited. She lay down
for a moment, collected herself, then went back out to the celebration. It

wasn't until the next day, after her daughter went away on her honeymoon and Sarah was still feeling terrible, that she finally went to the emergency room.

Unfortunately, says Dr. von Poelnitz, that's not quite the end of the story. "A *female* resident admitted the woman to the hospital because there were minor changes on the cardiogram. But I'm embarrassed to admit that she suspected the symptoms were caused by anxiety. She didn't even call in cardiology. The next day I was called to see the patient, and for me her cardiogram was classic for a heart attack—a small one. But the attending physician, the resident, all the people in the emergency room, passed off this woman's symptoms as if it must be anxiety because of her daughter's wedding." In spite of the delay, this woman was lucky. An angiogram detected a blockage in an artery, and an angioplasty cleared it. She quit smoking and recovered nicely.

This is not an especially unusual case. Cardiologists and women patients tell story after story of women who went to see their doctors for chest pain and were diagnosed with a variety of other illnesses, none of them related to the heart.

The stories all start the same: "This woman went to her doctor because she was having chest pains . . ."

The middle varies slightly:

- And the gynecologist thought it was a hiatal hernia
- And the female resident thought it was an anxiety attack
- And the family practitioner thought it was Lyme disease
- And the internist thought it was gallstones

But the endings are chillingly alike: "And then she went home and had a heart attack."

Dr. Legato, who wrote a book on women and heart disease several years ago, says, "If you could follow me around the country when I speak to women's groups, you'd be amazed by the stories women tell." Dr. Wenger says that each time she publishes an article on women and heart disease, she receives letters from women telling similar tales.

How is it possible that the leading cause of death in women is misdiagnosed so frequently? As one M.D. puts it, "You have to think of the diagnosis before you order the test." A proper diagnosis of heart disease in women requires a careful history from the patient, elicited by a physician who is informed enough to suspect heart disease and order the proper diagnostic tests if the history is suspicious.

"The biggest discrepancy occurs when a forty-year-old woman comes in complaining of something that could be heart disease, and a forty-year-old man comes in complaining of something that could be heart disease," says Dr. von Poelnitz. "Physicians react to the man, but tell the women it could be stress."

On the other hand, physicians can't order a battery of expensive tests for every woman, especially a premenopausal one, who walks in the door complaining of vague chest pains. Since not every chest pain is due to heart disease, ordering tests for everyone with possible symptoms would be enormously expensive and unproductive. Doctors are already under siege for ordering unnecessary tests to protect themselves from malpractice suits.

Physicians have to be skillful diagnosticians, not just at using technology but at really listening to women to find out if their pain is heart-related—not just where the pain is, but when it occurs, what it feels like. Says Dr. von Poelnitz, "If you take a careful history and really listen, 80 to 90 percent of the time you can determine who should be referred for cardiac testing. A lot of doctors who aren't listening just don't care and don't want to take the time."

Another problem is that half of all women see their gynecologists as their primary physicians, and when they have a chest pain, that's who they tell. The absurdity of this is obvious only when you switch genders: Consider how ridiculous it would be for a man to visit his proctologist complaining of chest pains. Physicians are most skilled at diagnosing illnesses that fall within their area of expertise.

Even when a woman is fortunate enough to recognize that her pain may be due to a heart problem, and she visits a qualified internist or cardiologist who takes a careful history, she is still not assured of proper diagnosis or treatment. Many of the high-tech tests that are used to diagnose heart disease are notoriously inaccurate in women.

The treadmill, or stress, test is the most widely used, and unfortunately it doesn't work very well in women. In this test the patient walks on a motorized treadmill, which gradually increases in speed, while small electrodes attached to the chest measure the heart's electrical output. "Thirty-five percent of women have false positives; 25 percent false negatives—so less than half of women have accurate treadmills (versus 70 percent of men)," says Linda Crouse, M.D., director of the Echocardiographic Laboratory at Mid-American Heart Institute of Saint Luke's Hospital in Kansas City, Missouri. "I don't think physicians are prejudiced, but I think the perception that heart disease is less common in women is primarily a result of the treadmill test."

Part of the problem may be the difficulty in interpreting the test results in women. "What we are calling a positive test is based on findings mostly for men," says Dr. von Poelnitz. "But, as we know, what is true for a male population is not necessarily true for women." Many women have a harmless heart condition called mitral valve prolapse, which can skew test results. Another reason for the test's inaccuracy may be the influence of the hormones in oral contraceptives and postmenopausal hormone replacement therapy. One theory holds that there is a similarity in structure of estrogen and digitalis (a heart drug), skewing the readings. Another hypothesis is that estrogen has a direct physiological effect on heart cells.

Some alternative tests are more reliable in women, but these tend to be expensive and may have other problems as well. For instance the thallium, or nuclear, treadmill is more reliable in women, but much more expensive than the regular exercise treadmill. Also the test was not initially considered suitable for women, because doctors found that female breast tissue often got in the way of the images, particularly on the left side. But now that the problem has been recognized, technicians are able to compensate. The test is now considered about 80 percent accurate.

Many experts feel that another new test, called exercise/stress echo testing, is the best hope for women. Unfortunately this test requires training and is not widely available yet. It, too, is considerably more expensive than the exercise treadmill test, as is PET (positron emission tomography) scanning, another option. What cardiologists are hoping for in the future is a cost-effective test that gives accurate information in both men and women.

Given the high number of false positives in the most commonly used test, the exercise treadmill, doctors must decide when to take the results seriously by referring women for more sophisticated testing such as angiography (cardiac catheterization). Studies have shown that women have a lower rate of cardiac catheterization than men with the same symptoms. "Everyone knows how inaccurate the treadmill test is in women, so they may discard positives when they occur," says Dr. Crouse.

In 1991 the American Medical Association Council on Ethical and Judicial Affairs issued a report on gender disparities in clinical decision making. They cited a 1987 study showing that in a group of 390 patients, of those with abnormal exercise radionuclide scans (nuclear treadmill), 40 percent of the men were referred for further testing—angiogram/cardiac catheterization—versus only 4 percent of the women. Even after the researchers controlled for the variables of abnormal test results, age, types of angina, presence of symptoms, and confirmed previous myocardial infarction, men were still six and a half times more likely than women to be referred for catheterization.

Of the patients with abnormal test results, women were more than twice as likely as men to have their symptoms attributed to psychiatric and other noncardiac causes than men. Once again, even with high-tech test results in front of them, physicians show themselves to be quick to believe that women don't have heart disease, they only *think* they do.

There is a small but vocal group of critics who wonder whether it isn't that physicians are undertesting and undertreating women—but *over*testing and *over*treating men. Just because men and women are being treated differently, they argue, doesn't necessarily mean that men are being treated better. "There's a lot of overcatheterization in this country, and we don't have the information on whether women are being undercatheterized or men are being overcatheterized," says Judith Hochman, M.D., director of the cardiac care unit at Saint Luke's–Roosevelt Hospital in New York. The answer may lie somewhere in between. In any event, cardiology research that includes women will eventually improve care for everyone.

■ TREATING THE FEMALE HEART

Not surprisingly, considering the obstacles to proper diagnosis, by the time women finally receive treatment for heart disease, their prognosis is worse than men's. The delay in obtaining care is one reason, but there are *many* other reasons as well. Because women in general are older than men when they develop heart disease, they may be more frail and may have other health problems that can complicate recovery. Also, women tend to have smaller coronary arteries than men, making surgical repairs more difficult. For all these reasons—and no doubt others that have not yet been recognized—women do not recover as well as men after a heart attack.

Nearly 40 percent of women's heart attacks are fatal, versus 31 percent of men's. In the first year after a heart attack, men's symptoms decrease, while women's increase, and women have a greater risk of death, cardiac distress, and a repeat attack. Age alone does not explain the difference; an Israeli study found that women have higher mortality than men even when they are matched for age.

Less aggressive cardiac care is partly to blame, but social factors may also be responsible. "Men come right out of the hospital to cardiac rehab, and their wives come with them—they want to learn how to cook low-cholesterol foods and take care of their husbands. But women come to rehab alone," says Jane Sherwood. "Sometimes husbands wait down in the lobby. Often the women are older, widowed. Very rarely do you get a call from the kids. The women come alone."

With no one to care for them, women recovering from heart attacks often continue to care for others. Sherwood describes a woman who came in with incisional pain from her bypass surgery. When Sherwood asked about her activities, it turned out the woman had been doing laundry for her twenty-five-year-old-son. "I'm amazed at how many women have bypass surgery and still vacuum the house and do major housework. And their families let them do it. Especially women in their sixties and seventies, who still identify with traditional roles and never worked outside the home."

As part of her research in the M.I. Onset study, Sherwood also found that when women have a heart attack and are admitted to a community hospital, if they have complications it takes them twice as long as men to get referred to a university teaching hospital for diagnostic testing, such as cardiac catheterization. "Women wait two days longer than men to get transferred to a tertiary center if there are complications," she says. "Part of the reason women have a worse prognosis after a heart attack, and part of the reason their long-term results from bypass surgery are not as good as men's, might be that they're not being treated as quickly. By the time they are treated, they're sicker." According to Sherwood, that leads to a vicious catch-22. "Physicians say they won't do these interventions, such as bypass, on women because they don't do as well. But they may not be doing as well because they're not having them soon enough."

Sherwood is quick to add that the fault isn't all on the part of the physicians. In some cases she found that local physicians had recommended that women be transferred to larger teaching hospitals, but the women themselves didn't want to be moved far from their communities. They didn't want to inconvenience other family members who would have to drive farther to see them.

Sherwood also found that even when women did get transferred, they weren't getting the same testing men were getting. "Even though there's more knowledge now, physicians are not necessarily acting on it," she says. "I'm hoping in the next couple of years they will. Women are becoming more aware and are demanding more cardiac assessments. It may help them get the intervention they need."

These interventions—clot-busting drugs and surgical procedures—are still being doled out with an uneven hand. Women who have suffered an acute MI (myocardial infarction, a medical term for heart attack) are less likely to receive clot-busting drugs, balloon angioplasty, and coronary-

artery bypass grafts. "In every type of coronary disease women have less diagnostic and therapeutic procedures than do men," says Emory University's
Dr. Wenger. "In general, because the patients are older, the physicians try
medication first. But when that doesn't work, then the patient is even older
and may have other problems. The surgery outcome is not as good, and it
becomes a self-fulfilling prophecy."

When women—and men—have heart attacks, there are several types
of treatment that may be offered, alone or in combination. The first therapy is generally a thrombolytic (clot-busting) drug to dissolve the blood
clot responsible for the heart attack and prevent further damage to the
heart muscle. These drugs—tPA and streptokinase are two examples—are
usually administered in the emergency room as soon as possible after the
onset of the attack, but no more than six hours later. Since women so often
ignore their symptoms, by the time they reach the emergency room the
lifesaving therapy may be off-limits to them. But even when they do reach
help in time, there's a prejudice in prescribing the drugs.

One study reported that 26 percent of men versus only 14 percent of
women received clot-dissolving drugs after a heart attack. One reason for
the disparity is that initial guidelines for using the drugs set an age limit
of sixty-five. "New research shows that these drugs have the greatest benefit
at ages sixty-five to seventy-five, but the guidelines haven't been changed,"
says Dr. Wenger. And most women who develop heart disease are older
than sixty-five.

Even when women do receive the drugs, they may not respond as well.
A Senate committee meeting reported a three-year study showing that
when men and women get the best care available and get it within four
hours of their heart attack, women are *still* more likely to die and more
likely to suffer a second attack within a year. One hypothesis is that men
and women react differently to clot-busting drugs. "Perhaps the fixed dosage that is used is too large for the average woman, and that's why women
have more bleeding," says Dr. Malloy. Women's blood may also contain
more fibrinogen, a substance necessary for blood-clotting.

Once their condition has been stabilized, men and women who have
suffered heart attacks usually undergo surgery—angioplasty or bypass—to
help prevent an attack from recurring. In both cases the fact that women
tend to be older, sicker, have smaller coronary arteries, and are more likely
to be suffering from diabetes and other health problems has a negative effect on their outcome.

In angioplasty a tiny balloon catheter is threaded into a blocked artery
and then inflated, flattening a blockage. Studies looking at gender differ-

ences in this procedure have found that women are at a disadvantage. According to the American Heart Association, women have more than a tenfold higher risk of dying in the hospital after undergoing coronary angioplasty.

These data might make any woman think twice before undergoing the procedure, but doctors claim the outcomes are improving. Angioplasty has been more successful in women in recent years now that machines have been scaled down and the inflatable balloons are smaller, more appropriate for women's smaller artery size. Many doctors now say women patients are doing just as well as men.

The same thing is beginning to happen with bypass surgery, which reroutes blood around a blocked artery. Once nearly twice as likely to die from the surgery as men, women now have better odds as surgeons have become more skilled. "Data from centers that do a lot of patients and a lot of women are not showing the same difference in mortality. The best centers, such as Cleveland Clinic and Mayo Clinic, are reporting they do equally well with men and women," says Dr. Legato. But it is still true that women are not being recommended for the lifesaving operation as often as men. More than 70 percent of bypass operations are done on men.

There are those in medicine who pooh-pooh any idea of gender difference in heart disease treatment. If you simply control for age, artery size, severity of disease, and so on, you'll find no difference for men and women, they say. Gender isn't an independent risk factor, they insist. However, how can these other risk factors be divorced from gender? Women do tend to be older and have other health problems; their coronary arteries are often smaller. What good is it to statistically turn women into men and then say there's no difference in outcome?

There's overwhelming evidence to show that women's and men's hearts *are* different. It's unfortunate, however, that there isn't overwhelming evidence yet to show how to take these differences into account and provide the quality of cardiac care women deserve.

■ AN OUNCE OF PREVENTION

Considering the inequities in diagnosis and treatment, women would be wise to do everything possible not to develop heart disease in the first place. Although public health authorities advocate the same lifestyle changes for men and women—minimizing fat in the diet, exercising regularly—these measures make definite heart sense for men, but the benefits in women aren't quite so clear-cut.

One of the strongest public health messages, ranking up there with "Don't smoke" in terms of importance, is that people should limit dietary fat. So it comes as somewhat of a shock to find out that low-fat diets may not have the same benefit in women as they do in men. That's because reducing the fat in the diet reduces total cholesterol—LDL *and* HDL. Since lowering LDL is the prime concern in men, the diet is clearly beneficial. But for women, maintaining a higher relative level of HDL is more important, so lowering total cholesterol this way may not reduce heart attack risk. In the summer of 1992 the cardiology journal *Circulation*, published by the American Heart Association, ran an article calling for a stop to the cholesterol campaign for women until more was known about the benefits. The campaign continues.

Several experts have questioned, without much publicity, whether a low-fat diet might not even be *harmful* to women's hearts. The British journal *Lancet* ran a piece by lipids researcher John R. Crouse III, M.D., professor of medicine and public health sciences at Bowman Gray School of Medicine in Winston-Salem, North Carolina. Crouse questioned the wisdom of recommending low-fat diets for women because of the possibility of lowering HDL. Dr. Crouse now doubts the diet is harmful, but still questions whether it has any benefits for women.

"If a low-fat diet had the same effect in women as it has in men—lowering HDL and LDL—then it might be risky for women," says Crouse. "But it's not clear anymore that the diet has as dramatic an effect in women as it does in men. It may be that a low-fat diet doesn't do anything to women's cholesterol and doesn't have a deleterious effect on cardiovascular disease. If a low-fat diet doesn't have any effect on lipids, then it might not matter what women eat."

Dr. Crouse criticizes the lack of data and the fact that there hasn't been a good review article putting the issue in perspective. He says that there's some evidence that only very low-fat diets, those containing just 20 percent of calories from fat, cause problems with HDL. "It may be that if you lower the diet from the American average—36 percent—to 30 percent you don't get as much of an HDL-lowering effect," he says. Unfortunately there simply isn't enough information to say right now.

The Women's Health Initiative study will test precisely this question. "If you can't show that diet is beneficial to cardiovascular disease in forty thousand women, then you're in trouble," says Dr. Crouse. But results from the Women's Health Initiative won't be known for fifteen years. What should women do in the meantime?

Most heart experts, including Dr. Castelli of Framingham, maintain that a low-fat diet *is* beneficial for women, and that even if the cholesterol-lowering benefits aren't clear-cut, lowering dietary fat can help control obesity, lower high blood pressure, and protect women from strokes. Dr. Castelli adds that it's important that women be included in the public health campaign "because we want them in the constituency that goes to the supermarket and buys low-fat beef, ham, and ice cream. These low-fat products will disappear from the shelf if we don't create a market for them."

Dr. Crouse, too, in spite of his doubts about the diet's cholesterol-lowering benefit in women, urges women to continue to make low-fat food choices. He, too, justifies the recommendation not on a scientific basis but on a public-policy one. "There's no room for flexibility in public policy; it has to tell everybody to do the same thing. You can't just tell women not to worry, because women don't live in a vacuum," he explains. "You can't have a woman eating one diet and her husband another. You can't have her cook fish and fruit for her husband while she's gorging on ham and cheese. And I do believe the low-fat diet is a good idea for men, so it doesn't make sense to tell a woman she can eat anything she wants but that her husband can't."

While Drs. Castelli and Crouse mean well, they're not being fair to women. Considering all the women who are constantly on weight-loss diets, eating rice cakes and grapefruit themselves yet still baking cakes and cooking steaks for their husbands, it seems ludicrous to say the tables can't be turned. Besides, what about women who live alone, are young and unmarried, divorced, widowed, or lesbian? When there's no man sharing meals, and even when there is, there's no justification for urging a woman to make such a drastic and difficult lifestyle change unless there are clear benefits for *her*.

That's not to urge women to start consuming massive quantities of cheese, butter, and meat, however. For a variety of reasons it probably does make sense for a woman to follow a low-fat diet; high dietary fat has been linked with breast and colon cancer, obesity, and other health problems. No one is saying that high-fat foods are healthy. But women have a right to know exactly what the benefits are before they adopt a diet that can be difficult and frustrating to follow.

Another ubiquitous public health message is the admonition to "go for the burn," to get up off the couch and get to an aerobics studio. Who would suspect that the evidence linking aerobic exercise and lowered heart disease risk in women is far from definitive?

Whether women's hearts benefit from regular exercise seems to depend on whom you talk to. Says Dr. Manson, "It's likely as protective in women as in men." Agrees Dr. Castelli, "One of the best studies, at the Cooper Clinic, found that just a modest amount of exercise resulted in a tremendous fall in heart attack and total death rate in women." Other researchers disagree. "Exercise doesn't seem to do it in women," says Trudy L. Bush, Ph.D., professor of epidemiology at the Johns Hopkins School of Hygiene and Public Health in Baltimore. "Studies have found that exercise raises HDL levels in men but not in women. Therefore exercise is not as protective."

So far the studies looking at the relationship of exercise and heart disease in women have been split, with half finding a positive correlation between a sedentary lifestyle and heart risks, and the other half showing no correlation between how much a woman exercises and her risk of heart disease.

Once again, even if the heart benefits are unclear, no one is condoning a couch-potato lifestyle. Exercise has many other benefits for women, including helping to maintain a healthy weight and prevent osteoporosis, the crippling bone loss that occurs in many older women as hormone levels fall.

In 1988 researchers triumphantly announced the results of the Physicians' Health Study: just one aspirin a day (later amended to half an aspirin tablet) can lower the risk of heart attack (although it raises the incidence of stroke). This was a prospective, randomized clinical trial, meaning that the twenty-two thousand men who participated were placed at random in a group that took aspirin, or a group that didn't, and then followed for six years.

But because no women were included in this study, physicians were at a loss as to what to tell their female patients when they asked if taking small doses of aspirin could help protect them from heart attacks, too. "It's very difficult as a clinician to say to a woman with cardiovascular disease, 'I can tell you what a large study of middle-aged white men and aspirin found' when the patient is an elderly black woman," says Pamela Charney, M.D., associate professor of internal medicine at the Albert Einstein College of Medicine in New York.

In an attempt to play catch-up and provide an educated answer without a randomized clinical trial, researchers at Harvard analyzed data collected from the 88,000 women in the Nurses' Health Study, an ongoing observational study of female nurses. The researchers found that nurses who reported using one to six aspirin per week had a lower rate of heart attacks than those who took fewer (or more), so it appears aspirin is protective in women, too. Since this was not a randomized clinical trial, the data were disturbingly inexact. The women were taking different doses of aspirin for different problems, such as headaches, joint pain, and menstrual cramps.

The Nurses' Health Study provided an interim answer. Women, however, have a right to more definitive medical advice. So after the aspirin results in men were published, researchers launched the Women's Health Study at Harvard in 1992. (Public outrage over the lack of data on women and aspirin, after the Physicians' Health Study results were published, helped get the new study funded. The Harvard researchers had been trying to get a women's study funded for the previous three or four years.) A prospective, randomized clinical trial like the Physicians' Health Study, the Women's Health Study will collect data on whether women would benefit from taking low doses of aspirin, beta carotene, or vitamin E to prevent cardiovascular disease and cancer. The researchers will collect data for at least five years before publishing any results. In the meantime women and their physicians must consider the existing data before making any decision about regular aspirin use. "It's a benefit-to-risk ratio," says Dr. Manson. "You have to look at the incidence of stroke compared to the incidence of heart attack. The ratio of stroke to heart attack is higher in women than in men; heart attacks are less likely for women, but strokes occur with about equal frequency. If aspirin increases the risk of stroke, then the overall benefit-to-risk ratio may be different for women."

Another benefit-to-risk ratio decision for women concerns alcohol. Several years ago studies showed that moderate alcohol intake, defined as one drink per day for women, two for men, may protect against heart disease. However, other studies showed that in women alcohol use might increase the risk of breast cancer. Most women worry more about breast cancer but are actually more at risk of heart disease. So to drink moderately or not? It's a decision that women must make individually, based on their own risks, fears, and lifestyles.

What the above discussion shows is that, for women, preventing heart disease isn't as straightforward a proposition as it seems to be for men. But public health officials shouldn't avoid sending any message at all for fear of its complexity. It is an injustice to women simply to include them in recommendations for men rather than to tailor advice based on whatever gender-specific evidence exists. Simplifying the message can only be done at the expense of women's health.

New studies have recently begun to examine the effects of hormones, diet, vitamins, and aspirin on heart disease; these studies promise to help close the knowledge gap. Already there are signs that more women are being included in cardiac research. A look at articles published in *Circulation*, the American Heart Association's journal, found that in 1973 there were seven men for every women included in studies reported by the journal. By 1993 the ratio was only three to one.

And there are a number of important new trials under way, such as the Women's Health Initiative, which will yield a wealth of data on women's health, including women's hearts. But this trial and others must last for years before they will yield any useful data. "I think we'll be lucky if we can say we know as much about women's hearts as men's by the turn of the century," says Dr. Malloy.

Until these trials begin to produce useful information, women will have to act on existing knowledge, which is sometimes sketchy and often inconclusive. And until the ratio of men to women included in heart studies is one to one, and until these unanswered questions about women and heart disease are addressed, women cannot afford to be complacent.

The subject of women and heart disease needs to be kept at the forefront of physicians' and women's consciousnesses. Physicians need the information for proper diagnosis and treatment, and women need the knowledge to protect themselves from heart disease as they age. Says Dr. JoAnn Manson, "The key point is that heart disease is a woman's disease at least as much as it's a man's disease." That's something that women, and their physicians, must always keep in mind.

5

BREAST CANCER
Malignant Neglect

When Lorraine Pace found the lump in her breast one day in 1991, her doctor told her not to worry, it was probably just scar tissue from a cyst she'd had removed a few years earlier. When nothing showed up on a mammogram, Pace was happy to let the subject drop. Married for thirty years, a fifty-year-old mother of three grown children, Lorraine Pace had been groomed to be compliant, a good girl. When her husband walked in the door after a day at the office, the house was clean, the clothes were ironed and folded, dinner was on the table. If Pace's doctor told her not to worry, she wouldn't worry.

Eight months later, on a flight from Florida back to New York, Pace struck up a conversation with the pleasant middle-aged man sitting next to her. He told her he was a mortician.

A mortician, yuck, Pace thought.

What he said next startled her even more: He was disturbed by all the young women he was being asked to bury—women who had died in their thirties and forties of breast cancer.

The next day Pace made a beeline for her doctor's office. "You told me not to worry about the lump. I want it out."

Certain the lesion was benign, her doctor performed the surgery on an outpatient basis using only local anesthesia. Fifteen minutes later he was standing in front of Pace telling her, "You have invasive breast cancer."

Recuperating from her lumpectomy in her home overlooking Long Island's Great South Bay, Pace received more bad news. The cancer had spread to her lymph nodes. She'd need radiation and chemotherapy. In her girlish, polite voice, she said, "Doctor, I did everything a lady is supposed to do to protect herself. I'm not a drinker. I'm not a smoker. I had my chil-

dren early. I don't buy any products with chemicals or preservatives. I went
for mammograms when I was supposed to. What did I do to get breast
cancer? What do I tell my daughters to do not to get it?"

Her doctor had no answers.

Pace soon learned that at least 70 percent of women with breast cancer
have no identifiable risk factors. She also learned that all too often doctors
don't listen to women. Pace had what is called a palpable lump. She'd had
numerous mammograms that same year for a variety of other breast problems, but not one X ray raised the specter of cancer. Yet Pace was fifty, the
age at which risk rises precipitously. Why didn't anyone take her concerns
seriously?

The experience radicalized her. Today, Lorraine Pace no longer plays
the good girl. Like thousands of other breast cancer survivors, she wants
answers. Driven by anger and the desire to protect their daughters and sisters and nieces, these women have formed the most visible political advocacy movement to hit Congress since AIDS activists took on the National
Institutes of Health in the 1980s.

Pace is president of Breast HELP (Healthy Environment for a Living
Planet), a Long Island advocacy group. Now when her husband comes
home from work, she's just as likely to be in Albany lobbying, out starting
a breast cancer support group at her hospital's new breast cancer wing, or
logging breast cancer cases on a map of West Islip in an attempt to identify
clusters that might point up environmental hot spots.

"Women have to speak up," Pace says, her voice a mix of girlish pro-
priety and determination. "We can't take a backseat anymore. A lot of
harm has been done by women being complacent. In 1960 one in fourteen
women had a lifetime risk of getting breast cancer. Now it's one in eight.
What is it going to be in ten years? Are we waiting until every other lady
gets breast cancer before something is done?"

Pace's West Islip group is one of 270 that have joined together under
the umbrella of the National Breast Cancer Coalition. Following the cue of
AIDS activists, who used their anger to raise awareness and money, these
women put breast cancer on the political map. At rallies around the country and in testimony before Congress, they demanded answers to tough
questions, such as why there wasn't a more reliable means of early detection, why up to 40 percent of women with negative lymph nodes would
have a recurrence, and why there were no alternatives to the standard
treatments—surgery, radiation, and chemotherapy—or what outspoken
breast surgeon Susan Love, M.D., calls, "slash, burn, and poison."

Breast cancer has become a symbol of women's fight for equal health care and, as such, is the focus of this chapter. It's telling that despite the fact that breast cancer is the most common malignancy in women—in 1994 an estimated 182,000 women will be diagnosed with the disease and another 46,000 will die of it—research efforts have been remarkably misguided.

■ DETECTION IS NOT PREVENTION

The mishandling of breast cancer begins with diagnosis. As far too many women can attest, even state-of-the-art methods for ferreting out the disease are inelegant at best. Women are told that if they practice breast self-examination (BSE) and get their mammograms, they will be able to catch their breast cancer early and ensure their survival. While finding a lump through BSE can mean the difference between having a mastectomy and a lumpectomy, not a single study has found an impact on survival. "By the time you can feel a lump, you've had cancer for a while," says Susan Love. "We oversell BSE and spread a lot of guilt. It's a little bit of blame-the-victim."

Mammography may be the best diagnostic tool available, but it too is far from perfect. The technology misses about 10 percent of breast cancers, often leading to misdiagnosis. And it has a false positive rate of 60 to 70 percent, meaning that areas that appear suspicious on the film turn out to be benign.

Susan Love hears too many stories about women who have lumps and have negative mammograms and think they're home free. "They don't seek help because they get a false sense of hope from the mammogram. We have to face the fact that mammography is not the ideal screening tool."

The sad story about mammography is that the women who can benefit most from it are not getting screened. In women ages fifty to sixty-nine, the technique reduces breast cancer mortality by up to 30 percent. But even though more than 75 percent of the breast cancer cases diagnosed each year are in women over fifty, older women have not gotten the message. A 1992 Mammography Attitudes and Usage Study found that only 47 percent of women between the ages of fifty and fifty-nine and 33 percent between sixty and sixty-nine were following recommended mammography screening guidelines. In contrast, 56 percent of women forty to forty-nine were getting regular mammograms.

The reason older women are not getting screened? Their physicians haven't told them they need to. According to the National Health Interview Survey, 30 percent of white women and 43 percent of black women in their sixties say their physicians never recommended mammography. Unless these women were radicalized by the early women's health movement, they tend to be passive about their bodies and their medical care. Physicians, too, are reluctant to talk. "We haven't educated physicians about how to talk to women about mammograms," says Barbara K. Rimer, a doctor of public health at the Duke Cancer Center in Durham, N.C. "Most older women don't feel comfortable bringing the subject up with their doctors." Some women believe that if they've had one normal mammogram, they don't need to go back again for screening. Others believe that by virtue of their age they're immune to breast cancer.

"You do have to die sometime," says Rimer. "But you don't have to die of breast cancer at sixty-five or seventy if you're otherwise healthy. You certainly shouldn't die of it because the medical profession didn't serve you well or because you didn't have access to a screening program."

Ironically women under fifty are the greatest users of mammography, even though there is little evidence that the technology saves lives. Studies conducted in Canada, Sweden, and Scotland showed no statistically significant reduction in mortality for women screened in their forties. What's more, false positives and false negatives are more common in younger women, whose denser breast tissue makes the X rays harder to read. Ruby Senie, Ph.D., an epidemiologist at Memorial Sloan-Kettering Cancer Center, worries about all the unnecessary biopsies that are occurring in this age group. Scar tissue from the biopsies may make it harder to identify tumors on future mammograms.

But despite questions about mammography's effectiveness in younger women, the American Cancer Society and eleven other groups have continued to defend the current screening guidelines calling for mammograms every one to two years for women in their forties. But in late 1993, after reviewing three decades' worth of breast cancer screening data, the NCI broke rank and announced plans to revise its guidelines. Rather than give advice, the NCI said it would recommend that women under fifty discuss with a health professional the advisability of screening, taking family history and personal risk factors into account.

This infuriated women's health advocates, who argued that the NCI should be taking a stand. "The NCI is the repository of public trust and public dollars," said Cindy Pearson of the National Women's Health Network. "As a consumer I want the government to say what they think the state of the science is."

If the medical community couldn't agree on what to do, how could women be expected to sort through the maze of information with their physicians, particularly when studies showed that their doctors weren't talking to them about cancer screening to begin with? This is particularly true in the case of black women, who have a lower incidence of breast cancer but are nonetheless dying at greater rates than any other group. Overall, in women under fifty, death rates have fallen by more than 10 percent between 1973 and 1990, with a decrease of 13 percent in white women. But in premenopausal African-American women, mortality has risen by 7 percent. And postmenopausal black women have experienced a 17 percent increase in mortality.

The higher death rates are probably not due to a biological difference in the disease in black women—although no one knows for sure since racial differences in breast cancer haven't been studied—but to the fact that the disease is diagnosed at a later stage in these women. "One reason we see women in advanced stages is that they're uneducated as to what a lump is," says Diana Godfrey, the administrative director of the Cancer Control Center at Harlem Hospital in New York. "If they feel a lump and the lump isn't bothering them, they're not going to bother that lump. And in those early stages, they don't feel any pain.

"Other patients who may have had cancer in their family feel that because the patient entered the hospital and was operated on, that caused it to spread. And fear alone will keep them away. We've had patients we've diagnosed, we've sent certified letters informing them, and we've even sent a tumor registrar to their homes, but they've refused to talk to us."

In Washington, D.C., Zora Brown has seen the same problems. Brown, who was diagnosed with breast cancer at age thirty-two, started the Breast Cancer Resource Committee with her sister Belva Brissett in 1989, a year before her sister died of the disease. Thanks to the support of physicians at Howard University Hospital and other medical institutions, there is now a place to send low-income black women who, after being diagnosed, would otherwise be shut out of the health care system.

Lesbians, too, face a quandary when it comes to diagnosis. To start, they may have a much greater chance of developing breast cancer compared to other women. A recent review of several studies by NCI epidemiologist Suzanne Haynes, Ph.D., suggests that lesbians may have two-to-three times the risk of getting breast cancer than the general population.

Asked to give a talk on lesbians and breast cancer, Haynes realized there was nothing in the medical literature on the subject. So she started from scratch, poring through the few lesbian health surveys and screening the data for risk factors. Haynes found that 80 percent of lesbians do not bear children (versus 11 percent of heterosexual women), that 25 percent are heavy drinkers (compared to 10 percent in the general population), and that they may be more apt to be overweight. In short, lesbians seemed to have more of the established risk factors for breast cancer.

They're also less likely to take advantage of early detection. Because lesbians have no need for contraception, they're less apt to see a gynecologist and, as a result, tend not to get routine breast exams and mammograms. Homophobia and the fear of being outed often make them feel uncomfortable in the traditional health care setting. One survey showed that up to 40 percent of lesbians have no ob-gyn provider. On average, they get gynecological exams every twenty-one months, versus every eight months for heterosexual women.

Susan Love, a lesbian herself, has said that it's a moot point whether lesbians are at a greater risk than other women. After all, she points out, "this is an epidemic."

■ THE YOUNG AND THE UNDETECTED

As we've discussed, routine screening does not guarantee a woman's breast cancer will be detected early, particularly if she is young. These defects in diagnosis are not only due to the fallibility of mammography in young women, but to the fact that doctors often believe premenopausal women are too young to have breast cancer and, therefore, dismiss a lump as nothing serious. Such was the case with Cass Brown.

After performing a routine Pap and pelvic, Brown's doctor offhandedly said, "You don't need a breast exam, do you?" Brown was taken aback. She certainly wanted an exam, but if her doctor didn't think she needed one, who was she to argue? Who was she to tell her doctor how to do his job?

Three weeks later Brown felt a lump above her breast on her chest wall. Although the mammogram showed a highly suspicious mass, the surgeon to whom Brown was referred didn't want to waste his time following it up.

"Who ordered this mammogram?" he barked. "You're too young."

By now Brown was angry. So what if she was only thirty-two. She wanted to have a biopsy. It didn't matter that her surgeon disapproved, that only 20 to 25 percent of biopsies came back positive. She wanted to be sure.

Brown remembers the day her surgeon called with the results. Uncomfortable and embarrassed, he couldn't choke out the word *cancer*. Instead he said, "It's something that can be handled short of mastectomy." As if that were some kind of consolation.

"Is it malignant?" Brown finally asked.

"Yes, but you don't need a mastectomy."

Brown was livid. "Everything about breast cancer is breast, breast, breast. The reason the emphasis is on the breast and not on your life is because it's men who lose your breast." But for Brown the biggest fear was of the cancer, of death.

Her experience exemplifies the problems faced by young women with breast cancer. Because the disease is rare in young women—between 1987 and 1989 only 6.5 percent of all breast cancers were diagnosed in women under forty—doctors tend to believe these women are not at risk.

Although the incidence among young women appears to have remained stable since the late 1980s, overall breast cancer rates increased by about 1 percent a year between 1940 and 1986, and 4 percent a year since 1987, indicating that the absolute number of young women being diagnosed is rising.

"It hasn't shown up in the national data yet, but clinically we're seeing a significant rise in younger women," says Amy Langer, a founding member of the National Breast Cancer Coalition, who was diagnosed at thirty. At the Marin County General Hospital, for instance, women under thirty-nine represented 6 percent of breast cancer diagnoses in 1992, up from 3 percent in the 1980s. The NCI estimates that in 1992, 12,600 women under the age of forty were diagnosed with breast cancer.

"Young women don't think they are at risk, and neither do their doctors," says Langer. "As a result they are diagnosed later or diagnosed incorrectly." Not only will these women have a longer time to worry about recurrence, but when they attempt to become pregnant, they will find that there are no firm answers on whether or not pregnancy after breast cancer is safe—for them or for their unborn babies. If they do have children, they'll live with the anxiety of wondering whether they will be around to see those children grow up. Chemotherapy will throw some women into premature menopause, putting them at increased risk of developing heart disease and osteoporosis. If they request hormone replacement therapy, either for the relief of menopausal symptoms or to protect their bones, they'll find its use has never been studied in breast cancer survivors.

Because breast cancer is so rare in young women, some researchers speculate that it is a biologically different disease than it is among older women. At an NCI conference on breast cancer in younger women, researchers reported that tumors in premenopausal women tend to be estrogen-receptor negative, which is associated with a poorer prognosis compared with tumors that contain estrogen receptors. Women under thirty are more likely to have larger tumors and more than three positive lymph nodes. These larger tumors tend to have more active cells in them, indicating they are more aggressive cancers.

Women under thirty are also at the greatest risk of dying of their disease, although the data here are sketchy. Because of the bias on the part of doctors that young women don't get breast cancer, few studies have enrolled a sufficient number of young women to yield statistically significant results. In a review of some four hundred articles published between 1990 and 1992 that addressed breast cancer survival, Marie Swanson, Ph.D., director of the Cancer Center at Michigan State University, was surprised to find that fewer than fifty included women under the age of fifty, and only about twenty specifically looked at women in their twenties and thirties.

Unable to draw any conclusions from these data, Swanson turned to the NCI's Surveillance, Epidemiology and End Results (SEER) Program. In a look at all women diagnosed with breast cancer between 1983 and 1989, she found that both black and white women between the ages of twenty and twenty-nine were at the highest risk of dying of breast cancer.

Perhaps the poorer prognosis in young women could be explained by younger women's unique—albeit misunderstood—risk factors, the most troublesome of which may be the early use of oral contraceptives. Safety questions have been batted back and forth since the birth control pill was approved for marketing in the U.S. in 1960. Results of the most recent study, published in the *Journal of the National Cancer Institute* in April 1994, are not considered to be too alarming. The authors, who studied 747 women with breast cancer and 961 without it, found that women under age forty-five who used the Pill ten years or longer, or who used it within five years of their first menstrual period, were 30 percent more likely to develop breast cancer than women who used the Pill for less than one year or began using it later in life. Women who used oral contraceptives containing high doses of progesterone for at least one year had a 50 percent greater chance of getting breast cancer, and women thirty-five or younger who used the Pill for ten years or more had a 70 percent higher risk.

Statistically speaking, these are modest risks, particularly because breast cancer is relatively rare in young women. But for women who used the Pill for a long period of time and have other known risk factors—for instance, they've never been pregnant or they had an early first period—the additional risk posed by the use of the Pill may prove to be important.

Danelle Butcher was diagnosed with breast cancer at age thirty-four when she was nursing her nine-month-old daughter. She'd had a three-year cycle of pregnancy and nursing followed by another pregnancy and had been on the Pill for fifteen years beginning at age twelve to control her irregular, painful periods.

Cass Brown was on and off the Pill for nine years beginning at age seventeen. "All of the women in our young women's breast cancer group were on the Pill," she says.

Despite the scores of studies published over the past twenty years, the final word on birth control pills and breast cancer remains elusive. "The current situation with the Pill and breast cancer is very complicated, and I don't think anybody really understands it," says Malcolm Pike, M.D., of the University of Southern California Medical School, who has been studying breast cancer risk factors for close to two decades. "There appears to be some increased risk in young women, but it doesn't extend to older ages, and we're not really sure what's going on."

Family history consistently shows up as a risk for premenopausal breast cancer. The younger a mother or sister is diagnosed, the stronger the risk. What's especially troublesome is that cancer occurs at a younger age with each successive generation. So you have grandmothers who got it in their fifties, mothers in their forties, and daughters in their thirties.

Some women are so terrified, they're having their breasts amputated rather than living in a state of perpetual fear. Margie Bernard, forty, has a strong history of cancer on both her mother's and her father's sides of the family. Her brother died of leukemia at age twelve, and her sister was treated for bone cancer at the same age. Bernard's mother, a paternal aunt, and her maternal great-grandmother all had breast cancer. In fact cancer was such a prevalent part of her formative years, "I wasn't aware that the kinds of serious illnesses that occurred in my home were not common in other families."

During her twenties Bernard had repeat cyst formations in her breasts that doctors believed would disappear as she got older. At thirty-two Bernard discovered a pea-size lump in her right breast. She waited two weeks to see if it disappeared. When it didn't she went for a mammogram, but the mass did not show up. Not long after the mammogram Bernard's physician found a second mass.

With a family history like hers, Bernard was not about to be cavalier. She knew all too well the dangers of taking a wait-and-watch approach. A colleague and close friend of hers had found a breast lump at the age of thirty-six. Because breast cancer was so rare in young women, her medical team had said that a biopsy was not necessary and put her off for more than a year. When she finally got the biopsy, not only was the lump malignant, it had already spread to three parts of her body. Five years later she was dead.

"I was not going to accept anyone passing over this lightly," says Bernard. "I've seen far too many women accept paternalistic pats on the head."

The pathology report showed that both lumps were benign, but three months later, in December 1986, Bernard noticed a bloody discharge from her right breast. In January and February she found two more suspicious masses. And in March three new masses. "No one in my peer group had ever gone through these things. Instead of being happy every time a test came back negative, it started to take an emotional toll. What was wrong with me? How come this doesn't happen to other people? Where's the support system? There was nothing I could do to stop the process that was changing who I was."

Bernard could no longer take it. She wanted a bilateral mastectomy—the removal of both breasts—with immediate reconstruction. The team of doctors—a general surgeon, medical oncologist, radiation therapist, and plastic and reconstructive surgeon—she consulted for a second opinion agreed that in her case a prophylactic mastectomy was appropriate. "You can only do so many biopsies," she says. "Follow-up is difficult because of the scar tissue. And they now know that even when breast cancer is found locally, every woman runs the chance it may have already metastasized at the time of diagnosis."

Bernard is aware that having her breasts removed is no guarantee she won't get breast cancer. The small amount of tissue that was left behind is still vulnerable to malignancy. "Even if, in ten years, I'm diagnosed with breast cancer, I'll never regret the interventions I took to keep myself well," she says.

Bernard has been most disappointed by the lack of support for women like herself who experience chronic benign breast conditions, some of which—such as lobular carcinoma in situ or atypical hyperplasia—are risk factors for breast cancer. "There's a tremendous amount of support available after a woman is diagnosed with breast cancer, but there's less understanding of how to help people through the emotional roller coaster of being at high risk. You have no idea of the fear you have to keep inside, what you undergo to live with that kind of strain."

■ TAMOXIFEN:
THE MEDICALIZATION OF PREVENTION

Prophylactic mastectomy might be justified in certain extreme cases among the 5 to 10 percent of women who are genetically predisposed toward developing the disease. But treating healthy women as if they already have a disease is science run amok. Nowhere is this more obvious than in the controversial Tamoxifen Breast Cancer Prevention Trial, which began in 1992 despite warnings from concerned researchers and advocacy groups that there were dangerous side effects that would overwhelm the benefits of the drug, especially in younger women. As of this writing, the study is showing every sign of becoming the female equivalent of the infamous Tuskegee trial.

The tamoxifen trial was announced to the public with a news release prepared by the National Cancer Institute and the National Surgical Adjuvant Breast and Bowel Project (NSABP). To be conducted at more than 270 sites across the United States and Canada, it was hailed as "the first large-scale breast cancer prevention study for women at increased risk for the disease."

In the United States the $60-million study of sixteen thousand healthy women age thirty-five and over was to be conducted in forty-six states plus the District of Columbia. Every day for five years half the women would take 20 mg of tamoxifen, a drug that blocks the tumor-promoting effects of estrogen in breast tissue. The other half would receive a placebo. NCI head Samuel Broder praised the Breast Cancer Prevention Trial as "an especially important investigation that may identify a practical method to prevent the development of this disease in certain high-risk women."

A "practical method"? Adriane Fugh-Berman, a medical adviser to the National Women's Health Network, hit the roof. Practical for whom? Here was a drug with a lot of unknowns—including its long-term effects on premenopausal women. And what was known about it wasn't exactly reassuring. Women who had taken tamoxifen as a cancer treatment or to prevent a recurrence of cancer in the other breast had experienced such menopausal symptoms as hot flashes and vaginal dryness as well as nausea and depression. Furthermore tamoxifen had been associated with eye disorders, endometrial cancer, blood clots, and in rats, liver cancer.

Why would the government consider subjecting healthy women to a drug with known toxicities? "There's a certain sense of desperation in the cancer establishment, because there's been so little progress in breast cancer treatment and in reducing breast cancer mortality," says Fugh-Berman.

Of course tamoxifen has shown some promise. Originally tested as a contraceptive, it turned out to stimulate fertility instead. Then it was noted that the drug worked primarily as an antiestrogen: It blocked the ability of cancer to combine with estrogen and continue to grow. In a worldwide collaboration of 133 randomized trials involving 75,000 women, tamoxifen plus chemotherapy was shown to reduce the risk of a breast cancer recurrence by 30 to 40 percent and significantly enhance ten-year survival.

It was easy to understand researchers' love affair with this chameleon-like compound. On some tissue the drug acted as an estrogen, lowering cholesterol and preventing bone loss. Based on its lofty track record in postmenopausal women—for whom it has been used since 1985 as adjuvant therapy and for some twenty years as treatment for advanced disease—the NCI estimated that tamoxifen would be able to reduce the incidence of breast cancer by one-third, heart attacks by 20 percent, and prevent osteoporosis. "If we can demonstrate the drug has three benefits, that would be quite remarkable," gushed Lawrence Wickerham, M.D., deputy director of the NSABP. "There's an incredible enthusiasm among investigators."

So far the study has found no shortage of volunteers. As of early 1994, eleven thousand women had signed up. Those who have seen generations of their families decimated by breast cancer would do almost anything to avoid getting this disease. For some women with a strong family history, the fear of breast cancer is palpable. The question for them is not whether they'll get it, but when.

According to the study protocol, any woman over thirty-five is eligible for the trial if her risk of getting breast cancer within five years is 1.7 percent or more, equivalent to the risk of a sixty-year-old woman. Risk factors include having a first-degree relative with breast cancer, first menstrual period under age twelve, no pregnancies or first child after age thirty, a history of benign breast biopsies, or a diagnosis of lobular carcinoma in situ, which by itself greatly increases a woman's chances of getting breast cancer. Any woman sixty and older is eligible based on her age alone.

Susan Granoff is one woman who joined the trial. She lost a mother, grandmother, and two aunts to breast cancer, and a third aunt has battled the disease. "Unless I can do something to weight the odds in my favor, there's a good chance that I'll be getting breast cancer too," says Granoff, who at forty-eight is the same age as her mother was when she died. Granoff is also thinking about her daughters, Johanna, twenty-two, and

Elizabeth, nineteen, who may have inherited a genetic propensity. "Breast cancer cuts women down when they should be living their lives to the fullest," she says. "I missed out on my mother. I don't want my children to be cheated out of theirs."

When Granoff heard about the tamoxifen trial, she jumped at the chance to participate. "Obviously if you're taking a powerful drug, there are going to be risks," she says. "But they seemed minimal compared with my chances of getting breast cancer."

Despite the eagerness of government researchers and study participants, serious questions were raised from the moment the trial was announced. Overlooked in the promise of tamoxifen are its potentially harmful effects in premenopausal women who, so far, make up half of the study participants.

At a congressional hearing in October 1992 chaired by Congressman Donald Payne (D-N.J.), researchers said they were worried about evidence that tamoxifen might stimulate the growth of tumors in premenopausal women. "I'm very concerned and very unhappy about including premenopausal women," says Richard Love, M.D., American Cancer Society professor of clinical oncology at the University of Wisconsin at Madison. Love, who had submitted a competing grant proposal for the trial, says he would not have recruited premenopausal women. "The objectives of the trial cannot be met by the way the study is currently being conducted."

Love believes tamoxifen may affect younger women differently than it does older women. In premenopausal women who still have functioning ovaries, tamoxifen has been shown to raise levels of total estrogens and estradiol, sometimes by as much as threefold. This may in turn diminish its antiestrogenic effects.

By the same token, tamoxifen may increase the incidence of ovarian cancer. The structure of tamoxifen is similar to that of the fertility drug clomiphene, which makes the ovaries work harder and often causes them to release multiple egg follicles. This hyperstimulation of the ovaries is theorized to be a contributor to malignancy.

Tamoxifen's unknowns have made it just as controversial in studies abroad. In the United Kingdom the Medical Research Council (MRC), Britain's equivalent of the NIH, decided not to fund a similar trial "on the grounds of liver toxicity in rats and the ethical issue of giving an anticancer drug to healthy women." The MRC is conducting a toxicology study on rats and human biopsy material to determine risk. Interim results presented in early 1993 suggested that the human liver may be less susceptible than the livers of rats to tamoxifen-induced tumors. As of 1994, the trial was going forward with support from two British funding charities, the Cancer Research Campaign and the Imperial Cancer Research Fund.

Richard Love believes the trial is justified only in women over sixty, but even with these women he would have taken a more cautious approach. In his grant proposal, he suggested conducting a pilot study of two thousand postmenopausal women before proceeding with the trial itself. "It's a canary-in-a-mine situation. Let's first investigate ways to minimize pulmonary embolism and other side effects. [NSABP director Bernard] Fisher completely stood in the way of substudies. The way the study is being done is treating women as chattel."

NCI estimates that of the 8,000 women receiving tamoxifen, sixty-two will be prevented from developing breast cancer. Love, however, did his own analysis of the risks and benefits and calculated that, of 10,000 healthy women taking tamoxifen, fifty-eight cases of breast cancer and ten cases of fatal and nonfatal heart attacks would be prevented, but close to three hundred women would experience such complications as blood clots, endometrial and ovarian cancers, depression, and eye disorders as a direct result of taking the drug.

"Even if major breast cancer 'prevention' benefits are assumed for premenopausal women, the costs are likely to be equivalent to or exceed these benefits," he concluded. "This is the first time a drug with such severe known toxicities has been considered for use in healthy populations. It's a dangerous trend toward medicalizing prevention."

From the beginning of the tamoxifen trial there were concerns about the risks, particularly to young women. There were also concerns that the risks of tamoxifen were not getting out to prospective participants. At Congressman Payne's hearing, women's health advocates said that at some of the trial sites investigators were placing more emphasis on the unproven potential benefits of tamoxifen and downplaying its potential risks, that the process of informed consent was a joke.

Indeed in England consent was a problem. When the study first started there, the participants received only an information leaflet that mentioned nausea and headaches as side effects and then said, "There are no long-term side effects which have been identified so far." After much protest the leaflet was withdrawn and rewritten to include the known toxicities.

In the United States informed consent appeared to vary by center and investigator. Sybil Fainberg, one prospective participant, had recently turned sixty. Two years earlier in 1991 her twin sister had been diagnosed with breast cancer. And Fainberg herself had had three breast biopsies, all of which turned out to be benign. Still, she says, "I was worried."

After a meeting with a nurse at the Georgetown Medical Center in Washington, Fainberg attended a seminar for women interested in joining the study. But most of the meeting was taken up with an overview of breast cancer, information she already knew. Tamoxifen was discussed only briefly, and as Fainberg recalls, "They talked only about the excitement of it. I don't remember hearing anything about drawbacks."

Meanwhile Fainberg had been doing her own reading on tamoxifen and had become "very unhappy with what we weren't being told." She decided not to join the trial. "If I were frantic about doing something to protect myself, I would have a prophylactic mastectomy," she says. "Major surgery is not going to kill me, but this drug might."

Fugh-Berman says it's one thing to study a toxic drug in sick people who stand to gain from it, quite another to subject healthy people to such a compound. There "has been a dangerous trend within the medical profession to elevate risk factors to the status of diseases, for which the inherent risks and side effects of medical treatment are thus acceptable. The medical profession has created a whole new category of 'patients' who have nothing wrong with them but a statistical possibility."

Bernadine Healy has defended the tamoxifen trial, however, calling it one of the most important ever undertaken in women's health. "We do not enter into clinical trials lightly," she said. "The most effective treatment of breast cancer is prevention." And by extension the most effective form of prevention is treatment.

But just as critics feared, by early 1994, some two years into the five-year study, trouble was on the horizon. Data from another breast cancer trial being conducted by the National Surgical Adjuvant Breast and Bowel Project found that twenty-three women with breast cancer who were taking tamoxifen to prevent a recurrence had developed uterine cancer. Four of those women died from the disease. Amazingly, Bernard Fisher had known about two of the deaths as early as September 1993 but delayed reporting them to NCI officials until November, presumably because he was concerned about the bad publicity that would be generated. Even more outrageous, it wasn't until January 1994 that the healthy women participating in the breast cancer prevention trial were told of the deaths.

Then in March, news broke about falsified data in the NSABP's lumpectomy trials, raising questions about the safety and efficacy of this surgical technique. Admitting its inability to monitor the quality of Bernard Fisher's research, in April the NCI temporarily halted recruitment in all fourteen NSABP studies, including the Breast Cancer Prevention Trial. Under pressure from federal officials Fisher resigned as principal investigator of the NSABP in what can only be described as a harsh public rebuke. In the meantime the National Women's Health Network has demanded that the tamoxifen prevention trial not be allowed to go forward.

Says Richard Love, "My view is that as time goes along, this trial will not just be a bust, it will be a total fiasco, because the net result will be that significantly more women will be harmed, in fact, probably killed, than will benefit from this trial."

■ DIET AND BREAST CANCER

"Treating" healthy women with a drug rather than investigating possible risk factors that are under their control, such as diet, seems ludicrous. But this is exactly what has happened in the race to find a cure for breast cancer. Like broken records, activists have been saying that less money should be thrown at treatment and detection and more at finding the causes of the disease. Diet was an obvious place to start. Since the 1960s, researchers had known that high-fat diets could promote breast cancer in animals. Even in humans, migration patterns showed that within a generation or two of moving to the United States, Japanese women's previously low breast cancer mortality rates rose to match the higher rates of American women, presumably as a result of changing from a low-fat to a high-fat diet. But cause and effect had yet to be proven. And the data were at best confusing.

Convinced of the breast cancer–fat connection, Dr. Maureen Henderson, of the Fred Hutchinson Cancer Research Center in Seattle, spent years trying to convince the National Cancer Institute to fund a study to answer this question definitively. What she wanted was a large clinical trial in which women were randomized to a low-fat or a normal diet and followed for a long enough period to detect differences in the incidence of cancer.

In 1983 the NCI approved the Women's Health Trial, which was to be a prospective randomized study of several thousand women between the ages of forty-five and sixty-nine. An intervention group would learn how to reduce their fat intake to 20 percent of total calories while a control group would eat a typical American diet of about 36 percent fat. But before the study began, the NCI wanted to conduct a pilot study of 300 healthy high-risk women to be sure the trial was feasible. The results were all the reinforcement anyone could need: By six months the women in the intervention group had achieved the dietary change. Not only that, most were able to maintain it over a two-year period. But whether larger numbers of women would volunteer was questioned.

Another feasibility study would have to be conducted. Maureen Henderson was among the investigators who received funds. Convinced the larger study could be done, she and her colleagues recruited an additional 1,700 women and successfully taught them how to follow a 20-percent fat diet. Henderson hoped the pilot would lead to funding of the most comprehensive study of diet and breast cancer. There was no reason not to move ahead.

But to accurately detect differences between the experimental and the control groups, researchers pointed out that the number of participants would have to be increased to 24,000, bumping up the cost of the study from $25 million to a hefty $107 million and making it one of the most expensive NCI trials ever conducted. In spite of the high cost, in July 1987 the NCI's Board of Scientific Counselors gave its interim approval. But the following January its special advisory committee recommended shelving the trial. According to Edward Sondik, M.D., deputy director of the NCI's Division of Cancer Prevention and Control, the board "was not convinced we had the methods to reduce fat to appropriate levels"—despite evidence to the contrary from the feasibility study. There were also concerns "that it was going to be difficult to maintain women at those levels."

A redesigned study was submitted. Although it won approval on scientific merit, it, too, was not funded by the National Cancer Advisory Board. In recommending that the trial not be funded, David Korn, M.D., then chairman of the advisory board, wrote to NCI director Samuel Broder that simply encouraging women to adhere to a low-fat diet should be enough to "reduce morbidity and mortality" from cancer.

The trial "could add to the body of existing knowledge about potential benefits of a low-fat diet," he conceded. "However, in the face of serious constraints on resources and the many important scientific opportunities in cancer research, it is not appropriate to fund a trial of this magnitude."

A third time around, the Board of Scientific Counselors again approved the trial, which included the effect of diet on heart disease and colorectal cancer, as well as breast cancer. But in December 1990 the advisory board recommended that, before the initiative went forward, investigators should show it was feasible in minority and low-income women. Yet a third pilot study was needed. How, the board asked, could these women be expected to stick to such a regimented diet?

"There's not a shred of evidence that anyone knows how to get a black population down to 20 percent fat," argued Korn. "It's one thing to develop behavioral changes in college-graduate, well-to-do white women, and quite another to talk to a bunch of high school dropout black women who worry whether they can get a bottle of milk on the table for their kids, let alone whether they're eating high-fat food."

The board was also concerned that there was no way to know whether the women were following the diet. As David Korn told *SF Weekly*, a San Francisco newspaper: "To this day, there is no way to measure fat intake. The only thing you can do is rely on memory. By the time you would've reached the latter part of the study, you would have a rather elderly population—how accurate would their dietary memory be? . . . Would half of them be in nursing homes with various kinds of senility or forgetfulness?"

It was as if the entire scientific community had had a collective memory lapse. No one pointed out that the men in the raft of cardiovascular trials had been asked to measure and report fat intake and had done so without problems. If the National, Heart, Lung, and Blood Institute could successfully conduct a diet study, why not NCI? Why not with women? What's more, the NIH had never before stopped a study over concerns that disenfranchised women were being underrepresented. Indeed for many years, studies didn't include any women at all—and no one had raised objections.

"Given the board's preconceived racist and classist presumptions, it was clear to most of the trial's advocates that the call for this feasibility study was a cynical ploy," wrote Susan Rennie in *Ms.* magazine. "For women health activists who'd strenuously lobbied for the inclusion of a full spectrum of women in NCI trials for years, having an investigation that promised to deliver information crucial to all women torpedoed for these very reasons was the ultimate irony."

Sheila Swanson, a breast cancer activist with the Y-Me Bay Area Breast Cancer Network in San Jose, was livid. "They're saying we're too stupid to follow a diet and write down what we eat. If it were a man's study, who do they think would be cooking for the men?"

Ultimately the message was that studying diet was not science and learning whether reducing dietary fat might prevent women from getting breast cancer was not important. More precisely, encouraging women to eat a low-fat diet was not a potential moneymaker. But pouring federal funds into the search for new drugs, into high technology, *that* spelled patents and profits. In the laboratory, with the test tubes and beakers and multi-million-dollar equipment, where the testosterone flowed, that's where real science happened. It was laughable to think that NCI, the quintessential old-boys' club, would study something as low tech as diet and breast cancer.

Ironically, in April 1991, a week after Bernadine Healy was confirmed as the new head of NIH, she proposed establishing the Women's Health Initiative, which would subsume the thrice-rejected Women's Health Trial. Eight years after the initial study was proposed and at six times the original cost, NIH was finally ready to fund a diet trial.

Then a bomb dropped. In October 1992 the largest study to look at the association between dietary fat and breast cancer concluded that reducing fat had no effect whatsoever. In monitoring the eating habits of 89,494 nurses over an eight-year period, Walter Willett, of Harvard's School of Public Health, reported that women whose dietary fat averaged 29 percent had the same incidence of breast cancer as those who consumed an average of 49 percent fat. In other words a low-fat diet did not reduce risk. Willett says the evidence is "strong enough to settle the debate about diet and breast cancer" once and for all. "Diet is not going to be the magic bullet for breast cancer. There is great consistency in the data and none of the associations [of fat and breast cancer] are considered statistically significant. We need to study non-dietary factors."

But many equally eminent epidemiologists argue that observational data such as Willett's cannot answer dietary questions. Ross Prentice, the biostatistician who would have headed the Women's Health Trial, points out that Willett's study lacked the statistical power to detect differences in breast cancer rates among the nurses. To reach statistical significance, he says, Willett would have had to enroll 360,000 women.

What's more, some researchers say that diets in which 25 to 29 percent of calories come from fat are not really low fat. It may be that 20 percent or less fat, particularly during adolescence, will prove a more important prognosticator. So far these hypotheses have not been examined.

Although the fat factor remains muddy, Susan Sieber, Ph.D., deputy director of the NCI's Division of Cancer Etiology, is convinced that diet plays some role in the development of breast cancer. "It might not be the addition of something to the diet in the United States that's absent in the Orient" that makes the difference, she says. "It might be the lack of something here that's present in the host country."

■ ENVIRONMENTAL TOXINS:
THE NEGLECTED RISK

The focus on diet as a possible contributor to breast cancer makes wonder-ful sense. However, it's also time to acknowledge that the problem may not be with women's bodies but with something in their environment.

Lorraine Pace thought about all the women in her community who had breast cancer. The day Pace was admitted to the hospital for her lumpectomy, one of her friends was exiting with a mastectomy. When Pace started chemotherapy, she learned that two other friends were also under-going treatment for breast cancer. Soon another friend was having a mas-tectomy. When she added it up, she could count at least twenty women who had breast cancer. They all lived in West Islip, New York, a town of green, manicured lawns along Long Island's Great South Bay, what Pace now calls Great Toxic Bay. Pace remembers looking out her window and seeing hundreds of clam boats tooling across the clear blue water. Now, ten years later, she's lucky to see any.

As Pace put the pieces of the puzzle together, she realized she and her friends had all used pesticides on their lawns. They all got their water from underground wells. (One of the wells is only a few yards from the South-ward Ho golf course, which is regularly treated with pesticides.) Their neighborhoods had overhead power lines. Was it possible, Pace wondered, that something in the environment had caused their breast cancer? Was it possible that "whatever got to the clams was getting to us?"

Pace knew that breast cancer rates were higher on Long Island than in the nation as a whole. Between 1983 and 1987 in Suffolk County, where Pace lives, there were 96.7 cases of breast cancer for every 100,000 women. In neighboring Nassau County the rate was 110.6 cases per 100,000, ver-sus 94.7 per 100,000 nationally.

Like Pace, Francine Kritchek wanted to know why. When she was di-agnosed with breast cancer in 1987 at the age of sixty, she learned that Marie Quinn, a friend from work, had had breast cancer several years earlier. A private person, Quinn had not told anybody about her disease. But the women decided breast cancer could no longer remain in the closet.

Kritchek and Quinn were catapulted into action in 1990 when the New York State Department of Health released a study addressing breast cancer incidence on Long Island. The report found a positive association between high incidence and high-income areas, and concluded that no fur-ther studies were necessary.

Outraged, Quinn contacted Barbara Balaban, director of the Breast Cancer Hot Line and Support Program at the Adelphi University School of Social Work. Together they put an ad in a local paper and sent out a mailing announcing a meeting. "Fifty-seven very angry, frustrated women showed up," says Kritchek.

Barbara Balaban, once a shy woman with a stammer, "screamed long and loud." The state study, she said, was irresponsible. Once again women were being put on the back burner. She knew that women on Long Island were not going to stand for it.

Not long after the release of the state report, Balaban, Kritchek, and Quinn formed 1 in 9: Long Island Breast Cancer Action Coalition. Among their major accomplishments was helping to pressure the Centers for Disease Control into holding a public hearing on Long Island to collect testimony about suspected environmental causes of breast cancer. In 1992 the CDC issued its report: The high incidence of breast cancer could be explained by the usual risk factors—the women's ages at first menstruation and menopause, their ages at the births of their first child, and the fact that most of the women are Jewish, another established risk factor.

This conclusion was not acceptable. Advocacy groups began popping up all over Long Island—in Babylon, Great Neck, Huntington, Long Beach, and West Islip. The women decided to take matters into their own hands. Each community started to map out breast cancer cases in an attempt to identify clusters, which might help point to an environmental cause, and the Long Island Breast Cancer Action Coalition announced that it would organize an environmental symposium of its own, to be led by Dr. Susan Love and Dr. Devra Lee Davis, now Senior Adviser to the Department of Health and Human Services' Assistant Secretary of Health.

A critic of the cancer establishment, Davis had long argued that the government was waging its war against cancer on the wrong front. Too much money was going into treatment rather than prevention. Davis contended that the scientific community was ignoring crucial issues that were all too apparent to women with the disease. It was serving science, not patients.

Davis asked, "Why is the generation of women now in their sixties, the generation that had more children and had them earlier in life, the generation that started out as Rosie the Riveter and ended up living out the Feminine Mystique, dying more of breast cancer? Based on all we know about the disease, these mothers of the baby boomers should have lower risks, as they had more children and had them earlier in life."

An obvious culprit is environmental toxins, in particular organo-chlorines: such synthetic chemicals as DDT, its by-product DDE, as well as dioxin and PCBs, all of which can get into the body through industrial exposure or the consumption of fish, meat, or dairy products. During the mid-to-late 1980s several studies suggested a link between exposure to high levels of organochlorines and breast cancer.

None of the studies, however, proved cause and effect. More research would have to be conducted. Unfortunately funding for a large controlled trial was not readily available. If researchers wanted to pursue these out-landish ideas, they would have to pick up the tab themselves. Intrigued with the data, Frank Falck, an epidemiologist at Hartford Hospital in Con-necticut, and Mary Wolff, Ph.D., of Mount Sinai Medical Center, decided to mount a pilot study.

Examining the breast tissue of twenty women with breast cancer and twenty controls, they found that the women with cancer had levels of DDE and PCBs that were about 40 percent higher than levels among women undergoing surgery for a benign breast condition. This study pro-vided one of the first potential links between exposure to environmental chemicals and breast cancer, but it had two major flaws: It had small num-bers and it did not adequately adjust for known risk factors.

Using these data, Wolff convinced the National Institute of Environ-mental Health Sciences to fund a larger study that would control for known risks. She speculates that she got the money because the study "was cheap, because it was a women's issue, and because a woman was the prin-cipal investigator." With the pressure on NIH to address gender gaps in biomedical research, it was suddenly fashionable to be a woman researcher studying a woman's disease.

Analyzing the blood serum of 58 women with breast cancer and 171 women without it, Wolff found that DDE levels were higher among the breast cancer patients. The women with levels in the top 10 percent had four times the breast cancer risk as women in the bottom 10 percent.

Critics have pointed to the lack of parallel animal data, but Wolff notes that other chemicals have been known to induce human cancer be-fore it was proven in lab animals. "Too little is known about breast cancer development to ignore the possibility that chemical exposures may play a role in this disease," she says. "This has got to be confirmed, and if it is confirmed, we need to figure out exactly when the effect takes place. Is it acting as an estrogen? Is it acting as a promoter?"

As an add-on to this study, Wolff hoped to get funding to measure the serum levels in women before they got breast cancer. But despite her earlier provocative results, "the NIH study section wasn't overwhelmed. They felt that it wasn't worth the extra $500,000. It pissed me off. We're not talking about a lot of money in terms of research grants. The epidemiologists who review breast cancer research represent a really entrenched point of view. They fund the same old things, the things that are a sure bet. It's a sure bet to tell you once again that diet is not related to breast cancer. This is one of the first new things to come along in breast cancer in twenty years. You have to take a chance sometime."

Then came another surprise. In April 1994 the largest study to look for a link between breast cancer and DDE failed to find one, although the study noted that DDE levels were significantly higher among black and Asian women compared to white women. This provocative finding has led many researchers to declare the DDE question far from settled.

Electromagnetic fields (EMF) are another potential contributor to breast cancer in women. Several studies have reported an association between occupational exposures to EMF and an increased risk of breast cancer in men working as electricians and utility linemen. Studies in women have been limited, and only one was suggestive of possible risk. Yet this, too, would appear to be a fruitful avenue of research.

The first double-blind, randomized, controlled trial of the effect of EMF exposure on women—titled Electric Power and the Risk of Breast Cancer—is currently under way at the Fred Hutchinson Cancer Research Center in Seattle. The results, which are not expected until 1996, hold special interest for Lorraine Pace. When she had the Long Island Lighting Company out to her house to measure the magnetic fields of her appliances, her electric stove was in the high range.

Could that have contributed to her breast cancer? Could some other danger be lurking in her environment? Pace got a stunning answer to this second question in April 1994. The New York State Health Department announced that women who lived about five-eighths of a mile from chemical plants had a sixty percent higher risk of developing breast cancer. Now it is up to researchers to try to prove that the chemical emissions actually caused the higher rates of cancer. If it can be shown that chemical emissions, pesticides, and other environmental toxins play a role in the development of breast cancer, as many researchers believe will be the case, Devra Davis wants to make the point very clear: "The issue is not what women can do but what society can do to limit women's exposure."

■ THE POLITICS OF BREAST CANCER

Diet, environmental toxins, attention to the unique problems of younger women—these issues would not have come to the forefront without the efforts of breast cancer activists. While Devra Davis attacks the environmental causes of breast cancer, others like Dr. Susan Love press the battle on the political front.

Love has become the medical conscience of the breast cancer movement. As a young surgeon she was well aware of the inequities women with breast conditions faced. At Boston's Beth Israel Hospital, where she joined the faculty as an assistant professor in 1980, her caseload consisted almost entirely of patients with breast problems. "They wouldn't send me men with gallbladders or hernias, because God forbid a woman would operate on a man," says Love. "But it was okay for me to take care of women. Breast problems were pretty much relegated to very junior faculty or people retiring who didn't want to do bigtime surgery anymore. So even clinically it wasn't considered very important. I realized this was an area where women received short shrift and I could contribute something that would be different."

In 1988 Love phased out everything in her practice except breast work and set up the Faulkner Breast Centre in Boston with five female surgeons. Traveling the country in 1990 to promote her book, *Dr. Susan Love's Breast Book*, Love discussed the shocking statistics—that 2.6 million women were living with breast cancer (1.6 million who knew it, 1 million who didn't), that breast malignancies were the second biggest cancer killer of women after lung cancer, that the breast cancer mortality rate had not changed in this country in sixty years. Everywhere she went, women asked one question: What can we do about this? As Love recalls, "I was in Utah . . . and gave a talk to six hundred women who were, by and large, straitlaced housewives. They were ready to storm the barricades. They would have marched on the White House the next day if I had told them to."

The year of Susan Love's book tour, breast cancer was receiving some $90 million in funding, compared to an incredible $1 billion for AIDS. Clearly breast cancer patients could learn something from the AIDS activists. Love got together with Susan Hester, president and founder of the Mary Helen Mautner Project for Lesbians with Cancer in Washington, D.C. Their goal was to unify the smattering of advocacy groups that were beginning to pop up around the country. First, they met with Amy Langer, executive director of the National Alliance of Breast Cancer Organizations. Then, with the help of Sharon Green of Y-Me, Ann McGuire from the

Women's Community Cancer Project, and Pam Onder from the Greater Washington Coalition for Cancer Survivorship, they organized a meeting in Washington in May 1991. More than 100 women representing 75 organizations showed up and the National Breast Cancer Coalition was born. The coalition's first project was a letter-writing campaign. Volunteers set out to collect 175,000 letters, one for every woman who would be diagnosed that year. In less than six weeks they had collected an astonishing 600,000 letters, which they delivered to members of Congress. As a result of the campaign Congress appropriated an additional $40 million for breast cancer research for 1992, for a total of $133 million. This accomplishment alone told them they had struck a nerve. The momentum was there for a national grassroots movement.

It took the activists, most of whom are breast cancer survivors, to point out what the scientific community seemed to be ignoring: In order to stop the death toll, it was crucial to get a handle on the causes of the disease. Tens of millions of dollars went toward developing new patentable drugs that represented not major breakthroughs but mere refinements in treatment. Yet the National Cancer Institute, with an annual budget of more than $2 billion, had little to show for its vast resources. Indeed, a 1991 General Accounting Office report concluded that "there has been no progress in preventing this disease." The report went on to note that, while "many breast cancer patients live longer and better than their predecessors, . . . we do not seem to be winning the war against breast cancer."

The breast cancer activists were angry, but they knew that anger alone wouldn't get them where they wanted to be. To gain credibility on Capitol Hill, they needed scientific data to back up their demands. So the coalition raised $20,000 and held technical meetings in Washington in February 1992 to which they invited fifteen top biomedical researchers, including Georgetown's Marc Lippman, Maureen Henderson of the Fred Hutchinson Cancer Research Center in Seattle, Graham Colditz of Harvard, and Darcy Spicer of the University of Southern California. The coalition took the data and developed a plan of how much money could reasonably be spent on breast cancer in 1993. They decided they needed an additional $300 million.

As a result of some skillful political maneuvering by Senator Tom Harkin, whose two sisters have died of breast cancer, the activists won an additional $210 million for breast cancer research, to be administered by the U.S. Army. This partnership with the Department of Defense was not as crazy as it appeared. Although few people knew it, the army had budgeted $25 million in 1992 for breast cancer research. The money was used

to buy new mammography machines, and to develop new high-tech diagnostic equipment.

Meanwhile the NCI's breast cancer budget had grown from $133 mil-
lion to $197 million. Now, between the two agencies, there was a total of
$400 million devoted exclusively to breast cancer. It was a stunning victory.
That the army had more breast cancer money than the NCI did not escape
the notice of NIH director Bernadine Healy and NCI director Samuel
Broder, M.D., who reportedly met with army brass in an attempt to get
the money shifted into their coffers. It didn't look good that the Department of Defense might be doing more to find a cure for breast cancer than
the nation's premier cancer institution. "We felt kind of gleeful," says Fran
Visco, president of the National Breast Cancer Coalition.

But the coalition wanted more than just money, it wanted a say in how
the money was spent. In a December 1992 meeting with the NCI's National Cancer Advisory Board (NCAB), Visco and Dr. Susan Love, now director of the UCLA Breast Center, called for representation by women
with breast cancer in all decision-making bodies. Among other things, they
asked that coalition members be included in groups that monitor data
coming in from clinical trials; they asked for a seat on the NCAB; and they
asked for the creation of a permanent Breast Cancer subcommittee of the
NCAB and for permanent breast cancer study sections with consumer representation.

Their chutzpah alienated some members of the scientific community,
in particular Frederick Becker, M.D., an NCAB member and vice president
for research of the M. D. Anderson Cancer Research Center in Houston,
who contends that earmarking money for breast cancer will squelch basic
biomedical research. But as Love explains it, "What we're saying is, too
much money is going into treatment research. We want basic research. We
can't afford to just say, well, the answer will come up if we just throw out
enough money and let scientists do whatever they want. So scientists are
objecting because it means they can't just study fruit flies' mating habits because they think they're interesting."

Critics say that politics have no place in biomedical research. When
the question is posed to Visco, she rolls her eyes. She's obviously answered
this question numerous times. "The scientific community is telling us,
'Fight for more money, but don't tell us where to spend it,' that politics
doesn't belong in breast cancer. But there's politics within the scientific
community, and those politics have worked in the past to the expense of
breast cancer and the expense of women's lives. There has always been a
limited amount of money to fund all the promising research that should

be funded. People make a decision to fund X at the expense of Y. And Y too often has been breast cancer."

The NCI appears to be responding, however. Samuel Broder, whose wife was diagnosed with breast cancer in 1993, has authorized the formation of an NIH breast cancer working group, consisting of some twenty-five representatives from the various institutes. Work-group head Susan Sieber says the group was formed to serve as a focus for breast cancer research at NIH and to forge new research collaborations among institutes. "Dr. Broder wanted the scientific community to know the Cancer Institute has put breast cancer as its top priority." Broder, who is maintaining an open dialogue with the activists—it was he who invited them to the NCAB meeting—notes that the NCI's breast cancer budget has grown 177 percent in recent years, versus an overall budget increase of 35 percent. By contrast, prostate cancer, the second leading cause of cancer deaths in men, receives only $40 to $50 million a year. Even some breast cancer researchers wonder whether giving the most funds to those who scream the loudest is the best way to spend scarce research dollars.

Some might argue that breast cancer funding is more than generous. But there is evidence that even this is not enough. In late 1993 the President's Special Commission on Breast Cancer, an independent panel of experts which between May 1992 and July 1993 held hearings on all aspects of the disease, called for even more money to eradicate breast cancer. "The National Institutes of Health and other involved health agencies must receive research funding of no less than $500 million per year . . . to make substantial progress in developing effective methods to cure and to prevent breast cancer, and to make current and future proven methods of early detection, treatment, and prevention universally available," said the group's report.

As the breast cancer activists stand poised to score another victory, some worry that their cause is going too mainstream. When breast cancer survivor Ellen Crowley and a group of demonstrators picketed a 1993 American Cancer Society meeting on breast cancer—carrying signs that read, "DDT, Are you killing me?" and "Haste, ACS, confront those polluters," members of the Massachusetts Breast Cancer Coalition quickly distanced themselves from the demonstrators. Acting up—or out—it seems is no longer politically correct.

Breast cancer survivor Ellen Hobbs has seen the changes and is less than thrilled. Addressing demonstrators at a Mother's Day rally in 1991, Hobbs unabashedly shoved her disease in the audience's face. She told the crowd that after her mastectomy and chemotherapy, her doctors said that her only hope of survival was a bone marrow transplant, that without it she'd be dead in a year-and-a-half.

"They gave me this," she said, and held up a breast prosthesis. "They said it would make me feel better, but I don't feel better."

"They gave me this," she said, as she plucked off a wig to reveal her bald head. "They said it would make me feel better, too. But I don't feel better."

Carried on TV stations throughout the country, Hobbs had become the poster child for breast cancer. But what started as a fearless grassroots movement—"nobody cared about offending anyone because we just wanted to make our point"—is now what Hobbs calls "the Suits," i.e., the bureaucrats.

"You go to these meetings and everybody's in suits with briefcases. There are a lot of aggressive, very ambitious people. You have women jockeying to be on the committees of these research panels and jockeying to go on these trips to Washington. We used to have a group of six people. If we had an idea for a project we'd just go ahead with it. Now if you do something, you get, 'Well, you didn't get board approval for that. You didn't clear it with so and so.' It's a bunch of bullshit. It's stifled a lot of creativity and activism in the movement.

"The early days were really exciting. We sent out this flyer [to members of Congress threatening to expose them if they failed to vote for a bill to increase funding for breast cancer]. It was really radical and people appreciated it. But now, if I were to send that thing out, I'd get fifteen phone calls the next day."

Perhaps not coincidentally, at the zenith of their success, the activists are also feeling a disturbing backlash from Capitol Hill. Emboldened after their stunning funding victory in 1992, they went back to Congress to ask for even more money. Says Fran Visco, "The response we got from some members was, 'Why are you here? We did our breast cancer thing last year. This isn't the Year of the Woman.' Congress would have you believe we only get one year. But we know that's not acceptable. They didn't believe us when we told them that a one-time jump-up in funding was not enough. We need a consistent high level of funding for breast cancer research. We told them, 'We're coming back year after year after year until the epidemic is ended. So get used to it.' "

6

AIDS
Women Are Not Immune

Mary Guinan was worried. A virologist at the Centers for Disease Control's sexually transmitted disease branch in Atlanta, she'd seen the reports that poor, young, inner-city women were dying of pneumocystis carinii pneumonia—the very same disease that was killing scores of gay men who had the new acquired immunodeficiency syndrome. One thing struck her: AIDS was a sexually transmitted disease. It was only a matter of time before large numbers of women would get this disease. Charged in 1982 with investigating AIDS, Dr. Guinan decided to interview all the heterosexual patients she came across.

She noticed that "there was just a minimal core of medical people who understood what sexually transmitted diseases were about. Physicians don't know, for the most part. They rarely take sex histories. They would stand up at meetings and say that women couldn't get AIDS or that they couldn't get it unless they had anal sex. I mean, who ever heard of a sexually transmitted disease that only one sex gets?"

Across the country Judith Cohen, Ph.D., then an epidemiologist at the University of California at Berkeley, was coming to the same conclusion. In 1984 Elizabeth Prophet, an AIDS-infected street prostitute and drug user, was brought by two prison guards to the AIDS clinic at San Francisco General Hospital. It was the first time that many of Cohen's colleagues had seen a woman with AIDS and Cohen had a disquieting feeling that it would not be the last.

But except for a handful of enlightened researchers, the rest of the medical community did not seem to share her concern. "Even in San Francisco, where AIDS consciousness was quite high, we only heard about the occasional odd case in women, and that was because we were asking and looking," she says. "Many of these diagnoses came very late in life or postmortem. A woman would show up with severe illness, but if she was a drug user and had a rapidly fatal pneumonia, nobody thought AIDS. If she was an older woman in poor health anyway, she got worked up for cancer and then died. No one ever thought AIDS. It didn't make any sense."

It didn't make any sense to Kathryn Anastos either. In 1982 Anastos, a feminist physician at Montefiore Hospital in New York City who had done her residency in social medicine, began seeing her first female patients with AIDS. "But whenever people talked about HIV in women, it was in the same victim-blaming terms. If you looked in the medical literature, the only discussion you saw involved two groups of women: mothers, who could infect their babies; and prostitutes, who might transmit the virus to their clients."

Guinan, Cohen, and Anastos felt like they were shouting into the darkness. No one seemed to notice that women were dying from AIDS. It didn't matter if IV drug users, prostitutes, or poor black or Hispanic women got AIDS. They were disenfranchised, dispensable. It was too easy to look the other way.

It still is, despite the fact that AIDS is now increasing faster among women than it is among men. In 1993 a total of 103,500 new cases of AIDS had been reported to the CDC, 16 percent of which were in women. Since 1992, cases among women have risen 151 percent, versus an increase of 105 percent among men. But even though half of all women with AIDS are acquiring it heterosexually, stereotypes about who gets this disease cause doctors not to think AIDS when they should. As a result, women with high-risk behaviors are not being identified, let alone referred for testing. Once diagnosed, they often have a hard time getting treatment. Incredible as it sounds, in some communities ob-gyns refuse to do pelvic exams and Pap smears on HIV-infected women.

But even for those practitioners who are willing to care for HIV-infected women, hard scientific data on therapy are hard to come by. Amazingly doctors don't know the best way to handle recurring vaginal candidiasis (yeast infections) or cervical dysplasia, a precancerous condition. They don't know whether HIV-infected women need to be treated more aggressively than men, whether all their gynecological conditions are related to immune suppression, or whether the use of oral contraceptives enhances or reduces the risk of HIV transmission. More than a decade into the epidemic, no one has definitive answers. The studies haven't been conducted.

The invisibility of women with AIDS stems from a mixture of institutionalized sexism and racism. If medicine revolves around the 70-kilogram Caucasian male, then AIDS diagnosis and treatment revolves around the 70-kilogram middle-class gay man. In such a clearly biased model, women are anomalies, not only by virtue of their gender but by their race and class as well: most women with AIDS are low-income blacks and Hispanics.

Historically, women have become visible in the AIDS epidemic only because of their capacity to bear children. As a result, although many more women than children are infected, there's been a disproportionate amount of research and scientific literature on pediatric AIDS. Equating women's health with maternal and child health has led to the labeling of women as evil vectors of transmission. It's easy to muster concern for their unborn children, the innocent victims, but lost in the battlefield of AIDS are the women themselves.

Perhaps most tragic is the realization that had public health officials recognized the threat to women, had there been strong leadership and a coordinated education and prevention effort from the beginning, women could have avoided this epidemic. That they haven't is an indictment of the entire public health response to AIDS, confirming our worst fears that women have been and still are second-class citizens when it comes to medical care.

■ TURNING A BLIND EYE TOWARD RISK

Since public health experts refused to recognize that women were at risk for AIDS, it's no surprise that women themselves were in the dark. Because women have been forced to fit a definition of AIDS tailored to men, the unique way in which they manifest the disease doesn't prompt doctors to suspect AIDS when they should. In June 1983, when Rebecca Denison began suffering from a variety of unexplained health problems, including fevers, fatigue, throat sores, and unexplained vaginal bleeding, the two doctors she consulted never thought of AIDS. Nor did any health care provider from whom she sought care during the next seven years. "No doctor ever asked me about HIV," she says. "I went into their offices and they saw a white, middle-class woman, not someone at risk for HIV. They had no idea what was happening to me so they told me it was all in my head."

The statistics bear this out. In a survey of 268 Washington, D.C., ob-gyns, only 40 percent said they regularly assessed HIV risk in their new adult patients. Forty percent of ob-gyns did not regularly recommend that women at risk limit the number of their sexual partners, and almost 30 percent did not regularly recommend the use of condoms for these women.

Close to a quarter of the physicians were not even familiar with the screening tests for the AIDS virus. Concluded the survey's lead author Bradley O. Boekeloo, of the Georgetown University School of Medicine, "This survey provides evidence that many obstetrician-gynecologists do not perceive HIV as a major threat to their patients and are not prepared to address the problem."

If ob-gyns are missing important warning signs in women, hospital staffs aren't doing much better. Wendi Alexis Modeste suffered from chronic vaginal yeast infections, endocarditis, recurrent bacterial pneumonia, and cervical dysplasia, which eventually became cervical cancer. Although she was homeless, was using intravenous drugs, and was having unprotected sex in exchange for drugs, none of the doctors she saw advised her to be tested for HIV. She was finally tested when she was hospitalized for a hysterectomy for the treatment of her cervical cancer, and then only because she told her surgeon that her ex-boyfriend had tested positive a month before.

Her situation is far from unusual. In a study of emergency room patients at an affiliated hospital of Montefiore Medical Center in the Bronx, Ellie Schoenbaum, M.D., director of the AIDS Research Program, found that women were less likely than men to be asked about any potentially risky sexual behavior or to be recognized as HIV positive. "There's a major window of opportunity to recognize warning signs early in the course of their infection so that they can get early treatment," she says. "At the moment we're not doing a very good job."

After women test positive, they often find their health care providers unable to address their questions and concerns. When Rebecca Denison finally learned she was HIV infected in June 1990, she had no idea what to do next—and neither did the counselor who broke the bad news. Denison asked the counselor what the chances were that she'd infected her husband. The counselor said she didn't know. Denison asked if she could have a healthy baby. The counselor had no idea. In lieu of guidance, she handed Denison a stack of flyers on AIDS, none of which pertained to women.

"There was no information, no services. It was difficult to get medical care," she says. "Support groups were not for women, just gay men. Even with excellent private insurance, I couldn't find a doctor who knew anything about women."

After Denison finally got the help she needed, she started the group WORLD—Women Organized to Respond to Life-threatening Diseases— and a newsletter of the same name to help other women like herself. Women from Argentina to Zambia wrote and shared their experiences with

HIV. For the first time they were able to break through the silence and the isolation.

But WORLD, like the handful of other women's groups—operates on a shoestring. The New Jersey Women and AIDS Network, for instance, has an annual budget of $200,000 and a staff of four. In contrast, Gay Men's Health Crisis in New York City, the grandaddy of AIDS service organizations, has an annual budget of $25 million and twenty-seven people sit on its board, including, in the past, socialites Judy Peabody and Joan Tisch. When GMHC, which has a staff of 280, does an AIDS walk, it raises close to $5 million in one day. "Whoopi Goldberg and Aretha Franklin have not taken on women and AIDS as a cause," Marion Banzhaf, executive director of the New Jersey Women and AIDS Network, says ruefully.

Although GMHC welcomes women, it prohibits anyone actively using drugs from interacting with clients and volunteers and does not allow drug users to join the recreation or buddy programs, effectively shutting out a large percentage of women with AIDS. "The AIDS movement as we know it has been defined by issues framed by gay white men," says Banzhaf. "The gay community's response to AIDS is the model," but women activists know that it doesn't always work for women.

Take the buddy program, a mainstay of the GMHC program. "We haven't figured out how to create buddy programs that work for women," says Banzhaf. "Some women clean up the house before their buddy gets there. Women are very particular about how their laundry is done. The whole concept of having someone come in and take care of them is foreign."

Organizations like WORLD and The New Jersey Women and AIDS Network can't solve all women's problems, but they can at least offer a safe haven: all-women support groups in which women can freely discuss sex and drug use and incarceration, and plan for their children's future.

■ ONE DISEASE—MANY RESPONSES

Despite the heinousness of AIDS, there are gender differences in the way the disease affects men and women. Early in the epidemic it was believed that women died faster than men after infection with HIV. But this turned out to be wrongheaded. Recent studies indicate that women do not fare worse. In a study at the Mount Sinai School of Medicine in New York, Henry Sacks, M.D., found that HIV-positive women had a higher survival rate than infected men, probably, he speculates, because the hospital routinely offers HIV testing to women being treated at its prenatal and gynecology clinics. "No recent data indicate women are dying faster than men—unless they're getting less care," says Kathryn Anastos.

Studies also suggest that women may have slower disease progression than men but more of the opportunistic infections that occur late in the course of the infection. "We don't know a lot about HIV in women because almost all the studies that were done originally were done on men," says Mitchell Maiman, M.D., associate professor and director of gynecologic oncology at the SUNY Health Science Center in Brooklyn. "We use the same antiretroviral therapy that we use on men. But such basic things as the dose of AZT and its side effects have not been worked out as well for women as they have for men. Medicine is fairly male dominated, and AIDS has been very male dominated, both in terms of researchers and patients, which makes it much more difficult to move forward on women's issues in this country."

While women are getting the same life-threatening AIDS infections as men—pneumocystis carinii pneumonia (PCP), tuberculosis, wasting syndrome, and mycobacterium avium—they seem to acquire some of them at increased rates. Women, for instance, have a higher incidence of chronic wasting, characterized by fatigue, weight loss, night sweats, fever, and diarrhea. One goal therefore would be to prevent these diseases in women. Whether this will prolong their lives or simply leave them vulnerable to other killer infections is unclear.

But there are also diseases that women with AIDS get that men can't. Most researchers have regarded women as men without penises, as if the female reproductive tract did not exist. And the ob-gyns who should have recognized the gynecological manifestations of AIDS seemed to be looking the other way. In fact it was a team of infectious-disease specialists in Rhode Island, led by Charles Carpenter, M.D., and Kenneth Mayer, M.D., director of the Brown University AIDS Program, who were among the first to notice that recurrent vaginal candidiasis was the most common initial manifestation of HIV infection in women, occurring in 38 percent of HIV-infected female patients. Carpenter and Mayer also saw higher than normal rates of pelvic inflammatory disease (PID) in HIV-positive women.

When Kathryn Anastos screened 250 women, she found that the likelihood of having an abnormal Pap smear went up as a woman's T-cell count went down. Fully half of her HIV-positive women had had abnormal Paps. There is concern that cervical dysplasia and cervical cancer, which are associated with the human papillomavirus (HPV), may be more common, severe, and rapidly progressing in HIV-infected women.

Even more perplexing, the usual therapies for cervical dysplasia often do not work in HIV-infected women. Tedd Ellerbrock, M.D., at the Centers for Disease Control and Prevention, found that despite treatment, 30 percent or more of the women were having persistent lesions or recurrences. Even the new loop electrosurgical excision procedure, in which infected tissue is scraped away via an electrical current, does not appear to be effective in HIV-infected women with cervical disease. To better treat these conditions, scientists need a true understanding of the role of HPV, cervical cancer, and PID in women with AIDS. They need a natural history study. Without it they are just taking shots in the dark. But throughout the 1980s no large-scale studies were funded.

Although research showed that STDs conferred a sixfold increase in the risk of HIV transmission, few people considered the unique problems STDs posed for women. For instance, a woman who has unprotected sex is twice as likely as a man to contract an STD. (Adolescent girls are particularly vulnerable because their immature cervical tissue predisposes them to infection.) Or the fact that STDs tend to be symptomless in women, which means they often go undiagnosed. Even the public health service underestimated the risk to women. For the last decade the bulk of the federal funds to diagnose and treat STDs has been directed toward clinics that primarily serve men, rather than to the family planning clinics where many women go for their reproductive health care.

■ THE FIGHT TO CHANGE
A DISEASE'S DEFINITION

By the end of the 1980s, with little attention being paid to the gynecological manifestations of AIDS, it was obvious that the disease was characterized around men. For years women's health advocates and researchers such as Judith Cohen and Kathryn Anastos had been pressuring NIH to take a stand. Finally, in the summer of 1990, James Hill, the deputy director of the National Institute of Allergy and Infectious Diseases (NIAID) phoned Caitlin Ryan and asked her if she was interested in organizing a conference to identify research priorities on women and AIDS. The meeting, to take place December 13 and 14, 1990, in Washington, D.C., would be the first national conference on women and HIV infection.

A lesbian and a feminist, Ryan had been involved in the women's health movement since the 1970s and had done AIDS work since the early 1980s. Now she had a whopping $300,000 budget for the conference and she intended to make every penny count.

The conference, the planning committee decided, would deal with vulnerable populations such as the homeless. It would be racially and ethnically diverse. There would be funds to enable women with HIV to travel to Washington, where they would be put up in community housing. There would be child care and sign language provided. Presentations would discuss epidemiology, biomedical research, psychosocial issues, gynecological manifestations, access to research trials, alternative therapies, sexual behavior, and substance abuse—in short all the issues that had long been ignored in women.

From the start it was obvious this conference was going to be a clash of cultures. "Is this AIDS 101? You're preaching to the converted," one woman yelled as Anthony Fauci, the director of NIAID, tried to discuss the pathogenesis of HIV infection.

Daniel Hoth, then director of NIAID's Division of AIDS, discussing current therapeutics, said, "We can say very little about the treatment of women with HIV infection because we don't have information."

A woman shouted back at him, "I won't be ignored no more," and the audience erupted in cheers, catcalls, and hoots.

Later another woman said, "You come to our poor black and Latino communities and you use us and you're gone."

And still another: "Will you offer clinical trials in long-term drug treatment facilities?"

On the one hand there were public health officials trying to hold a civilized medical meeting, on the other HIV-infected women were spewing out years of pent-up frustration and anger. Caitlin Ryan felt chills. "For years these women had been ignored, patronized, abused, and discriminated against. We were trying real hard to develop a research agenda, but at the same time there was a profound need to testify, to stand up and be counted."

James Curran, M.D., associate director, HIV/AIDS, at the CDC, said he wanted to begin his talk with a moment of silence for the men, women, and children who had died from HIV infection. People started shouting, "Silence equals death."

"We need to have a better understanding of the impact of HIV infection on gynecological conditions, including those that have long been underemphasized in our society—PID, cervical dysplasia, and cancer," he said. Someone shouted, "Put them in the definition," a reference to the CDC's AIDS surveillance case definition. People started clapping and chanting, "Women die faster, change the definition."

In fact much discussion centered around the AIDS definition, a list of twenty-three disabling infections that occur almost exclusively in people with severe immune deficiencies. For years activists such as New York City attorney Theresa McGovern had been trying to get the CDC to expand the case definition to include diseases HIV-infected women get—such things as invasive cervical cancer, recurrent PID, and vaginal candidiasis. The CDC had long maintained that there were not enough scientific data to justify adding these conditions. But there was a paucity of data because institutions such as the CDC had refused to fund the studies that could provide answers. It was a horrible catch-22.

Some public health experts were also worried that adding gynecological conditions commonly seen in women without AIDS would scare the general population of women. McGovern says that by not broadening the definition the CDC is "responsible for women being the fastest-rising group of people with AIDS."

McGovern was angry because she knew that women who were gravely ill but who did not have CDC-defined AIDS were being denied Social Security and Supplemental Security Income benefits. The law provided monthly cash benefits for people who were unable to work due to a physical or mental impairment, or combination of impairments, which were expected to last at least one year or result in death. A presumptive disability regulation enabled people with CDC-defined AIDS to be paid benefits while they awaited a decision on their application for ongoing benefits. But time after time women's claims were delayed for years and then, finally, denied. Often women died homeless and poor before getting an AIDS diagnosis.

In October 1990 nineteen New York State residents filed a class action suit against the Department of Health and Human Services charging they were unlawfully denied benefits even though they were unable to work because of AIDS-related disorders. "The lawsuit really translated what HIV-positive women were saying all along, that this disease in our bodies is doing different things to us," says McGovern. "If your immune system is destroyed, you're obviously going to have gynecological problems, and they're going to be more aggressive, resistant, and lethal."

One of the plaintiffs, thirty-one-year-old M.C., had been disabled since May 1984 by a combination of gynecological and pulmonary impairments. Her medical records included two hospitalizations for PID, a hospitalization for the treatment of cystic carcinoma of the ovary, treatment for pneumonia, a hospitalization for a total abdominal hysterectomy, two separate hospitalizations for the removal of her ovaries, and treatment for vomiting blood for five days. Yet despite her severe and often recurrent illnesses, M.C.'s claims for benefits were turned down.

While awaiting a decision on her appeal, M.C. was hospitalized several times for pneumocystis carinii pneumonia. In April 1991 the Appeals Council finally determined she had been disabled since 1984. "Ms. M.C. is gravely ill at the present time and it is quite remarkable that she has managed to stay alive the six years it took for the SSA to properly adjudicate her claim," McGovern wrote in an amended complaint in 1991.

With the class action suit on behalf of thousands of people pending, McGovern turned her attention to the CDC. She and other AIDS activists were convinced the CDC's case definition was undercounting women by 40 to 50 percent. This was important for other reasons. The numbers were used to calculate how much money states got under the federal Ryan White funding program. Places such as New York were losing a lot of money.

Like the women at the AIDS conference, McGovern knew the definition had to be changed. The CDC suggested calling it AIDS when anyone had a T-cell count of 200 or less and leaving it at that. But McGovern was not sold. "Lots of women who show up at hospitals don't get T cells taken," she said. "No one knows they have HIV. I knew how many of our clients were dying of AIDS and not counted."

On September 2, 1992, the CDC held an open meeting to discuss the expansion of the AIDS surveillance case definition. Marion Banzhaf read a consensus statement prepared by, among other groups, the New Jersey Women and AIDS Network, the American Civil Liberties Union, and McGovern's HIV Law Project. They proposed adding fifteen conditions including invasive cervical cancer and cervical dysplasia, pulmonary tuberculosis, and recurrent bacterial pneumonia.

As McGovern explains it, "Opportunistic infections in the AIDS definition drive the research agenda. For infections not considered to be AIDS, there's no attempt to develop alternative treatments. The government has been really passive. I feel pretty outraged about the whole thing. We made progress due to the courage of HIV-positive women who stood up against the Bush administration. AIDS is a microcosm of women's health care generally. If there's a place to save money, it's going to be on women."

The new definition, adopted in January 1993, added T-cell counts under 200 as well as cervical cancer, tuberculosis, and recurrent pneumonia. By the end of the first quarter of 1993 the total number of reported

AIDS cases increased 204 percent over the first quarter of 1992, exceeding McGovern's estimates by 150 percent.

Then in June 1993 the Clinton administration issued new rules making it easier for people with AIDS to get disability benefits. The new criteria for evaluating HIV infection included a variety of conditions specific to women: PID, cervical cancer, and vaginal yeast infections. Finally something had been done.

■ AIDS RESEARCH: WOMEN NEED NOT APPLY

The delay in adding women to the AIDS definition put research back years, but the CDC cannot take all the heat for the lack of information on HIV in women. The AIDS Clinical Trials Group (ACTG) could have independently redressed many of the imbalances in the research agenda. A nationwide network of more than 50 medical centers, the ACTG was established in December 1987 by the National Institute of Allergy and Infectious Diseases to test the safety and efficacy of new AIDS therapies. In 1994 the ACTG, which accounts for 67 percent of all NIAID-funded AIDS clinical trials, received funding of $100 million. (NIAID, with an annual budget of more than $1 billion, gets the lion's share of federal AIDS funds.)

But the ACTGs have a long history of underrepresenting women. As of April 1994 the ACTGs had enrolled a cumulative total of 32,174 men, women, adolescents, and children. Women made up 12 percent of the adult participants, slightly less than their 12.7 percent of the cumulative CDC-reported AIDS cases. But these figures are misleading. On paper women may appear to be fairly well represented, but their numbers aren't sufficient to provide definite answers to questions about drug toxicity. Constance Wofsy, M.D., codirector of the AIDS Program at the University of California, San Francisco, and San Francisco General Hospital, says that even a large study may need at least 15 percent women to enable researchers to draw conclusions that reach statistical significance.

A closer look at the different classes of drugs reveals more inequities. For instance, of the 28 trials of drugs designed to fight the virus, only 131 of 2,634 participants were women. Although studies of drugs that treat HIV-related bacterial, viral, and fungal opportunistic infections accrued 4,273 patients, women accounted for only 7.65 percent of adults. Women were sorely underrepresented in studies testing drugs for: cytomegalovirus retinitis (5.3 percent women), mycobacterium avium complex (7.1 percent), and pneumocystis carinii pneumonia therapy (7.9 percent). This is a real shortcoming because, as we noted above, women succumb to these infections at the same rate as men.

Women with AIDS were initially excluded for the same reasons most clinical trials have excluded women, most notably because of their child-bearing potential. (Studies, however, no longer exclude women for this reason.) Some studies required participants to meet the CDC's AIDS case definition. But since, up until January 1993, that definition did not include a single gynecological manifestation, women with a host of disabling conditions who were too sick to function were not sick enough to be included in a clinical trial.

As a result of this negligence, doctors are still guessing at drug dosing in women. Everyone had hoped that the long-awaited study comparing the benefits of AZT to the drug deoxyinosine would provide much-needed answers. But when the results were released in August 1992, it turned out that only 4 percent of the participants were female—again too few to draw any conclusions.

Because these AIDS drugs have not been proven safe and effective in women, doctors are sometimes reluctant to prescribe them, particularly during pregnancy. As Howard Minkoff, M.D., director of maternal-fetal medicine at the State University of New York in Brooklyn, explains, "What happens is, drug X goes through a clinical trial on only nonpregnant people, and now a pregnant woman gets AIDS, for which drug X is normally used. And the clinician says, 'It's never been tested in pregnancy, so I'm not going to use it. I'll go to some older drug.' And so the exclusion of women carries on long after the drug is approved."

The exclusion of women from research may partially explain why women with AIDS are not prescribed drugs at the same rate as men. Studies suggest that women are less likely than men to receive AZT even after taking into account such factors as race, insurance status, and mode of transmission. In analyzing data from the Robert Wood Johnson Foundation's AIDS Health Services Program, researchers found that 65 percent of the men but only 30 percent of the women were offered AZT. Similarly Ruth Greenblatt, M.D., associate professor of medicine and epidemiology at the University of California, San Francisco (UCSF), found that women with T cells under 500 were less likely than men to receive antiviral treatment and women with T cells under 200 had a relatively low prevalence of being on PCP prophylaxis, a treatment to prevent the development of pneumocystis carinii pneumonia. "And these were women who actually were attending clinics. There are so many layers of things that inhibit women from getting care," Greenblatt laments.

The boys' club that makes up this country's research community is one such layer. When Judith Feinberg, M.D., of Johns Hopkins University, reviewed two hundred AIDS studies, she found that the gender of a study's principal investigator made a difference in the number of women recruited. When the principal investigator was female, women comprised 10.8 percent of study participants. When the principal investigator was male, women made up only 5.3 percent of subjects.

Perhaps this should come as no surprise. Most AIDS researchers are men who, for more than a decade, have had the ideal research subjects: gay men who are generally affluent and motivated when it comes to their health care. As Constance Wofsy says, "If a clinic announces a promising new study, gay men will line up at the door."

Women, in contrast, are diverse. They don't bond around a single social group. Women with AIDS tend to be indigent and unemployed. Their health is often not a priority. "We often fail to think about women's day-to-day reality," says Georgetown's Mary Young, M.D. "When you have two children at home, the phone is about to be disconnected, the food stamps have run out, and there are rats in the bedroom, HIV disease and clinical trials drop way down in life. These women are not going to take a bus four hours in the rain to get their bloods drawn, especially if you're just doing research and providing primary care."

It's easier for researchers to buy into the myth that women with AIDS don't want to participate in clinical trials than it is to try to understand the cultural forces that keep them away, in particular the shameful legacy of Tuskegee. But women researchers seem to understand it's their job to go the extra mile to get these women to participate. "We reimburse people for their time and travel costs," says Ruth Greenblatt, M.D., of UCSF. "If someone comes in for a colposcopy [in which a microscope is used to look for cell changes on the cervix], and they're there a long time, we have a volunteer take care of their children and give them a meal ticket. If they have kids and they're not feeling well and they're due to come in, we give them a taxi voucher. We offer reimbursement because their time is valuable. They may have to pay for a baby-sitter. Somebody who has to take four buses to come in, I don't think it's fair to ask them to do that for your study, which is of obvious benefit to you as a researcher but of unclear benefit to the patient.

"We do reminder calls. That's not part of the normal protocol for clinical trials. We check back to see how people are doing. We try to establish a rapport. For many of our women it means a lot if the study clinician calls up and says, 'How are you doing? Did you have any spotting after your

Pap smear?' They may have no one else to talk to. We're flexible that way. We've recruited 150 women so far. It definitely can be done."

The ACTGs have resisted providing these ancillary services. Most don't reimburse women for participating, nor cover child care or travel expenses. Indeed, shockingly, only one of the more than two hundred ACTG studies provides gynecological care. "Researchers tend to feel that they shouldn't have to do anything more than offer these experimental drugs," says Greenblatt. "In San Francisco they haven't had to because for most male patients it doesn't matter. For women, having a gynecological exam makes a very big difference."

For too long it was a policy of fetal protectionism that kept women out of clinical trials. So when the first drug trial for women was announced, it was to everyone's surprise a study of pregnant women. It wasn't a study to determine how the drug in question—AZT—affected the mother. It was a study to determine whether AZT would halt transmission of the HIV virus from mother to fetus. "What was left out was the women," says Georgetown's Mary Young. "They were just looking at women as vectors for disease transmission, as carriers."

From the beginning AIDS Clinical Trials Group #076 was fraught with controversy. The goal was to enroll 748 pregnant women, but the original protocol included no evaluation of the mothers' health or the drug's impact on them. When AIDS activists protested the study's design, NIAID revised the study to include a maternal health component. AZT would be given to the mother in the second trimester. Then continuous AZT would be administered intravenously to the mother during labor. The newborn would get AZT for six weeks.

On the one hand activists were upset that there was a placebo arm, that only half the women would receive AZT. On the other they were worried about toxicity to the fetus. How ethical was it to give a toxic drug to a child who had only a 25 percent chance of becoming infected anyway?

At the ACTG meeting discussing the study design, activists charged that the study was immoral. HIV-infected African-American and Latino women, meanwhile, screamed that the activists were racist. Stop speaking for us, they said, we want this trial.

Activists also objected to a federal rule that got dusted off and resurrected for this trial: Pregnant women were required to get the permission of the father before they could enroll in the trial. But Johns Hopkins's Judith Feinberg knew this rule "could potentially damage women. Suppose the father didn't know she was pregnant?" The irony of the situation didn't escape Howard Minkoff: "A woman can choose without the consent of the father to terminate a pregnancy but she can't try to spare her baby with a research protocol."

As of February, 1994, 076 had enrolled 477 women. An interim analysis found that the treatment under study reduced the risk of transmission from mother to infant from 25.5 to 8.3 percent. Unfortunately, for all the time it's taken to get it right, the study wasn't designed to answer questions about how and when infection from mother to fetus occurs. And despite the decision to offer the mothers treatment, most clinicians still refer to it as the "fetus-bearer trial." "The resources that go into studying perinatal transmission dwarf the research dollars going into the way women get sick," says Kathryn Anastos.

To date, most of the emphasis has been on the effect of the mother's infection on the health of her fetus. But what about the effect of pregnancy on the mother's HIV disease? A few studies support an association between pregnancy and the clinical progression of AIDS. It is known that in women as well as men, decreasing CD4 counts, a measure of the number of disease-fighting white blood cells, is an important predictor of the development of opportunistic infections and progression to AIDS, and that pregnant HIV-infected women with low CD4 counts may be more likely to develop a serious infection during pregnancy. Even so, a 1992 study found that 33 percent of obstetricians did not test their patients' T cells as part of routine prenatal care, although this appears to be changing.

Pneumocystis carinii pneumonia is the most common cause of pregnancy-associated death due to AIDS in the United States. Preventive pentamidine therapy has been shown to delay both primary and recurrent episodes in nonpregnant women—and to extend lives—but the CDC states that the use of this therapy during pregnancy is "inadvisable." Noted Howard Minkoff in a 1990 paper in the *American Journal of Obstetrics and Gynecology*, "When some clinicians are confronted with this fairly strong caveat, it is probable that they will withdraw the drug from their patient's consideration until delivery has occurred. The appropriateness of this approach has not been formally considered." Minkoff and others argue that all pregnant women should be offered informed consent; that is, they should be counseled about the risks, benefits, and uncertainties of therapeutic options and be allowed to make their own decisions.

But all too often pregnant women—and HIV-infected women who hope to have children—are not offered options. Throughout the epidemic, infected pregnant women have been told that abortion is the only rational choice in their situation, and HIV-positive women of childbearing age are told not to conceive, despite the fact that there is only a 20 to 30 percent chance of transmitting the virus to their fetuses. But looked at another way, a woman has a 70 to 80 percent chance of not infecting her baby. As Hortensia Amaro, Ph.D., of Harvard, writes, "For many HIV positive women, a 70 percent chance of having a child who is not infected may be the best odds they have ever had." One HIV-positive pregnant woman who was a recovering heroin addict told Amaro she wanted to have her baby because "maybe" it would not be infected. "For her the pregnancy provided hope," says Amaro.

Curtailing women's rights in the name of fetal rights is a worrisome trend. Writes Amaro, "Notions of moral superiority and their application to AIDS are important . . . because they support a new approach to the limitation of women's reproductive choice." Especially troublesome is the fact that this patriarchal attitude toward women and their bodies is coming from the highest reaches of our federal government. In 1985 the CDC recommended that "infected women should be advised to consider delaying pregnancy until more is known about perinatal transmission of the virus." There was no discussion of how long these women, whose life expectancy was drastically reduced by AIDS, should "delay" childbearing. In 1987 the Surgeon General's Workshop on Children with HIV Infection and Their Families recommended that infected women be "advised to defer pregnancy." That same year the American College of Obstetricians and Gynecologists issued a report saying infected women "should be strongly encouraged not to become pregnant and should be provided with appropriate family planning assistance," although this recommendation was wisely withdrawn in 1988.

The attitude toward HIV and pregnancy was in sharp contrast to the way physicians were counseling women who carried the genes for Tay-Sachs and cystic fibrosis, both of which can also prove fatal to children. These women received nondirective counseling that explained, in an unbiased way, the risks and benefits of carrying their child to term. Most of these women, according to the medical literature, opted to have their children.

But with AIDS the whole concept of nondirective counseling flew out the window. Concern over the potential danger to the fetus—the innocent victim—took precedence over reproductive choice. And why wouldn't it? The majority of HIV-infected infants are born to black or Hispanic women, most of whom are uneducated, poor, and under- or uninsured. The underclass, the disenfranchised. Their physicians, primarily white middle-class men, couldn't understand that these women's ability to reproduce might be their only link to normality. If anyone had bothered to look at it from the mother's perspective, they would have understood why an HIV-infected woman would choose to carry her baby to term.

There was also the sexist and racist belief that these women, even if presented with the facts, couldn't be depended on to make intelligent decisions. Yet when Kathryn Anastos discusses the issue of pregnancy in a nondirective way, many of her patients choose to terminate.

"We're consultants," she says. "Our job is to tell a woman what the perinatal infection rate is—that a woman who's sicker has a higher transmission rate. We should not go around choosing for moms. We don't share their culture or their lives. People always exaggerate the perinatal transmission rate, but even that's not a cogent reason to take away a woman's rights around this issue."

Ironically those women who do decide to terminate their pregnancies may find it's actually not an option. Except in cases of rape, incest, or the endangerment of a woman's life, federal funds can no longer be used for abortion services, and some states permit the use of Medicaid funds only to save the mother's life. What's more, even where abortions are covered, doctors often refuse to perform them on HIV-infected women. One study in New York City found that 64 percent of abortion clinics refused appointments to HIV-infected women who sought abortions.

Pregnant women who are substance abusers face even more barriers. Learning they are HIV-positive often makes them want to clean up their act. But all too frequently they find themselves barred from drug rehabilitation programs. A survey of New York State substance abuse programs found that 67 percent refused to provide services to pregnant women and 87 percent refused care to pregnant women on Medicaid whose addiction was to crack cocaine.

■ CARE DELAYED, CARE DENIED

AIDS is a social and political barometer and it highlights what is wrong with our country's health care system. Men with AIDS may be part of an ostracized minority—homosexuals—but they are educated and affluent and they have the clout and dollars to fight the system, to act up for change. The women being decimated by AIDS, mostly inner-city African-Americans, are not in a position to make demands. They're disposable. And when you're dealing with disposable members of a society, it's okay not to study them if you think it might be too much trouble and cost too much. It's okay not to treat them. At least that has been the attitude of many of this country's ob-gyns and infectious-disease specialists where HIV-infected women are concerned.

One of the saddest legacies of the AIDS epidemic is the degree to which physicians have felt justified in refusing gynecological care to HIV-infected women. In one national survey of 2,545 primary care physicians, only 29 percent said they would provide prenatal care to women with HIV and 33 percent would provide elective gynecological services. In many instances physician assistants and nurse practitioners say they are doing pelvic exams and Pap smears on women no one else will touch. In a review of one hundred women with AIDS who were seen at Detroit's public hospital, for instance, Paula Schuman, M.D., found that only three had had pelvic exams, and in two of those cases the lab results had been lost. Says Schuman, "The house staff examines every nostril and ear, under the eyelids and toenails, but no one does pelvics. When we ask why, they say, 'Well, we didn't have time.'"

Disgusted by her colleagues' neglect, Schuman, an internist and infectious-disease specialist, took it upon herself to get an appointment in obstetrics and gynecology so that she could treat the women no one else would. Now she's teaching other doctors how to do Pap smears and perform colposcopies.

The same battles are being waged at other hospitals and clinics throughout the country. On Ward 86, the AIDS clinic at San Francisco General Hospital, up until a few years ago nurse practitioners were still running around looking for speculums with which to perform pelvic exams. Many of the examining rooms were not even equipped with stools or lamps. "For a long time, we had one single instrument tray," says nurse practitioner Catherine Lyons. "There was no pressing concern about gynecological issues."

When nurse practitioner Pat Kelly started working at the AIDS clinic at University Hospital of SUNY Brooklyn in 1988, she realized that women weren't getting Pap smears, so she dutifully sent them to the gynecology clinic for care. "It was a zoo," she says. "You had to be the first twenty on line or you'd wait there half the day." So Kelly suggested that the infectious-disease doctors at the AIDS clinic, mostly men, begin doing pelvic exams and Paps. "Everyone was grossed out by the idea," she says. "I finally said that I'd do Paps on their patients in addition to the patients I saw."

Over at Bronx Lebanon Hospital in New York, nurse practitioner Risa Denenberg had the same problems. "A lot of clinics, particularly those that have traditionally served gay men, don't provide gynecological care. Doctors send me patients to do Pap smears. I've seen cases where four years go by and the woman's got invasive cervical cancer because she never got a Pap. That's criminal. Cervical cancer is totally preventable. Primary care doctors should be doing their own Paps."

Denenberg often gives lectures to doctors about HIV management in which she discusses Pap smears. At one lecture a male doctor looked at her and said, "Really, we shouldn't be doing that. Nurse practitioners should be doing that." Denenberg was dumbstruck.

Over and over one hears the same stories of neglect. "I got a call from a hospital administrator who said they had an AIDS clinic in their hospital and a woman had cervical dysplasia and they couldn't find anyone who would treat her," says Ruth Greenblatt. "Most people who provide care in AIDS clinics do not have gyn expertise, unless they're people with an STD background."

This truly is outrageous. As Denenberg says, "Ob-gyns are in a unique position to see the gynecological complications of HIV. They have seen it and they've ignored it. They persistently looked in one hole and not the other. They would see women with oral thrush and not consider vaginal candidiasis. All over the country gynecologists have ignored the epidemic in women when they could have been at the forefront. Now there's money to study HIV in women and suddenly ob-gyns are interested and that's disgusting. They haven't shown leadership. At Bronx Lebanon we have a department that doesn't know there's an epidemic going on, and this is not uncommon."

Why have doctors looked the other way? In general, physicians go into infectious diseases to avoid primary care. "This is an area in which you give people magic bullets and you don't have any further responsibility for them, because they're cured," says Schuman. But as women survive longer with AIDS, they may no longer need acute care but rather long-term primary care. Infectious-disease people are generally not prepared—nor interested in—dealing with AIDS as a chronic condition.

Gynecologists and gynecological oncologists, meanwhile, are trained as surgeons. Although these physicians, who can make upward of $300,000 a year, should be providing primary care to women with AIDS, there's not much incentive to care for patients who have no health insurance and can't pay their tabs.

Amazingly, of the ninety researchers at NIAID, none are gynecologists. "This is why there ends up being a gap in women's health research," says Pamela Stratton, M.D., obstetric medical officer at the National Institute of Child Health and Human Development. "The reason that gynecologists are not engaged in this research is partly due to the fact that women who are HIV-infected are fairly asymptomatic. They identify themselves in the course of screening during pregnancy."

Frustrated by the lack of participation by ob-gyns, in December 1989 Stratton, the only ob-gyn at NIH working in the area of AIDS, met with a group of one hundred ob-gyns from the ACTG sites and public health service agencies. A survey of these doctors revealed that 18 to 32 percent of HIV-infected pregnant women in the United States delivered babies at an ACTG site in 1989. Clearly ob-gyns were in a unique position both to care for and to conduct research on HIV-infected women.

Stratton was encouraged. The physicians agreed that clinical trials for the prevention of mother-to-child transmission must include the care and treatment of HIV-infected women. In March 1990 Stratton helped form the Obstetric Gynecologic Working Group within the ACTG. Its first project was the redesign of Trial #076 to include initiation of AZT and placebo in the second and third trimester of pregnancy. So far the group of sixty doctors has developed a research agenda to answer such questions as the effect of HIV infection on pregnancy outcome, the timing of mother-to-child transmission, which women will and will not transmit HIV infection, and the most useful predictors of HIV disease progression in women postpartum. The group has also developed treatment guidelines in pregnancy, collected data on AZT use during pregnancy, and developed gynecological standards of care for women participating in the ACTGs.

As an outcome of this, the ACTG formed a Women's Health Core Committee, initially cochaired by Constance Wofsy and Arlene Bardequez. It's working to develop clinical trials for women, both pregnant and non-pregnant, to increase the enrollment of women in studies, and to provide recommendations for gynecological assessments of women participating in ACTG trials.

And there has been more encouraging news. In 1992 the CDC and NIH announced the establishment of a natural-history trial of women. Drs. Ruth Greenblatt, Kathryn Anastos, Paula Schuman, and Mary Young were among the researchers who received grants. This national study of 2,500 HIV-infected women will attempt to determine the occurrence of such non-AIDS-defining illnesses as the human papillomavirus, cervical dysplasia, chronic vaginitis, STDs, urinary tract infections, and gastrointestinal infections. It will attempt to define the rate of progression of HIV infection in women and will look at the effects of oral contraceptives, drug use, and such medications as antibiotics and antiretroviral drugs. By the turn of the century, some two decades into the epidemic, the medical community may finally have a few answers about women and AIDS.

LESBIANS WITH AIDS: A FORGOTTEN GROUP

If heterosexual women find it difficult to realistically gauge their risk and protect themselves, lesbians have it even tougher. Intravenous drug use and sex with men are known routes of HIV transmission into the lesbian population, but these behaviors are so stigmatized within the lesbian community that many women keep them a secret. "If you're a lesbian, shooting drugs and fucking men are not considered appropriate," says Amber Hollibaugh, director of the Lesbian AIDS Project at Gay Men's Health Crisis in New York.

Throughout the epidemic lesbians have tended to view themselves as God's chosen people. They truly believe they can't get AIDS. "HIV-infected women whose only risk was female-to-female sex have encountered incredible anger from other lesbians," says Hollibaugh. "There's this attitude: 'What are you trying to cover up?' Everyone says transmission is impossible. But I know of women who started out HIV-negative, who never shot drugs, maybe slept with a man twice. When she finds she's HIV-positive, everyone assumes it was heterosexual sex. Meanwhile she's sleeping with a woman who's HIV-positive every night.

"As women we're so demonized around our sexuality. We're trying to prove we're innocent. We believe there are good women and bad women. If you slept with a lot of women but no men, we say, 'I'm not a whore like you.' Even though the mythology is so extraordinarily pervasive, that lesbians are not supposed to be at risk, I'm meeting more and more lesbians who are HIV-positive and more and more women who partner with HIV-positive women."

So far only a few cases of possible woman-to-woman transmission have been reported to medical journals. Constance Wofsy and Judith Cohen found HIV does grow in vaginal secretion and therefore could be transmitted through mucous membrane exposure. Cohen's research also determined that women who have female sexual partners tend to engage in a greater number of high-risk behaviors—for instance intravenous drug use—than women who do not sleep with women. "But given the way the CDC counts people who have AIDS, this will never show up in their statistics," says Cohen. In fact the CDC has not kept statistics on lesbians as a group.

In a review of 18,199 cases of AIDS in adult women reported over an eleven-year period, Susan Chu of the CDC found that almost one percent said they had had sex only with other women. Chu could not document any cases of female-to-female transmission. But her study was limited by its narrow definition of lesbians: She eliminated all women who said they had had sex with men since 1977.

Several unpublished studies, one by Nancy Warren at Montefiore Medical Center, found that in prisons 40 percent of women with AIDS had slept with other women. Applying these results to the general population, lesbian activists now estimate that 30 percent of women with AIDS have slept with other women.

For lesbians, assessing risk is particularly difficult. "There's an assumption that oral sex is all lesbians do," says Hollibaugh. "The idea of sex toys, fisting, and rimming is never placed in a lesbian context. For the most part we don't know what each other is doing, what they call it, and when they do it."

Hollibaugh's mission is "to crack the invisibility and denial and bring support to lesbians who are HIV-positive so that they're not marginalized outside the lesbian community." Currently, some two hundred HIV-positive lesbians attend programs at GMHC. "Our job is to try to remove the bias that women are heterosexual unless they self-identify as lesbian. The starting point is that there should never be a burden placed on an HIV-positive person to identify her risky behavior to access service."

For the first time in our nation's history lesbians appear to be gaining a sympathetic ear in the White House. In April 1993 Mary Beth Caschetta and a group of fifteen HIV-positive lesbians from the ACT-UP New York Lesbian Caucus and the National Women's ACT-UP Network went to Washington to meet with Health and Human Services Secretary Donna Shalala. As the meeting took place, some of the women remained outside, marching and carrying placards with the names of lesbians who were homeless and incarcerated. The guards looked at the street-smart dykes and refused to let them in the building without IDs. "We don't have IDs," the women shouted. Meanwhile out walked a group of white gay men with short hair and designer ties, the kind of AIDS activists bureaucrats have become accustomed to dealing with. "It was a very stunning example of what we think of AIDS and how we don't really think about women," says Caschetta.

During the meeting with Shalala, "a lot of the women said they were sex workers or they were shooting up but they also considered themselves lesbians so they figured they were immune to HIV," says Caschetta. "Studies show that if you don't educate a specific target population about their health care risks, they're more likely to get infected. Everybody since the beginning has been saying that if AIDS is God's wrath against gays, how come lesbians don't get infected? Unfortunately lesbians are getting infected.

"Shalala assured the women that when she addressed women's policy issues, she would include lesbians. She used the *L* word. It was a big moment in history that someone that high up in government would meet with a bunch of lesbians with these concerns."

■ HOW CAN WOMEN PROTECT THEMSELVES?

That prevention efforts haven't been geared to lesbians is no surprise. Even heterosexual women have been neglected when it comes to protecting themselves against AIDS. This is all the more shocking when one considers that 11.4 million women are thought to fall into the two highest risk categories for AIDS: IV drug use and heterosexual contact with an infected partner.

After her fourth child was born, Marlena had her tubes tied. Married and faithful to her husband, John, she never considered using condoms. Despite John's infidelities, she truly believed she was immune from AIDS. Yet on February 17, 1991, she tested positive for HIV. Looking back, she realizes she caught the virus from John, who not long before had been sick with a high fever and severe diarrhea.

Marlena's inability to recognize that she was at risk and to take steps to protect herself represents the complete failure of the prevention programs in this country. Ultimately no one was telling women like Marlena—like most of us—that they could be at risk. No one was saying that the virus is much more easily transmitted from male to female than from female to male. The safe-sex messages on billboards and in subways, on TV in the wee hours of the night, weren't warning women that having sex with their husbands and steady boyfriends might be their ticket to AIDS.

In short the public health system ignored the threat to heterosexual women, so they didn't get the kind of counseling and education they needed to avoid illness. Even though it was obvious to infectious-disease specialists that the AIDS epidemic would eventually hit women, no one bothered to investigate contraceptive methods for their AIDS-preventiveness. And no one tried hard enough to develop a female-controlled microbicide that would simultaneously permit pregnancy and kill HIV.

But consider: In 1992, for the first time ever, more women contracted AIDS from heterosexual intercourse than from intravenous drug use. Nearly 60 percent of infected women were sex partners of men who were

IV drug users. Some 3 percent had male partners who were bisexual. Women are being put at risk primarily by the behavior of their partners, behaviors of which they are often unaware.

Bisexuality is a case in point. Because many bisexual men do not consider themselves gay, they may ignore the safe-sex messages targeted to gay men. In a paper presented at the International Conference on AIDS in Berlin in 1993, Joseph Stokes, Lynda Doll, and colleagues reported that of 350 men who had had sex with both men and women, 30 percent had had unprotected anal sex with a male partner in the preceding six months. Sixty-one percent had had unprotected vaginal or anal sex with at least one female partner in the same time period. An appallingly high 71 percent of the men had not told their female sexual partners that they had had sex with men.

"The lack of disclosure to female partners is especially disturbing if the men are engaging in unprotected sex with both their male and female partners," the authors noted. "It is not the case, in these data at least, that men who have unprotected sex with women are careful to use condoms when they have sex with men."

Cultural mores also influence how a bisexual man views his sexual orientation. In the Latino community, where homosexuality is highly stigmatized, only the passive receptive partner in anal intercourse is considered gay. The active insertive role is viewed as "machismo," super macho rather than homosexual. If these machismo men do not view themselves as gay, they're less apt to protect themselves when having sex with men. And they're certainly not going to wear condoms with their steady female partners and risk revealing their infidelities. Worries Lynda Doll, "How can women protect themselves if they don't know the risk behaviors of their sexual partners?"

Certainly many women can refuse to have sex. But for those who won't or can't abstain—due to a coercive partner—public health experts offer this advice: If women would only use condoms, all their problems would be solved. But there's a major flaw in this logic. Until the female condom came on the market in 1994, women couldn't wear condoms, and they can't necessarily control their use. A variety of social, economic, and cultural forces often limit a woman's ability to negotiate condom use on her behalf. Raising the issue of condoms in an ongoing relationship often brings up painful issues of fidelity and trust.

In a study conducted in Haiti, which has been ravaged by AIDS, researchers found that women felt powerless to protect themselves by demanding condom use. A substantial proportion of Haitian men have more than one female partner, while women are more likely to have a series of monogamous relationships, each providing her with one or more children and the hope of financial support. Women who refuse sexual relations or who require condoms sometimes face physical retaliation or abandonment. One man told researchers, "If the woman does not want to make love, well, I will go out. If you do that and get AIDS, who is responsible? Your wife is responsible if you get AIDS." A woman said, "If I don't want to have sex, I know I send my man to the streets to get AIDS and bring it to me."

Lost in the whole debate is the fact that women shouldn't have to be responsible for men's sexual behavior. Besides, like men, many women find condoms unpleasant to use and view unprotected sex as a sign of intimacy. For women who want to protect themselves from AIDS but who also want to conceive, there's another major hitch: Condoms prevent pregnancy. All of which adds up to a low rate of condom use. In one national telephone survey, researchers found that 71 percent of respondents with partners at high risk for HIV had not used condoms in the previous six months.

Interestingly studies show that women who use such female-controlled methods as contraceptive sponges and diaphragms have a lower risk of gonorrhea, trichomoniasis, and the hepatitis-B virus. While these studies did not address HIV infection directly, the findings provide strong circumstantial evidence that a female-controlled method could play a significant role in averting HIV infection, says Christopher Elias, of the Population Council. Yet prevention efforts have failed to focus on methods women can control.

The spermicide nonoxynol-9 should have been a serious contender. A number of studies show the compound is able to reduce transmission of such STDs as gonorrhea and chlamydia. Only a handful of studies have been designed to test whether nonoxynol-9 can prevent transmission of HIV in humans. Of those that have, the results have been mixed. Some suggest that consistent use of nonoxynol-9 can reduce the risk of HIV transmission by 60 to 80 percent. But another study, among prostitutes in Nairobi, found that daily use of the nonoxynol-9-containing Today sponge appeared to be associated with almost twice the risk of HIV transmission.

These worrisome results have halted further research into the possible usefulness of nonoxynol-9, even though the Nairobi study had serious design flaws. Elias speculates that nonoxynol-9 may be an appropriate HIV prevention strategy for many women, but not for women who have highly active and dangerous sex lives, such as prostitutes.

Given the conflicting data, public health officials have remained noticeably silent. In 1992 the New York State Health Department took something of a stand and recommended nonoxynol-9 as a last resort for women, hardly a ringing endorsement. Yet research has revealed that many women have already come to rely on nonoxynol-9 as their primary HIV-prevention strategy, under-scoring the need to conduct studies to clarify its safety and efficacy.

In the meantime people like Columbia University's Anke Ehrhardt and Erica Gollub keep telling public health experts that the existing methods to control the spread of HIV are proving inadequate for many of the world's women. Since 1989 Ehrhardt has been calling for the development of a tasteless, odorless virucide women could use without their partner's knowledge. The Population Council's Elias has argued for a microbicide that could prevent transmission of HIV as well as bacterial and viral STDs but not necessarily stand in the way of pregnancy.

Despite the desperate need for prevention methods under a woman's control, the federal government has been slow to pick up the gauntlet. In 1993 the National Institutes of Health spent only $8.6 million on micro-bicide research, versus an $84.9-million investment in HIV vaccine re-search. Thanks to some hard work by Congresswoman Connie Morella (R-Md.), the NIH is raising its microbicide research budget to $24.8 mil-lion for fiscal year 1995. By the end of 1994 ten new compounds may come under investigation in the United States. At the same time, the World Health Organization has announced plans to develop a safe and ef-fective vaginal microbicide. So far, however, funds have not been ear-marked for noncontraceptive microbicides.

"Why have the needs of women been overlooked?" wrote Elias. "The answer lies in a complex interplay between gender bias within the medical research community and the entrepreneurial factors that drive private-sector research. The neglect of microbicide research in the public sector has been matched by an even greater disinterest among private pharmaceutical companies. Microbicides are largely perceived as not profitable, due to the difficulty in securing patent protection for such products and an extremely complex regulatory environment."

Development is also being stymied by the lack of knowledge of the exact biological mechanism of HIV transmission. "We don't know which cells in the female reproductive tract are the primary targets of infection," says Elias. "We don't know whether it's the cervix. We don't know what the role is, if any, of the upper reproductive tract. If we knew the answers to those ques-tions, we could better focus our efforts. If, for instance, we knew that trans-mission across the vaginal wall was a rare event and that cervical transmission was a common event, then we could develop something that could be used with a diaphragm that would provide a physical barrier as well. But we don't even know if the primary site is the vagina or the cervix or the uterus.

"People who follow the funding priorities say that this is a late recognition of AIDS as a woman's disease in America and a late investment of significant funds for women and AIDS as opposed to other AIDS research issues."

The way things are going, Elias guesses, it will be another five to ten years before researchers identify an effective microbicide. In that time thousands more women will needlessly die of AIDS.

7

SURGERY
The Unkindest Cut

A Seattle physician remembers an incident from her medical residency that not only made surgeons' regard for women crystal clear to her but nearly ended her medical career before it began. "We were making rounds in the hospital," she recalls. "I was the only woman, and we were discussing the case of a woman who had checked into the hospital for a hysterectomy. 'She doesn't really need it,' said the physician who was leading the rounds, 'but let's do it anyway, because you can all use the practice.'" Outraged, the young doctor couldn't stop herself from blurting out, "And while we're at it, why don't we remove your testicles for practice, too!" She nearly got kicked out of the training program.

Or consider another incident: A woman who had just moved from a large northern city to a small southern town went to a local doctor for a mammogram. She explained to him that she had a benign cyst that was being carefully watched for signs of change. "I told my new doctor that I'd have my old records sent so that he could compare the images," she remembers. She told him the cyst had been there for years and was considered harmless as long as it didn't change. She had the mammogram, and was called several days later by a surgeon who told her that the doctor had scheduled her for a biopsy. "He hadn't listened to anything I told him, hadn't waited to see the old pictures, and hadn't even called to tell me he was recommending a biopsy," she said furiously. "He just went ahead and scheduled me for a surgical procedure." She canceled the appointment, found another doctor, and learned there was no change in the cyst, no need for a biopsy.

Incidents like these illustrate a cavalier attitude toward cutting into women's bodies that is disturbingly widespread. "We learned in medical school that if you get an abnormal result on a Pap smear, you do a cone biopsy, which is removing a big chunk of the cervix," says Wayne Burrows, M.D., assistant professor of maternal-fetal medicine at the University of South Carolina School of Medicine. "And then, if that's abnormal, you do a hysterectomy. No one would ever remove body parts like that from men without more tests, other treatments."

Twenty-five years ago a prominent medical journal covered a cancer conference where surgeons agreed that they didn't hesitate to remove an ovary, but thought twice about removing a testicle. "The doctors readily admitted that such a sex-oriented viewpoint arises from the fact that most surgeons are male," reported the journal. Said one of the surgeons, "No ovary is good enough to leave in, and no testicle is bad enough to take out!"

With the exception of circumcising boy babies, doctors do seem particularly reluctant to operate on male genitals. Hysterectomies may be performed for the flimsiest of medical reasons, but even cancerous prostate glands are often left in place to be observed or treated with medication. And when couples choose surgical sterilization, more often than not the woman submits to a tubal ligation, sparing her partner a vasectomy, even though female sterilization is a riskier and more expensive operation. Approximately two tubal ligations are performed in this country for every vasectomy.

In operating suites and physicians' offices around the country, the vast majority of bodies being cut and sutured belong to women. Nearly fifteen million American women have surgery performed in the hospital every year, versus eight and a half million men. Millions more have outpatient procedures performed in physicians' offices.

Surgery itself is not the villain. Done appropriately and skillfully, it saves lives. But performed unnecessarily, surgery exposes patients to risks unjustified by the condition being treated. And when the patient is a woman, chances are good that the operation is unjustified.

A list of the country's most common inpatient operations is dominated by surgery performed exclusively on women. Seven of the twelve most frequently performed surgical procedures are operations unique to women, including episiotomies (an incision made between the vagina and the rectum intended to hasten vaginal childbirth), cesarean sections, and hysterectomies. (Only one of the top twelve surgeries, prostatectomy, is unique to men.) That the most common operations in the country are procedures for which only half the population is eligible, is truly astonishing. A large percentage of these operations are elective and may even be medically inappropriate. Depending on which expert is consulted, anywhere from 20 to 90 percent of the nearly 550,000 hysterectomies performed in this country every year are medically unjustified. And one-third to one-half of the nearly one million cesarean sections could be avoided without harm to mother or child.

Some of the medical biases *against* operating on women have already been discussed. In chapter 4, for example, studies show that women with cardiac symptoms and disease equivalent to men are less likely to receive potentially lifesaving bypass surgery or angioplasty to clear blocked arteries. Chapter 3 documents a report from the American Medical Association's Council on Ethical and Judicial Affairs that women with kidney failure are 30 percent less likely to receive kidney transplants than men.

But when it comes to elective surgery, the vast majority of surgery performed in this country, all reluctance to operate on women seems to disappear, whether or not the surgery involves the reproductive organs. For instance, women have twice as many appendectomies as men, despite the fact that they are less likely to develop appendicitis. Approximately one in four women will have their appendixes removed, compared with just one in eight men. Yet the risk of developing appendicitis is just 6.7 percent for women and 8.6 percent for men. Many women's appendixes are removed "incidentally" during other abdominal surgery, such as gallbladder removal or hysterectomy. Women ages thirty-five to forty-four—well past the age when their appendicitis risk is greatest—have the highest rate of these incidental appendectomies.

Women also lead the numbers in foot surgeries, often the result of wearing fashionable but crippling footwear (which could be a whole other topic of discussion). More than three-quarters of all foot operations are performed on women, including 94 percent of bunion surgery, 87 percent of neuroma surgery, and 81 percent of hammertoe surgery.

Finally, women far outnumber men in sheer numbers of purely cosmetic procedures, such as liposuction and facelifts. In these cases particularly, the surgery may be exposing women to risks that far outweigh any benefits.

Women seem to bear the brunt of the unofficial credo of American surgery that more is always better and all is preferable to none. The unnecessary surgery performed on women is an extension of the same quick-fix mentality that leads physicians to prefer writing a prescription for medication rather than dispensing the information necessary for patients to make lifestyle changes. And when a pill doesn't work, a knife or laser will.

This line of reasoning continues with the same specious logic. If you're going to do surgery, why not go all the way? Why take out a fibroid tumor when you can take out the entire uterus? Why remove just a cancerous lump when you can remove the entire breast? Even women in perfect health do not easily escape the knife. Physicians seem loath to let a baby be born without interference when they can slice a woman's body open to remove it or, at the very least, make an incision between the vagina and rectum.

With their advanced surgical techniques and high-tech equipment, American surgeons pride themselves on providing the best care in the world. But too much surgery is as dangerous and detrimental as too little. Americans, and specifically American women, won't be getting the best surgical care until the number and types of operations are appropriate to the conditions being treated. While nearly 25 percent of American babies are delivered by cesarean section, only 7 percent of Japanese are. Almost 40 percent of American women will eventually have their wombs removed, but fewer than a quarter of French women will. Yet infant mortality rates are lower in Japan, and female longevity is higher in France.

Even within the United States, there are vast differences in surgery rates for different geographical areas, racial and ethnic groups, and income and educational levels. These variations have little to do with the health of the patients, but everything to do with the attitudes and practices of the local medical community.

The propensity to perform unnecessary surgery is deeply ingrained in American medicine. Even when the media publicizes the unjustifiably high numbers of specific operations, surgeons don't change their practices. Medical journal articles for the last few decades have shown concern with the high rate of hysterectomies, for example, but the concern doesn't seem to translate into fewer operations. Instead of the old medical saw "If it ain't broke, don't fix it," advocating conservative treatment to expose people to as little risk as possible, surgeons seem to say, "What the hell, fix it anyway."

Part of the problem is the way American health care is structured. A fee-for-service system means that doctors are paid for the services they perform. Performing a cesarean rather than simply waiting around for the baby to be born not only means an obstetrician can go home and get some sleep but promises to bring in an extra thousand dollars or so. Why wait?

Another problem is that physicians are trained to practice medicine a certain way, and resist changing their methods even when faced with compelling reasons for doing so. Says John M. Smith, an obstetrician-gynecologist and author of *Women and Doctors*, "Doctors who do unnecessary operations on women almost always genuinely believe that they are acting in the best interest of the women. Because their behavior is not the result of a conscious decision to do harm, but rather the result of psychosocial conditioning that leads to the behavior, we cannot simply ferret out the bad guys and eliminate them."

"Physicians practice medicine based on professional knowledge that is obtained in medical school and residency," says Joseph C. Gambone, D.O., associate professor, and director of the fertility program, department of ob-gyn, University of California, Los Angeles. But medical school training does not include teaching in how to constantly update and improve skills, something many doctors neglect. "It can be threatening for a physician, who has spent a lot of years training to handle a problem by taking a woman's uterus out, to be told there's a better way."

Women's dubious status as the more operated-on gender unfortunately doesn't carry over into surgical research. A case in point is chronobiology, the field of studying body rhythms that affect both susceptibility to disease and response to medical treatments. This field seems particularly applicable to women, with their monthly cycles, yet so far this aspect of the field has received scant notice. Researchers have concentrated on such factors as what time of the day specific drugs are most potent in the body and why heart attacks are more common in the morning. And, of course, they've studied mostly men.

For women, however, chronobiology may have dramatic implications. Some recent research has indicated that the survival rate of premenopausal women with breast cancer may be related to the timing of their surgery. Because of changing levels of estrogen and progesterone, surgery may be most effective during the luteal phase (days fifteen to twenty-seven of a twenty-eight-day cycle). The findings are intriguing enough to suggest that other surgical procedures may be similarly affected by the timing of the menstrual cycle. But few studies are being done, and few doctors are paying attention to the earlier findings.

While the oversurgicalization of women has many reasons, three stand out: the all-or-nothing philosophy responsible for so many hysterectomies and mastectomies; the surgicalization of childbirth, which leads to cesarean sections and episiotomies; and the selling of cosmetic surgery. Following is a more extended look at all three.

■ HYSTERECTOMY: ALL-OR-NOTHING SURGERY

Surgeons in this country seem to believe that the more tissue removed, the better. Nowhere is this more evident than in surgery on the female reproductive organs and breasts.

The statistics on hysterectomy are mind-boggling: Each year approximately 550,000 women have their wombs removed. More than one-third of women will not have a uterus by age fifty.

The numbers of these operations and the often insubstantial medical rationale behind them bear a chilling parallel to the useless ovariotomies and clitoridectomies of the last century. "Many gynecologists feel that the uterus is a disposable organ, one that bleeds, cramps, carries babies, and gets cancer. These doctors seem to believe that it can be removed with no more effect than to make them heroes to their patients for having taken this miserable organ from them," writes Dr. John Smith.

Another gynecologist author, Stanley West, of St. Vincent's Hospital and Medical Center in New York City, adds, "No man would agree to have his sexual and reproductive organs removed for anything short of a life-threatening illness. And no doctor would suggest such a radical course of action except when the alternative is certain death." Yet women in America, advised by their physicians, agree to just such radical surgery for less-than-solid medical reasons all the time.

Eighty to 85 percent of hysterectomies in America are elective, meaning that at least one reasonable alternative for treatment exists. And the surgery is recommended and performed for such vague symptoms and common conditions as fibroids (which approximately one-third of premenopausal women have), pelvic pain, uterine prolapse, stress urinary incontinence, abnormal bleeding, and cervical dysplasia (changes in cervical cells that may progress to cancer). Before age fifty-five the leading reasons for hysterectomy are uterine fibroids and endometriosis. After age fifty-five the surgery is most commonly performed for uterine prolapse and cancer.

Many woman have hysterectomies when they are approaching menopause, a time when fibroid tumors naturally shrink and heavy bleeding problems often end. But instead of waiting for symptoms to abate naturally, physicians may recommend hysterectomy for an instant cure.

Enlarged uteruses are also removed, although the benefits of the surgery are questionable. "Traditionally in gynecology, women are told that if their uterus is above a certain size, it is medically necessary to remove it, because they could have cancer there," explains Gambone. "But women are *not* told that the chance of cancer is one in two thousand. And the death rate for hysterectomy for benign indications is one in one thousand. If women have the information explained to them that way, a great many of them don't want to have surgery."

And many perfectly normal uteruses are removed. Very little research has been done on healthy menstruation, including what type of bleeding is normal in perimenopause, the several years before the last menstrual period. Many women whose heavy bleeding at this time may represent only a temporary, transitional phase wind up with hysterectomies to end the flow.

When one New York City health care professional reached her mid-forties, she noted that her menstrual cycle was changing, as is typical during the perimenopausal years. When her bleeding became constant and heavy, she worried that her fibroids were to blame. She consulted her physician, who recommended a total hysterectomy. "The doctor's attitude was that I had this troublesome uterus, and by removing it and my ovaries I'd be cleaning house and sailing into a healthy midlife."

But the woman couldn't reconcile herself to the idea of a surgical menopause. "Even though I obviously was not going to bear children at that point, I felt oddly attached to my uterus, not to mention my ovaries," she says. "Did I have a choice? I asked my doctor if I had options." A laparoscopy (to look at the pelvic organs) and a D&C (dilation and curettage, to obtain a tissue sample for diagnosis) ultimately solved her problems. Having averted major surgery, she reached a natural menopause four years later.

Several years ago hysterectomy used to be routinely "tacked on" to surgical corrections for urinary incontinence. But studies showed that the additional surgery provided no benefit to the patient. Also, many women have their normal uteruses needlessly removed while having diseased ovaries or fallopian tubes taken out. The additional surgery more than quadruples the postoperative complications. Women who have hysterectomies along with their surgery for benign ovarian growths lose twice as much blood and must spend twice as long in the hospital. (Conversely, more than one-third of women having a hysterectomy have their normal ovaries and fallopian tubes removed too.)

Alternative treatments exist for all of these noncancerous conditions. Fibroid tumors, the leading reason for hysterectomy (accounting for about 30 percent), are rarely dangerous and often asymptomatic. If they cause pain or bleeding, they can be treated with hormones or myomectomy (surgery to remove the fibroids rather than the uterus). One reason many surgeons do not offer this procedure is simply that they have not been trained to do it. Because the uterus has so many blood vessels, myomectomy can be a trickier and bloodier operation than hysterectomy, and requires a skilled surgeon. But this surgery is becoming more and more common as women balk at having their wombs removed.

Some bleeding problems can be treated with hormonal therapy or with endometrial ablation, a new procedure in which the uterine lining is electrically coagulated. Uterine prolapse, a condition in which weakened muscles fail to hold the uterus in place, can often be successfully treated with a pessary (a ring inserted into the vagina to help support the uterus and keep it in its proper position), or with exercises to strengthen the abdominal and vaginal muscles.

Less than 15 percent of hysterectomies in the United States are done to treat uterine (endometrial or cervical) cancer, the most absolute and compelling reason for the surgery (although even these cancers can sometimes be treated with radiation or less drastic surgery). The uterus is also usually removed during surgery for cancer of the ovaries or fallopian tubes. And emergency hysterectomies may be performed to save a woman's life if her uterus ruptures during childbirth, an abortion, or after a trauma such as a stabbing or shooting.

Some women's health experts now believe that, with the exception of emergency surgery, cancer is the *only* justification for a hysterectomy. Others believe conditions that aren't life-threatening but affect quality-of-life can make hysterectomy a reasonable option. For instance, when heavy bleeding does not respond to other treatments it may cause severe anemia. Also, very large benign tumors may not be easily treated with medication or womb-sparing surgery, and can cause extreme pain and uncontrollable bleeding. Serious infections of the uterus and fallopian tubes may also be just cause for a hysterectomy.

But the vast majority of hysterectomies do *not* fit the above criteria, and the women who are agreeing to the surgery are undoubtedly basing their decisions on information their physicians feed them. Patients with painful cramps or heavy bleeding may accept a doctor's opinion that surgery is a better option than alternative treatments, such as hormones or other drugs. These patients sign a so-called informed-consent form after a physician explains the situation, often in an extremely biased and misleading way. As Dr. John Smith writes, "A physician can say to a patient, 'I can take out your uterus and you will never have another period, never have to worry about birth control or cancer of the cervix or uterus, and all it means is perhaps five days in the hospital . . .'"

Women might feel differently about the operation, believes Smith, if a physician said instead, "You should know that if you have a hysterectomy

done you could die from a pulmonary embolus, you could hemorrhage after surgery and have to have a second operation to save your life, you could
get a permanent passage of feces through your vagina, you could have a
ureter inadvertently tied or cut and wind up losing a kidney, you could develop an infection that would require the subsequent removal of your ovaries, and you could conceivably end up with your vagina shortened so
much that you may never experience comfortable intercourse again."

Presented with such comprehensive and honest information, no doubt
many women would choose to avoid hysterectomy, and there is some evidence that more informed women are less likely to agree to the operation.
Rates of hysterectomy do vary by race, education, and income level: poor
women, women without a college education, and African-American
women are all more likely to have the surgery. (Hysterectomy is rarely performed for sterilization anymore, since tubal ligation is a simpler and safer
operation. But it wasn't too long ago that poor black women, who never
signed a proper informed-consent form, had what came to be called Mississippi appendectomies—sterilization by hysterectomy, usually done while
they were in the hospital giving birth.)

There is also some evidence that female gynecologists perform fewer
hysterectomies than males. Swiss researchers looking at statistics for 1983
found that female gynecologists performed half as many hysterectomies as
male gynecologists. As the researchers explained, "Women seem to perceive
this procedure as signaling a 'loss of womanhood and of attractiveness.' Female gynecologists may perhaps identify more easily with this position and
thus be more restrictive in their indications."

Whether the physician is male or female, hysterectomies are performed
much less frequently in Europe than in the United States. An American
woman has two to three times the chance of having a hysterectomy as her
counterpart in England, France, or West Germany. Author Lynn Payer, in
her book *Medicine and Culture*, talks about her personal experience with
European attitudes toward the operation. While working as a medical journalist in France, she had a myomectomy to remove a fibroid tumor. Later,
after she had moved back to the United States, the tumor recurred. She
writes, "In France, where great value is put on the woman's ability to bear
children, hysterectomy was not even suggested as an option. Instead, the
French surgeon told me I *must* have a myomectomy, a major operation in
which the fibroid tumor is removed while the ability to have children is
preserved." The French doctors told Payer that up to six myomectomies
could be performed while still sparing her childbearing ability. When Payer
consulted American physicians about her condition, however, she was told

that a second myomectomy would be impossible, and was pressured to have a hysterectomy.

Not only do French surgeons try to avoid performing hysterectomies, but when they feel the surgery is unavoidable—generally for cancer or abnormal uterine bleeding that cannot be controlled any other way—they do a less radical operation than American physicians. French surgeons prefer doing "subtotal" hysterectomies, which remove the fundus (the large upper end) of the uterus, but leave the cervix intact. According to Payer, this is because French physicians believe the cervix plays a role in maintaining a woman's sexual responsiveness and the stability of the pelvic floor. Painful intercourse and lack of sexual desire are common complaints after total hysterectomy.

Why aren't subtotal hysterectomies offered here? According to Dr. Gambone, it's more a matter of convention than science. "In the thirties, prior to the acceptance of the Pap smear, a woman could develop cervical cancer if you left the cervix," he explains. "And there wasn't any good way to screen for that. So a rule was set up that a total hysterectomy was a better operation than a subtotal. But no one ever studied it."

Even though the Pap smear is now in widespread use, detecting cervical cell changes before cancer develops, surgeons have not changed their practices. As if the sexual health of millions of American women was too trivial a matter for research, there are still no studies being done to convince doctors that perhaps a change to subtotal hysterectomies is in order.

Rather than trying to avoid performing hysterectomies, or even performing less radical surgery, American surgeons seem determined to convince women that new technology is the answer to their problems. A publicity packet for a new surgical technique called laparoscopically assisted vaginal hysterectomy (LAVH) begins with the quote "I know I can't avoid the hysterectomy. I just want to avoid the long recovery and pain." Surgeons using LAVH do not remove the uterus through an abdominal incision. Instead they insert a tiny telescope—the laparoscope—into the abdomen. Then, using tiny surgical tools guided by an image transmitted to a television monitor, they remove the organ through the vagina. A woman is left with smaller scars, less pain, and less recovery time—but still no uterus.

For the most part, surgeons see no need to alter their philosophy; often they feel they are doing women a favor by removing an organ that causes nothing but trouble. After childbearing and menopause, all the uterus can do, they feel, is develop cancer. These doctors seem to ignore some of the possible health consequences of living without a uterus, consequences that far outweigh the risks of most benign fibroid tumors. For instance, when the ovaries are removed along with the uterus, a premenopausal woman is forced into a premature menopause, complete with hot flashes, insomnia, and an immediately increased risk of heart disease and osteoporosis. And there is even some evidence that removing the uterus, even while leaving the ovaries in place, increases the risk of later heart disease and osteoporosis, because the ovaries often stop functioning after hysterectomy.

Also, much about the uterus, including basic knowledge about menstruation, is still poorly understood. Without a full understanding of what hormones or other substances the uterus produces and exactly what roles it plays in the body, it is arrogant and foolish for physicians to decide that it is a useless organ after menopause. After all, it wasn't too long ago that children's tonsils were routinely removed to prevent sore throats—until it was discovered that the tonsils play a role in the immune system. Who can possibly say that women's bodies are better off without the uterus, a lifegiving organ?

■ MASTECTOMY VERSUS LUMPECTOMY: WHOLE VERSUS PART

Women's breasts are another common casualty of the surgeon's knife. There's no denying that breast cancer rates are alarmingly high in this country: the latest figure from the American Cancer Society is that one in eight women will develop the disease during her lifetime. But performing a mastectomy—an operation to remove all of the breast tissue—is only one option among an arsenal of treatments. Less drastic surgery, called a lumpectomy, to remove just the cancerous tumor and a margin of tissue around it, is a vastly underused option.

In 1985 a landmark study was published showing that lumpectomy followed by radiation is as effective as total mastectomy for treating early cancer. Numerous other studies with the same conclusion followed and added proof that the more conservative surgery was also appropriate for treating most women with large breast tumors as well (after the tumors have first been shrunk by chemotherapy). Psychiatric research showed that there were psychological (and sexual) benefits to sparing women's breasts.

But rather than accept the findings as good news for women, many physicians refused to believe the evidence or to change their surgical practices. In spite of the growing body of evidence demonstrating lumpectomy's advantages over mastectomy, between 1985 and 1989 the percentage of women who received lumpectomies actually went *down*. Although there was no medical justification for amputating the breast, surgeons persuaded women that mastectomy was a safer option. "Very often what a surgeon does is say: 'You have two options. If I were you or if you were my wife, I'd choose a mastectomy,' " says Susan Love, M.D., director of the Breast Center at the University of California, Los Angeles. Many women believed that their only options were either to save their breasts or to save their lives.

Physicians were initially so resistant to breast-conserving surgery that one proposed study comparing lumpectomy and mastectomy nearly had to be scuttled because doctors balked at participating. Two years after the trial was announced, only a fraction of the patients needed for the study had been enrolled. The project was in jeopardy. Medical researchers attempted to determine why physicians were refusing to include their women patients in the trial. In a 1984 article published in the *New England Journal of Medicine*, researchers found that 73 percent of the physicians who refused to participate said that they were concerned that the doctor-patient relationship would be affected (although earlier trials comparing radical mastectomy and total mastectomy did not elicit these fears). Thirty-eight percent cited "difficulty with informed consent," as if women could not be made to understand the potential risks and benefits of participating in this research.

Even today surgeons in this country still seem hesitant to perform the less radical surgery. Based on the medical evidence, up to 90 percent of women with breast cancer may be eligible for lumpectomies. But the reality is far different, and what type of surgery a woman receives depends on such nonmedical factors as where she lives, and her age, income, and race. In one study, 41 percent of Seattle women were treated with breast-conserving surgery, versus fewer than 20 percent of women in Iowa. Older women were more likely to have their breasts removed than younger women.

For Medicare patients the numbers are even bleaker. Nationwide an average of only 12 percent of women on Medicare have lumpectomy, with a low of 4 percent in Kentucky and a high of 21 percent in Massachusetts. Black women are 20 percent less likely to have lumpectomy than whites. The rate of surgery also varies with the size of the metropolitan area: the larger the town or city, the higher the rate of lumpectomies.

The breast surgery rates, like those for hysterectomy, vary even more internationally. According to Payer, one study found three times as many mastectomies in New England as in England or Sweden, even though the rate of breast cancer was similar in all three places.

As a lifesaving therapy, removing the breast does not always make sense. Women do not die because there is a malignancy in their breast tissue; they die because cancer has spread to the bone marrow or to a vital organ such as the lungs. The spread can sometimes occur before a breast tumor is even palpable. Removing a cancerous tumor and then irradiating the area around it to kill any stray cancer cells is usually just as likely to stop the disease's progress as removing the entire breast. As of this writing, many physicians are still resisting the switch to lumpectomy surgery, and the procedure is still underused.

In 1994 the public was shocked to discover that some of the data from the landmark 1985 study that helped establish lumpectomy as a safe alternative to mastectomy had been falsified. The flawed information came from only one of the eighty-eight institutions (L'Hôpital Saint-Luc in Montreal) that had participated in the National Surgical Adjuvant Breast and Bowel Project (NSABP), and involved 328 of the 1,855 women who took part. Scientists rushed to assure the public that the study's conclusion was still valid and had been confirmed by more recent investigation: both a re-analysis of the research minus the questionable data, plus a newer California study of nearly six thousand women that was rushed to publication in order to reassure women and their doctors. In spite of the confirmation, many physicians and their patients may find renewed grounds for doubting lumpectomy's safety.

Of course there are legitimate medical reasons for a woman to opt for a mastectomy. And there are legitimate psychological reasons, too. Renee, a woman in her mid-thirties, says that if she is ever diagnosed with breast cancer, "I'd rather have the breast removed than even consider a lumpectomy." In fact, Renee says, she'd be tempted to have *both* breasts removed, and then perhaps reconstructed. While her statement may seem shocking, Renee has family precedent on her side. Both her mother and her grandmother were diagnosed with breast cancer at a young age, had mastectomies, and then lived for many decades afterward. Although Renee is familiar with the studies showing that lumpectomy and mastectomy have similar cure rates, "I just wouldn't want to have a lumpectomy, have the cancer recur, and then think I'd jeopardized my life for a breast."

Some women with family histories like Renee's are opting for an even more drastic solution. Although the hereditary risk of breast cancer is not well understood, some women who have several close relatives with the disease are choosing not to delay surgery until their own diagnosis. Rather than waiting for the disease to strike, these women are choosing prophylactic mastectomies—removal of healthy breasts to prevent cancer from developing. These operations are still uncommon, and surgeons, to their credit, seem hesitant to recommend them in all but the most compelling cases, such as when a woman has watched several close relatives die of breast cancer at young ages. The value of this surgery is being hotly debated, with some physicians charging that women are being needlessly mutilated and others defending the operations as justified in certain high-risk cases. "It's not an operation you want to offer without a lot of soul-searching and careful explanation of options," says Henry Lynch, M.D., president of the Hereditary Cancer Institute at Creighton University.

Another factor upping the number of mastectomy operations is the availability of reconstructive surgery. When women are told they can have their breasts reconstructed at the same time as their surgery, they may accept mastectomy more easily. These women leave the operating table with two breasts, although not the same two they came in with. To keep the numbers of mastectomies down, however, the decision to have breasts removed should not depend on the availability of cosmetic surgery; the two surgeries should be considered and performed separately. Now that the risks of breast implants are coming to light (see the implant section at the end of this chapter), lumpectomy may become a more popular alternative for those who previously would have opted for reconstructive surgery.

■ THE SURGICALIZATION OF CHILDBIRTH

It was November 1991, and Diana St. James was in labor. "Oh my god, oh my god," she moaned, as waves of pain rolled through her body.

"You don't need to feel the pain. We can give you something for the pain," a nurse kept repeating.

Before she knew it, St. James, then twenty-seven, was getting epidural anesthesia, which not only numbed the pain but made it difficult for her to use her abdominal muscles when it came time to push. After four strenuous hours her doctor said she'd been pushing too long. She needed an emergency cesarean section. She gave birth through a surgical incision in her abdomen.

Several years later St. James, a community theater director in Pasadena, California, is convinced that her son, Joshua, did not require a surgical birth. For one thing, she says, her hospital had a C-section rate of 40 percent, well above the national average. What's more, it was her first delivery, and those normally tend to take longer.

Although obstetrics-gynecology is often thought of as a primary care specialty—and there is a strong movement among these physicians to be thought of this way—the field is really a surgical subspecialty of medicine, and the doctors who opt to become gynecologists are trained in surgery of the reproductive organs. And, as the saying goes, "When you only have a hammer, everything looks like a nail." In obstetrics and gynecology this means that doctors trained in this subspecialty will not hesitate to look for surgical solutions to reproductive problems. Not surprisingly, this attitude has carried over to dealing with *non*problems as well.

When attending to a normal childbirth, a surgeon might as well be a cabdriver. No matter what he or she does, the baby will emerge, healthy and crying, on its own. Fewer than 10 percent of deliveries require some kind of surgical intervention to ensure the health of the child, yet doing *something* has become routine. One in four babies is now born by cesarean section. Those mothers fortunate enough to be left alone to deliver vaginally will not escape suturing. Three-quarters will have an episiotomy, although study after study has shown this procedure to be useless.

The rate of cesarean sections began to rise in the 1970s, about the same time that women began to spurn anesthesia and other then-routine childbirth practices (enemas, shaving the pubic hair) in favor of natural childbirth. The cesarean section rate quadrupled in twenty years, up from just 5.5 percent in 1970. Not content to let nature take its course, obstetricians seem to believe that some form of intervention, often in the form of cesarean section or episiotomy, justifies their presence.

The coinciding rise of doctor-preferred cesarean sections and mother-preferred natural childbirth is especially ironic. One in four women, after spending hours taking childbirth preparation classes and discussing their preferences with their physicians, will be told while in labor—not the easiest time to make decisions—that a cesarean is recommended for the health of the child. Only a small percentage of cesareans are performed for the health of the mother; in fact they pose a significantly higher risk of death than a vaginal birth.

"When I started out in obstetrics, the average C-section delivery rate was 7 or 8 percent," says Dr. Gambone. "Now the average has gotten as high as 25 percent. It would be one thing if you saw a decrease in perinatal mortality, some benefit, but that's not the case. Just more cesarean deliveries."

There are four main medical reasons for an obstetrician to perform a cesarean section: because a woman has had a previous cesarean birth (35 percent of cesareans), because the baby is presenting in the breech position (11.7 percent), because of dystocia (a medical grab-bag term for a variety of complications, mainly the vague "failure of labor to progress"—this is responsible for 30.4 percent of cesareans), and fetal distress (9.2 percent). The remaining cesareans, nearly 14 percent, are due to miscellaneous other complications—for instance, a mother's outbreak of genital herpes at the time of birth.

But none of these reasons are as clear-cut as they seem. Studies have shown that three-quarters of women who have had a previous cesarean can safely deliver a child vaginally. And a breech presentation can often be recognized before delivery, so that an obstetrician or midwife can turn the baby, guided by ultrasound. A diagnosis of labor not progressing can simply mean that the doctor is tired of waiting and anxious to get the delivery over with. And fetal distress has been much overdiagnosed since the widespread use of electronic fetal monitors (EFM), whose readings are often misinterpreted.

It's been known for more than fifteen years that EFM leads to an increase in cesarean sections with no increase in fetal survival, but efforts to lessen physicians' reliance on the technology have not been successful. A 1989 bulletin to ob-gyns from the American College of Obstetricians and Gynecologists, for example, advised that listening intermittently to the fetal heartbeat with a stethoscope is as effective at diagnosing true fetal distress as continuous electronic fetal monitoring. But still the inappropriate and routine use of EFM continues, with countless women being operated on as a result. And even herpes outbreaks may not require cesarean sections; one study found that more mothers would die from the cesarean sections than babies would be saved by the surgery.

Other proposed reasons for the astronomically high C-section rate are the decreased use of obstetrical forceps, the trend toward bigger babies, the fact that cesareans are safer than ever before, and requests for the surgery by mothers-to-be who want to be able to schedule their deliveries in advance or shorten painful labor.

But overriding all of these reasons is another, more disturbing one: Doctors do cesarean sections because they fear being sued for malpractice if something goes wrong at the delivery, or if the baby has problems unrelated to the birth and the parents blame the doctor. To defend themselves, physicians feel they must show they did everything medically possible to get the baby out quickly, and that means a cesarean.

A 1993 study published in the *Journal of the American Medical Association* found that cesarean section rates do seem to be influenced by fear of lawsuit. The researchers found that physicians who paid the highest malpractice insurance premiums and perceived the greatest risk of lawsuit also had the highest cesarean section rates. Another 1993 study found that money plays a role in the surgery rate, too. Low-income, uninsured women received fewer cesarean sections than women with private insurance (17 percent versus 23 percent).

Interestingly, the gender of the doctor does not seem to influence cesarean rates; male and female obstetricians have similar surgery rates. But older, more experienced doctors of either sex have lower rates than younger obstetricians. These veteran physicians perform fewer operations for dystocia and breech presentation and are more comfortable using forceps in difficult births. A woman who had her first child in the 1950s recalls being in labor for over twenty-four hours, fed by intravenous line. Her baby was finally helped into the world with forceps. "If that were happening now, I'd probably have a cesarean," she says. "And then my next two children would have been cesarean deliveries too."

Cesarean sections are also more common among older mothers, regardless of pregnancy complications. Women over thirty-five have twice the chance of delivering by cesarean as teenage mothers. "Many times, a hospital staff looks at a thirty-seven-year-old first-time mother coming in the door and says, 'Get the cesarean room ready.' Their mind-set is, 'She's not going to do it because she's too old,' " says Patricia Burkhardt, a certified nurse-midwife and doctor of public health who manages the Nurse-Midwifery Service at Columbia-Presbyterian Medical Center in New York.

There is a feeling among obstetricians that, having waited longer for parenthood and perhaps battled fertility problems, these women are more anxious about delivery. Doctors feel that these women want a perfect baby because they may have only one. Physicians coined the phrase *premium baby* to describe these later-in-life children. But aren't all wanted children premium babies? And shouldn't all pregnant women be premium mothers, not subjected to unnecessary surgery?

"Women are interesting people," says John Goldkrand, M.D., director of resident education in ob-gyn, and associate director of perinatology, at Memorial Medical Center, Savannah. "I wouldn't lie down to get operated on any more than I had to. I don't know about you, but I don't think it's any fun. But women are willing to pop right in, lie down, and get operated on under the stimulus of protecting their babies versus *themselves*."

Perceiving the mother's interests as separate from the child's is a recent obstetrical innovation. The risk of death and complications from a cesarean, which is major abdominal surgery, is very real for the mother. Complications such as urinary tract and wound infections are common, and women must spend longer in the hospital, and a longer time recovering from the surgery, than they would if they delivered vaginally. The expense is greater as well.

Women willingly subject themselves to this surgery to give their child the best start, yet the presumed benefits to the baby are unconvincing. The United States has not only one of the world's highest cesarean section rates but also one of the highest perinatal and infant mortality rates in the developed world. These mortality rates have been attributed to drug and alcohol abuse, HIV infection, poverty, and lack of prenatal care. But women affected by these problems are not, for the most part, the women who are having cesareans. The women who make up the bulk of cesareans are older, better educated, wealthier, and usually receiving good prenatal care— precisely the women who should have less complicated pregnancies and easier deliveries.

In Japan, where the cesarean section rate is just 7 percent, infant mortality is among the lowest in the world. European cesarean rates are lower, too, with lower infant mortality. In England, for example, the cesarean rate is about 13 percent, and British medical journals are already showing concern that the number is too high. The United States ranks twenty-fourth in infant mortality yet has the third highest cesarean section rate in the world after Brazil (32 percent) and Puerto Rico (29 percent). In Brazil women often choose cesareans because they erroneously believe that a vaginal delivery makes normal sexual relations impossible after childbirth.

There are some signs that the American C-section rate is dropping, although the change is small: down from a high of 24.7 percent in 1988 to 23.5 percent in 1991. The less-than-2-percentage-point reduction translates to a savings of $322 million in health care costs, money that could be far better spent on prenatal and child care than on unnecessary surgery.

Much of the tiny drop is attributable to a rise in VBACs—vaginal births after cesarean. In 1982 the American College of Obstetricians and Gynecologists issued guidelines to its members urging them to attempt VBACs. Again in 1988 they released guidelines stating that repeat cesareans should no longer be routine (as per the old saying, "Once a cesarean, always a cesarean"). A study at California hospitals found that 75 percent of women who have had a previous cesarean are able to deliver vaginally. Yet in spite of these official pronouncements and medical evidence, currently only about 24 percent of women who have had a cesarean go on to deliver vaginally. Repeat cesareans are still the leading reason for the surgery. That wouldn't surprise one Manhattan woman, who had to visit several different obstetricians before she found one who would agree to let her try to deliver her second child vaginally.

The overriding fear about letting women who have had cesareans attempt labor and vaginal delivery is that the old uterine scar would rupture, endangering mother and child. But this fear is largely unfounded. "The risk of having a [uterine] rupture after a previous cesarean is the same whether you have a cesarean or a vaginal delivery," says Dr. Gambone. "It's less than one percent."

While the rate of repeat cesareans is slowly dropping, the rate of primary cesareans has not dropped in nearly a decade. It's unlikely that the country will meet the Centers for Disease Control and Prevention's goal of reaching an overall C-section rate of 15 percent (12 percent or fewer for primary cesareans) by the turn of the century. (Other experts feel that even 15 percent is too high, and a more appropriate goal would be a rate of 10 percent or less for normal pregnancies, and 17 percent for women considered high risk.)

Sidney M. Wolfe, M.D., of the Public Citizen's Health Research Group, says the goal of 15 percent is achievable *now* if only physicians followed commonsense guidelines. Some hospitals, for instance, have instituted quality-control programs that have helped drop their cesarean rates dramatically. At Mt. Sinai Hospital Medical Center in Chicago, for example, the cesarean rate dropped from 17.5 percent in 1985 to 11.5 percent in 1987 to 10.2 percent in 1989 after the hospital began requiring second opinions before surgery and instituting objective criteria for the four most common reasons for the procedure.

Other solutions are more woman-centered, including using midwives for uncomplicated pregnancies, and providing women in labor with "doulas," trained labor companions who have experienced a normal labor and vaginal delivery themselves. A Texas study found that the mothers with doulas had a dramatically lower cesarean section rate: 8 percent versus 18 percent for the controls.

But too few hospitals and too few individual obstetricians are seriously attempting to lower the surgery rate. "The incentives are all in the direction of doing more, not fewer," says Wolfe. "[If you were a doctor,] would you rather stay up all night and wait through labor or would you rather schedule it a couple of months in advance? Would you like to make more or less money? Nothing is going to change unless the incentives are changed and people start being disciplined and people start getting sued. We would strongly encourage women who have been injured during unnecessary C-sections to sue their doctors."

When the surgery is done, the baby is healthy, and the mother is healed, few women are interested in suing, even if they believe that the operation was unnecessary. But health care reforms may succeed where women have failed. A few insurance companies now reimburse physicians the same amount of money for either a vaginal or a cesarean delivery. Faced with earning the same amount of money for less work (although perhaps more waiting), more physicians may decide that many cesareans are not really necessary after all.

A 25 percent cesarean rate still means that three-quarters of births in this country are vaginal deliveries. But even uncomplicated vaginal births now involve surgery. Today obstetricians routinely perform an episiotomy—an incision from the vagina to the rectum—on the theory that it will speed up the delivery and in the long run be more kind to a woman's body, leaving a clean, sutured cut rather than a messy, jagged tear. So even these new mothers must deal with uncomfortable stitches that turn walking into a painful experience and make it necessary to use a squeeze bottle of water rather than toilet paper after urinating.

The problem with performing routine episiotomies is that the practice is based on a false assumption made early in the century. And study after modern study has found the surgical procedure to be not only unnecessary but perhaps even harmful. The nearly universal use of episiotomy in childbirth can be traced to Dr. Joseph DeLee, an obstetrician who in 1920 recommended the use of forceps, episiotomy, and the early removal of the placenta even in uncomplicated deliveries.

Today, in spite of studies showing that Dr. DeLee was wrong, obstetricians seem loath to abandon the practice. "I've been doing research into episiotomies for years," says Nancy Fleming, Ph.D., CNM (certified nurse-midwife), who practices in Hensdale, a Chicago, suburb. "In spite of every study showing that they don't help with the outcome, and that even women who tear have less discomfort and faster healing time than women who have episiotomies, practitioners continue to do them routinely. They really shouldn't do them unless it looks as if a tear is imminent, or if it's necessary to have the baby come out quicker." The problem, says Fleming, is that "obstetricians tend to practice by the three C's—convention, convenience, conjecture."

One of the most recent studies was a 1992 Canadian study of over one thousand mothers, divided into two groups. One group received routine episiotomy, the other group only had the incision if there was a clear medical need. The authors found that the routine use of episiotomy was so ingrained in doctors that it was difficult to get them to withhold the surgery in the restricted group, much like the doctors who wouldn't participate in the trial of lumpectomy versus mastectomy. Many of the doctors were unwilling or unable to reduce their episiotomy rate.

When the study was finished, the results showed no advantages of routine episiotomy. Not only were there no medical benefits, but the surgery, by making the recovery from childbirth even more difficult, caused more harm than good.

While obstetricians persist in performing this procedure, women's best hope of avoiding surgery in an uncomplicated birth lies with nurse-midwives. Studies conducted for the American Nurses Association at the University of Texas–Houston Health Science Center School of Nursing show fewer cesareans and episiotomies with midwives, with less physical trauma for the mothers, and babies as healthy as those delivered by physicians.

The lower cesarean section rate can be at least partially explained by the fact that midwives handle more uncomplicated births, and refer high-risk or complicated cases to obstetricians. But the lower episiotomy rate represents a real difference in philosophy.

One woman, who had her first child in a hospital attended by an obstetrician, and her second two at home attended by a midwife, says, "Midwives show women how to massage the perineum, to stretch and soften the skin and minimize the risk of tearing. And they're willing to spend time easing the baby out."

Today the surgicalization of childbirth extends beyond cesareans and episiotomies in delivery to *terminating* pregnancy too. Even though European women have access to RU-486, a safe, hormonal way to end a pregnancy, American women who wish to terminate a pregnancy must have a vacuum aspiration or dilation and curettage procedure. Keeping abortion legal yet denying women access to the latest, safest nonsurgical procedure is just one more way to subject women's bodies to unnecessary surgery.

■ BREAST IMPLANTS:
   WHAT PRICE VANITY?

Gloria Westly (not her real name) was twenty-nine years old when she had her breasts augmented with silicone implants in 1990. An actress and singer, she had always been thin, athletic, and flat-chested, but she went from "not even fitting into an A-cup" to a 36C after her surgery. "I felt great, and I could wear costumes without a padded bra underneath," she says. A year and a half after her surgery Gloria woke up one morning with a severe pain in her back. She hasn't been well since.

"I used to work out every day, but for months I couldn't even get out of bed without assistance," she says. Doctors checked for kidney infections, muscle pulls, muscle tears, appendicitis, and ulcers, but the test results were all negative. Finally, after she lost consciousness one day at home and was taken to the emergency room, doctors diagnosed pelvic inflammatory disease. "My entire pelvic area was infected, but no one could ever figure out why," she says. "PID is usually caused by a sexually transmitted disease, or sometimes by an IUD (intrauterine device) infection, but I'd been sexually celibate for over a year and had never had an IUD. They never identified the bacteria that were responsible, and when I had an emergency laparoscopy, they never found any of the scarring on my fallopian tubes or uterus that I should have had with PID." After massive doses of antibiotics she began to feel better and soon tried to resume her career.

Several months later Gloria began to feel dizzy and light-headed all the time. One day she passed out on the street on the way to a doctor's appointment and was taken to the emergency room. Blood tests showed she had mononucleosis. But because she'd had mono twice before (most people are immune after one infection), and because she did not get better as quickly as she should have, Gloria's diagnosis was recurrent, chronic Epstein-Barr infection.

At the hospital a sympathetic woman internist listened to Gloria's story and was the first to make the connection between her two years of physical agony and her breast implants. "She told me, 'I think your implants are somehow related to your immune system being totally out of whack. I think they have to go.'"

The surgeon who had originally done the implant surgery agreed to remove the implants free of charge, and Gloria has finally started to recover. "I'm still not 100 percent, but I'm feeling better every month," she says. "I don't miss the implants at all. When they came out, it was as if my body was sighing a big, huge sigh of relief."

Information is still emerging about the risks from silicone-gel breast implants, which threaten the health of an estimated one to two million women who received them before the FDA limited their use in 1992. Surgeons may not have much compunction about removing female breasts, as evidenced by the continuing preference for mastectomy over lumpectomy, but they seemed more than willing to replace missing breasts, or augment perfectly normal ones, with implants. One surgeon likened performing the expensive surgery to squeezing a marshmallow into a piggy bank; slits are cut under a woman's breasts and then squishy bags are stuffed into the pockets.

The Food and Drug Administration didn't have the authority to regulate medical devices, including breast implants, until 1976. A "grandfather" clause allowed products already on the market to skip the approval process unless there was reason to believe they were hazardous. Breast implants had been around since 1964.

Some FDA scientists tried to get breast implants put in a category that would require proof of their safety as early as 1978, but the agency didn't request that manufacturers register any reports of serious health problems until 1984, didn't begin classifying the implants as potentially dangerous until 1988, and didn't require manufacturer's safety data until 1991. In the meantime surgeons were free to insert these toxic pillows into hundreds of thousands of women's bodies.

The surgeons felt they were correcting a deformity. "One of the petitions from the American Society of Plastic and Reconstructive Surgeons said that small breasts were a disease that required medical intervention," says Jane Sprague Zones, Ph.D., chairman of the board of the National Women's Health Network, who was on the FDA panel that was regulating breast implants in the early 1980s. But Zones says that far from being abnormal, most of the breasts that were augmented "were normal, healthy, attractive breasts. When you look at before-and-after pictures of women with breast implants, it's often difficult to see any significant differences."

The silicone gel that filled the majority of implants was first used as a sealant, then sold as Silly Putty. The polyurethane foam used to cover one type of implant was industrial grade, used in furniture, upholstery, oil filters, and carburetors. At first the company manufacturing the foam had no idea it was being used for medical applications. "My eyes popped out when Powell [Tom Powell, a vice president at Cooper Surgical, manufacturer of a foam-covered implant] explained his company was buying the foam from a jobber in Los Angeles and using it as a covering for a breast implant," said Ed Griffiths, product manager at Scotfoam Corporation. "I wanted him to know that we had no expertise in determining the suitability of the foam in medical applications. . . ." Manufacturers were free to make the devices any way they liked; one small company applied foam to implants with a type of bathtub caulk and a waffle-iron device.

The most common complication of silicone gel-filled implants is capsular contracture—a buildup of scar tissue and contraction of the muscles around the implant, which can make the breasts feel hard and look misshapen. Dow Corning, the leading manufacturer of breast implants, estimated that no more than 15 percent of women suffer from this reaction. Today it's thought the percentage is much higher. "In the package insert it says that a capsular contracture is a complication. Now the doctors are trying to say it's not a complication because it happens so often. But yes, it is a complication, and I believe it happens in 95 percent of the cases," says Sybil Goldrich, cofounder and codirector of the Command Trust Network, an information clearinghouse for women with implants.

To remedy capsular contraction, surgeons grab women's breasts and squeeze them in an attempt to break down the hardened tissue. Sometimes the torture treatment works, and sometimes it simply ruptures the implant, releasing silicone into the chest, allowing it to migrate to other parts of the body.

In the 1980s, studies were published showing that the implants obscure mammography, making it difficult to detect early breast cancer. There was some evidence that silicone itself was a breast cancer risk. Then it was found that the foam coverings on some implants released a chemical called 2-toluene diamine, a known animal carcinogen.

For women who had reconstruction after mastectomy, the news that silicone might be a cancer risk was particularly cruel. The very implants that were supposed to restore their bodies and their self-images after cancer surgery were threatening their health. "It's like somebody playing a dirty trick," said one woman who had received implants after double mastectomies. "They were supposed to be emotionally and physically a help, but they're another set of time bombs, another poison in your body." When women with implants are diagnosed with breast cancer, they are more difficult to treat. Radiation can cause scar tissue to contract and can leave the breasts looking deformed.

As women began to report further physical reactions to the implants, an even more ominous picture emerged. Allergic reactions to the foam, including itchy rashes, caused some women to scratch themselves until they bled. Silicone seeped through nipples or migrated throughout the body. "When I had a hysterectomy, it showed that I had silicone in my uterus, my ovaries, and my liver," says Goldrich. "When they tell you that silicone is inert, you know they're lying."

Some women reported breast and joint pain, excessive fatigue, mental confusion, and short-term memory loss. Finally, severe autoimmune reactions began to be acknowledged as women's bodies produced antibodies to the silicone and to collagen, attacking its own tissues in the process.

Women suffered from illnesses such as rheumatoid arthritis, systemic lupus, scleroderma, and Sjögren's syndrome. Now doctors suspect that all these immune reactions are symptoms of a disease unique to breast implants.

Reading of these risks, thousands of women with implants—those already suffering from symptoms and those who decided they didn't want to wait around for them to appear—decided to have the devices removed. But the "explantation" operation is expensive and tricky. The removal surgery carries the risks of bleeding, infection, and permanent scarring. When a surgeon opens up a woman's chest to remove the implant, he may have trouble finding the silicone envelope, which may have ruptured or fallen apart. Gel can be stuck in irregular lumps throughout the chest. One woman described the mess inside her chest as looking "like an oil spill." The operation can take hours, with the surgeon painstakingly scraping silicone from the chest wall. "Once breast implants have been put in you, they can never be totally removed," says Goldrich. And after having implants removed, a woman's breasts will not necessarily look the way they did before the surgery; they may be disfigured, misshapen, or droopy.

As the information about implant risks emerged, rather than express appropriate horror at the dangers they were exposing women to, surgeons vigorously defended breast augmentation. And the manufacturers, reluctant to lose such a lucrative product, dug in their heels. Dow Corning took out newspaper ads late in 1991 with the copy "If you want accurate information about breast implants . . . instead of innuendo and half truths . . . call the Dow Corning Implant Information Center, where the information is based on thirty years of valid scientific research." Although some of that research had been rejected by the FDA, Dow encouraged women to call and find out "the truth." One of these ads appeared in the *New York Times* on the same day as the report of a woman who had won $7.34 million against the company because her silicone breast implant had ruptured, causing a painful immune disorder called mixed-connective-tissue disease. The six-member jury found that the implant was designed and made defectively and that Dow Corning had failed to warn the woman of the risks of the device, breached its warranty, and committed fraud. That same month the FDA began investigating assertions that Dow had improperly withheld documents raising safety concerns about the implants. (In April 1994, lawyers representing women in a class action suit against the manufacturers of breast implants said they had discovered a 1975 Dow Corning study showing that the silicone in the implants harmed the immune system of mice.)

Then Dow's phone line came under attack. The FDA charged that operators on the consumer information telephone line had been making false statements, such as "Scientific data and research show that breast implants are 100 percent safe." Women were also told that silicone leaked less than half a teaspoon over decades and that the substance "doesn't go anywhere."

In early 1992 the FDA said it could not assure women of the safety of these devices and asked surgeons to stop using them. While professional surgeons' organizations pledged to abide by the ban, they still asserted that the devices were safe and that women were being unnecessarily alarmed. Dow continued to insist the products were safe, too, but by March the company announced it was out of the implant business. In April the FDA formally banned silicone-gel implants, with limited exceptions. The only women who can now receive silicone-gel implants are those having reconstruction after mastectomy or serious injury and others who meet specific criteria (for instance, women suffering from congenital breast deformities). These women will be part of a clinical trial to answer basic questions about the implants—questions that should have been answered before they were implanted in anyone's body. Said FDA commissioner David Kessler, "We know more about the lifespan of automobile tires than we do about breast implants." Saline-filled implants have still not been regulated by the agency.

Now hundreds of lawyers are handling thousands of lawsuits brought by women whose health has been damaged by silicone, but some medical authorities are *still* defending the implants. In late 1993 the *Journal of the American Medical Association* carried a report from the AMA's Council on Scientific Affairs, urging that the AMA "support the position that women *have the right to choose* [italics added] silicone gel-filled or saline-filled breast implants for both augmentation and reconstruction."

The article appeared one month before researchers reported a possible link between silicone breast implants and damage to the esophagus in breast-feeding infants. The author of the *JAMA* article, Donald R. Bennett, M.D., Ph.D., was a former employee of Dow Corning Corporation, who was still receiving a pension from the company. Referring to the journal's emphasis on women's choice, Jane Zones says, "They're trying to co-opt the language of feminism to defend products that are actually harmful to women."

■ THE SELLING OF COSMETIC SURGERY

The American obsession with large breasts, translated into millions of risky operations for American women, is not a harmless sexual fixation but a real health risk. Cultural standards of beauty and femininity are often arbitrary, but they can determine the surgical risks that women are exposed to. In Brazil—another nation obsessed with beauty and plastic surgery—women more commonly opt for buttocks implants or lifts, and breast *reductions*. In France, also, breast reduction is performed three to four times more often than breast augmentation; eight reductions for every two augmentations. "Many breasts reduced in France would be considered quite beautiful in America," said one French surgeon. Face-lifts are also much more rare in France, where a woman's face as she ages is still considered attractive.

Besides desiring bigger breasts, American women also seem to want slimmer hips and thighs. Yet liposuction, the "fat-sucking" procedure most commonly used to achieve these results, is hardly risk-free. Marketed as a quick and easy way to thinner thighs, it has resulted, albeit rarely, in death from postoperative infection or from a fat embolism that enters the blood-stream and lodges in the lungs. Even as women died, mostly as a result of surgery performed by unqualified doctors inadequately trained in the technique, liposuction continued to be urged on women dissatisfied with their bodies. Naomi Wolf, author of *The Beauty Myth*, posed as a prospective client and visited "counselors" to inquire about liposuction. In spite of the deaths, she was told by five different professionals that the operation was virtually risk-free.

Although plastic surgeons' advertisements present liposuction as simple and safe, the procedure is actually quite violent and destructive. A surgeon removing fat from the thighs, for example, must use brute strength to shove a hollow tube over and over again beneath the skin, moving it from side to side to loosen and "vacuum" away the fat. Worst of all, there is little known about the long-term effects of the procedure, or even whether the results are permanent.

Plastic surgeons today advertise themselves in popular magazines much like beauticians, hairstylists, and facialists, promising a more youthful appearance, a "whole new you." What they can't promise is a completely safe and complication-free procedure, because no surgery fits that bill. A bad haircut grows out in a few months, a bad facial may make the skin break out temporarily, but a bad face-lift may result in facial paralysis, permanent tightness or pain, or eyes that won't close properly.

Feminists may debate the merits of all these operations but whatever a woman's motives, if she chooses to have elective surgery of any kind, she has the right to make an informed decision based on knowledge of the risks involved. Unfortunately, women are often denied that right.

8

REPRODUCTIVE HEALTH
Fertile Ground for Bias

Reproductive health is a major part of women's medical care; the need for contraception and prenatal counsel bring most young women into the health care system. Yet women's reproductive concerns have been given short shrift by the medical establishment. The degree to which this is so was driven home to gynecologist Sally Faith Dorfman, M.D., chair of the American Medical Women's Association's Reproductive Health Initiative, when attending grand rounds at a major academic medical center. At a talk on new forms of birth control, the chairman of the department proceeded to introduce the junior faculty member assigned to give the presentation by saying, "We'd like to thank Dr. [So and So], who's taken on the thankless task of running our family planning clinic."

Dorfman's jaw dropped. "In that one sentence he sent a message to residents and medical students and faculty that this is not something that has any future in it, that it's not interesting, exciting, or important, and if you really want to get on with your career and make it in an academic institution, you'll train in one of the other areas.

"I remember standing up and saying, 'I hope you all realize this was probably the single most important lecture of the entire year, because there's nothing else we deal with that affects such a large percentage of our clientele. Everything else we deal with affects one percent of the population or five percent of the population. Few people have twins or triplets, yet how many lectures do you get on multiple birth in ob-gyn residency?'

"Only 15 percent of the population has fertility problems, yet we spend inordinate amounts of time teaching residents assisted reproductive technology and how to treat infertility."

Looked at another way, up to 85 percent of women of reproductive age may be trying to control their fertility. According to The Alan Guttmacher Institute, women spend an average of twenty-seven of the thirty-six years between menarche and menopause trying to avoid unplanned pregnancy. But medical students get the message that attending to the contraceptive needs of women is a thankless task.

■ CONTRACEPTIVE RESEARCH: CONTROLLED BY A MEDICAL "MAFIA"

Contraceptive research still hasn't recovered from the highly charged antiabortion politics of the Reagan and Bush presidencies. "We are a nation that supposedly prides itself on the primacy and the ingenuity of our science, yet the policies of the Bush and Reagan Administrations have increasingly limited American women to the most narrow contraceptive and family planning options," said Oregon congressman Ron Wyden.

Sterilization is now the most commonly used form of contraception for married couples in this country. According to some experts, there's a disturbing implication that women opt for sterilization because they are simply too frustrated with the lack of adequate contraceptive choices. A 1992 report by the Institute of Medicine estimated that at best only 50 percent of contraceptive users are happy with their method. And reliance on female sterilization has increased dramatically—from 12 percent of married contraceptive users in 1973, to 31 percent in 1988.

Since women's bodies, and not men's, are affected by contraceptive failure, clearly the lack of acceptable contraceptive options affects women more. "Women in Bangladesh have more contraceptive choices than women in the United States," says David Grimes, M.D., professor and vice chairman of the Department of Obstetrics, Gynecology and Reproductive Sciences at the University of California at San Francisco. "The United States went from being the undisputed leader in contraceptive research to a Third World nation." The reason, he says, has to do with government reluctance to encourage research and dwindling funding—fifteen minutes of the government's military budget equals a whole year of contraceptive research. "There's little research going on now, and there will be little coming out in the next five to ten years. The United States is in the backwater."

Time magazine reported that Europe was years ahead of the United States in terms of contraceptive research. There, pharmaceutical companies are aggressively pursuing male birth control pills, reversible vasectomies, and long-lasting contraceptive vaccines. Said Carl Djerassi, Ph.D., a

Stanford University chemist who helped develop the first Pill, "The U.S. is the only country other than Iran in which the birth-control clock has been set backward."

But politics alone can't explain medical and pharmaceutical company disinterest in developing new methods and products that would potentially be used by millions of adults. Because federal funds are so scanty, much contraceptive research is funded by public agencies and private foundations. But a variety of market factors are causing private companies to lose interest. Currently only two major pharmaceutical companies are conducting research into new contraceptives. It takes an estimated fifteen years and $50 million to get a new contraceptive on the market. And the threat of product liability lawsuits hovers over every attempt at development: the pharmaceutical company A. H. Robins, for example, declared bankruptcy after a spate of lawsuits by women who were injured by the Dalkon Shield IUD.

All these factors leave women longing for more contraceptive options for themselves and their partners, yet skeptical of anything new, unsure whether to accept the safety data trotted out with every new product. The birth control pill, after all, was approved in 1960 after being tested on only 132 Puerto Rican women who took it for a year or more, and 718 other women who took it for less than twelve months. Five of the women died during the course of the study, yet the Pill was declared safe.

The Pill's risks were deemed acceptable for social reasons—the importance of controlling population growth—even if it was risky for individual women. But if population control were the primary motivation for contraceptive research, the focus should be almost exclusively on *male* contraception. A woman can have only approximately one child per year. But an individual man can theoretically father hundreds of children in that same time.

Research into new male contraceptives is being blocked by what one disgusted NIH researcher calls the contraceptive Mafia. "Their attitude is that men won't take a pill because it may lower their libido," says this researcher. "But that's sixty-year-old men talking. Have they asked eighteen-year-olds who don't want to support a child? If I were a man, I'd be angry that I weren't being given the choice. The assumption is that men are irresponsible."

It is said that when a woman asked British playwright George Bernard Shaw (who was also a campaigner for women's equality) to define the difference between the sexes, he replied, "Madam, I cannot conceive." Because of that biological difference men may be unwilling to take any health risks at all for contraceptive purposes. Women's birth control pills contain sex hormones that affect nearly every organ system in the body. Because men do not risk pregnancy from contraceptive failure, they may be less likely to ingest contraceptive chemicals or hormones. One way to make men accept the kinds of reversible hormonal methods (oral contraceptives, Norplant, Depo-Provera, hormone-releasing IUDs) that women use would be to convince them that the contraception has health *benefits*, much as physicians have been selling women on the Pill by touting its ability to lower the risk of endometrial and ovarian cancer.

"There's no data yet, but it's possible that hormonal contraception for men might reduce cardiovascular risk or the incidence of prostate cancer," says Gary D. Hodgen, Ph.D., president of the Jones Institute of Reproductive Medicine in Norfolk, Virginia. "And [stressing these benefits] might be one way to make men accept it."

Some of the (scanty) research into male contraceptives includes the search for a male Pill. One possibility is gossypol, an oil derived from cottonseed. Also under investigation are implants or injections of hormone combinations: gonadotropin–releasing hormone (GnRH) antagonist or luteinizing hormone-releasing hormone (LHRH) antagonist, both of which can lower libido, supplemented with an implant releasing male hormones to restore the sex drive. Researchers are also investigating new sterilization methods such as reversible vasectomies in which silicon plugs are inserted into the vas deferens, injections of a sclerosing agent into the vas deferens, and "no-scalpel" vasectomies where occlusive clips are placed on the vas deferens.

While doctors stress safety in their search for a male contraceptive, they've been more concerned with effectiveness in preventing pregnancy when devising methods for women. The IUD carries a risk of reproductive tract infection, the Pill may increase the risk of breast cancer, the cervical cap smells (and some studies have linked it to Pap-smear abnormalities and toxic shock), and Norplant causes prolonged or irregular bleeding in one-third of users. These are considered acceptable side effects for female contraceptives.

Most of the current contraceptive research aimed at women consists of alternative formulations of hormones and birth control pills—variations on methods that are already available. But according to the Institute of Medicine, what's really needed are the following:

- Contraceptives that protect women against breast and cervical cancer
- More choices to increase user satisfaction

- Contraception for groups that are currently underserved: men, lactating mothers, teenagers, premenopausal women
- Contraceptives that protect women against sexually transmitted diseases

Says the report, "If contraceptive research is to be successful, it must be conducted with the cooperation of women who wish to have new and better methods of family planning. Departments of obstetrics and gynecology are in an almost unique position to develop new contraceptives since many young women seek advice from gynecologists for reproductive health care, including contraception. Thus, the gynecologist can study the desires of women and conduct appropriate clinical research into new contraceptive methods." In other words, *ask women what they want.*

For years now women have been waiting for the new contraceptives that the media keeps reporting are "on the horizon." These include:

- New delivery systems, such as transdermal hormone patches, vaginal rings that release steroids, and injectable microspheres, microcapsules, or pellets
- Vaccines against sperm or early pregnancy (one uses a genetically altered salmonella bacteria that causes the immune system to reject sperm)
- Implants that, unlike Norplant, would biodegrade and would not need to be removed
- New IUDS and new (smaller) contraceptive sponges
- Spermicides that are also virucidal—that is, kill chlamydia organisms and even HIV
- A disposable diaphragm coated with spermicide

Not only are these options years away from availability but right now many physicians are not even properly trained in prescribing the contraceptive options that are already available. One study found that 38 percent of ob-gyn residents had never inserted an intrauterine device; nearly half of the physicians in a California survey admitted to lack of knowledge about IUDs. Many physicians also don't know how to prescribe currently available oral contraceptives for use as morning-after pills, which one study estimated could cut the number of surgical abortions in half if they were more readily available after unprotected intercourse. With the lack of acceptable contraceptive options and morning-after protection, it's no wonder that 1.6 million abortions are performed in this country each year.

■ NO SUCH THING AS ABORTION ON DEMAND

A combination of politics, economics, and male medicine may limit women's contraceptive choices, but a more volatile mix limits women's access to abortion. The topic of abortion is so charged that even at professional medical conferences the atmosphere can be tense. At the 1993 annual meeting of the American Medical Women's Association, armed guards stood outside the conference room door as women glanced nervously around the hallways before entering. Inside the room the tension increased as the women scrutinized the crowd. Then, as a well-dressed middle-aged woman walked into the room and began speaking, the room grew hushed.

The speaker was Elizabeth Karlin, a forty-nine-year-old feminist with grown children—and a physician who has risked threats on her life to provide abortions. She spoke fervently to a room of young women, many of them doctors-in-training, about why she did what she did and why she found it so rewarding.

"Most women say they want about two children, which means we spend about thirty years trying *not* to get pregnant. And birth control is not perfect," she began. "I want to make a difference in women's lives, and I love my work. The abortion controversy is all about the control of women and the lack of respect for body boundaries."

Dr. Karlin described how antiabortion demonstrators tell women going into her clinic that they will die and go to hell, that abortion is an unclean procedure because the same instruments are used over and over again without sterilization, that the death rate is high, that the ambulance just left, that they will never be able to have children again, and that they will get breast cancer from the procedure. "What difference does it make after that what the government says?" asks Karlin, commenting on the Clinton administration's support for abortion services.

At one point, after the March 1993 shooting death of Florida physician David Gunn by a fanatical antiabortionist, Dr. Karlin was the subject of a vicious campaign by abortion foes, who circulated postcards reading, "Elizabeth Karlin is an abortionist," with her name and home address. It was an open invitation for someone to harm her. Yet while this campaign of harassment was going on, "not one doctor called in support," she said sadly. "Physicians have put their heads into the sand. It was the lawyers in town who sprang into action—for free—to protect me."

Dr. Karlin ended her talk with an impassioned plea to the women medical residents in the room to consider being trained in abortion procedures so that they can go on and provide the service to women nationwide.

■   ■

While a woman's right to a legal abortion has been assured since the *Roe* v. *Wade* decision in 1973, there are still formidable obstacles facing women who choose to abort a pregnancy. *Roe* v. *Wade* established that states cannot ban abortion, but the 1992 Supreme Court decision in *Planned Parenthood of Southeastern Pennsylvania* v. *Casey* held that states may impose restrictions on abortion as long as they do not have the "purpose or effect of placing a substantial obstacle in the path of a woman seeking an abortion."

"We talk about abortion on demand, but I don't know anywhere where a woman can just walk in off the street at any stage of her pregnancy and have an abortion," says Lynn Paltrow, director of special litigation for the Center for Reproductive Law and Policy.

Although abortion is currently a legal medical service, it is not a readily available one. Currently 83 percent of the nation's counties have no abortion provider. Seventy of the country's 305 metropolitan areas—more than one-quarter of the nation's cities—have no abortion provider. (While many women in the United States must travel to another county—or state—to obtain their abortion, in Europe women often have to visit another country. Women from Ireland and Poland, where abortion is prohibited, may visit England, France, the Netherlands, Sweden, or Norway for the procedure. Such "abortion tourism" is unlikely to abate unless the twenty-six member states of the Council of Europe can agree to make abortion equally available for all European women.)

In many areas of the United States restrictions such as twenty-four-hour waiting periods or parental notification or permission rules are in place. Seventeen-year-old Becky Bell died in 1988 because she did not want to tell her parents—or a local antichoice judge—that she was pregnant. Instead she sought an illegal abortion and died a week later of a lung infection. Twenty-five states currently have parental notification or permission laws in effect. Yet the Supreme Court does not find the parental notification requirement an impediment.

Seven states currently have waiting periods—twenty-four hours in Mississippi, Nebraska, Michigan, North Dakota, Pennsylvania, and Utah; eight hours in Kansas. Lynn Paltrow tells of women paying for their abortions with rolls of quarters and sleeping outdoors on the plastic chairs outside of discount chain stores because they could barely afford the abortion, let alone a place to stay overnight. Yet this restriction, too, does not qualify as a substantial obstacle.

While the Clinton administration has announced that it wants abortion services covered under any new national health plan, so far the Pres-

ident has not even succeeded in getting Medicaid funds to cover abortions
for poor women. In the fall of 1993 both the House and the Senate voted
to continue to prohibit Medicaid payments for most abortions, with the
exception of cases of rape or incest, or when the woman's life is endangered
by the pregnancy. Well into 1994, even these scanty provisions were being
challenged by Medicaid officials from at least half a dozen states, who
flouted the law by refusing to pay for *any* abortions for low-income
women.

The Clinton administration's push toward health care reform may also
be inadvertently limiting women's access to abortion by encouraging institutions to reorganize for cost-efficiency. "We're beginning to see a trend of
hospital consolidation that's happening both as a result of health care reform and in anticipation of it," says Kathryn Kolbert, vice president of the
Center for Reproductive Law and Policy, whose attorneys have been counsel in virtually every major U.S. Supreme Court case about reproductive
rights. "Catholic hospitals merge with nonsectarian hospitals, and they
then refuse to provide abortion services. When religious and nonreligious
hospitals merge to form alliances or HMOs, there may be obstacles placed
in the path of women who need confidential reproductive-health care."

But perhaps the biggest obstacle women face in obtaining the safe, legal abortions they are entitled to by law is the lack of physicians trained
in the procedure and willing to provide it. Only 12 percent of the nation's
medical schools *require* abortion training as part of an ob-gyn residency,
and nearly one-third do not offer any abortion training at all. Between
1985 and 1991 the number of medical programs that taught doctors how
to perform abortions dropped by half. Since 1982 the number of abortion
providers declined by 11 percent overall, 19 percent in rural areas. Yet the
1.6 million abortions performed yearly make it one of the most common
surgical procedures for women.

Many of the physicians who currently provide abortions are older,
committed to their work by memories of the women they saw in emergency rooms, mutilated from self- or backstreet abortions before *Roe* v.
Wade. Younger doctors accustomed to legal abortions may not feel the
same drive to provide a service that pays poorly and carries the added risk
of harassment and even death threats. When the Feminist Women's Health
Center of Atlanta, looking for a physician to provide abortions at its clinic,
sent out three thousand letters to ob-gyn residents about to graduate, not
one of the new physicians was willing to take the job.

Ironically, the efforts of family-planning organizations and feminist
groups in the 1970s to make abortion readily available may have contrib-

uted to the current crisis. Twenty years ago it made sense to establish separate clinics to offer centralized family-planning and abortion services. Now those clinics have become targets for antiabortion groups. And physicians in private practice have become accustomed to referring their patients who want abortions to those clinics rather than performing the procedures themselves. Today few women can obtain an abortion from the physician who also does their Pap smear and pelvic exam. And only 13 percent of abortions are performed in hospitals. Instead most women must visit special clinics, where they are easy targets for antiabortion protesters who harass women, trace their license plate numbers, and call their families and employers in an attempt to talk them out of the abortion. Where are those protesters when a desperately poor woman finally has her child and cannot afford the food to feed it?

If more physicians were trained and willing to provide abortions, perhaps the reliance on centralized clinics would be lessened. When abortion is finally a part of every ob-gyn practice and clinic, every HMO and hospital outpatient service, then women will not be singled out for harassment and doctors will not receive death threats.

In 1993 Planned Parenthood of New York City instituted its own training program for physicians. In announcing the program, Alexander C. Sanger, president and chief executive of New York's Planned Parenthood chapter (and grandson of Margaret Sanger, the founder of the American birth control movement), said, "Most teaching hospitals find it easier to leave abortion training to someone else. We have decided to become that someone else." Planned Parenthood's program is the first large-scale effort aimed at increasing the number of doctors who do abortions nationwide.

Why aren't physicians' groups, such as the American College of Obstetricians and Gynecologists (ACOG), undertaking such efforts? "The vast majority of ob-gyns in this country do not want to do abortions," says Allan Rosenfield, M.D., professor and dean of the Columbia University School of Public Health. Although a 1985 survey of ACOG members found that 84 percent supported a woman's right to an abortion, only about one-third of that group said they provide such services. Most of these doctors performed four or fewer abortions each month. Only 5 percent of the physicians who perform abortions (fewer than 2 percent of all ob-gyns) perform more than twenty-five a month.

Instead of supporting women's rights, ACOG seems determined to divorce itself from the controversy. In early 1994 the organization came out with a statement supporting training *non*physicians as well as physicians to perform abortions. Said ACOG president William C. Andrews, M.D., "I think the ideal would be that physicians would be performing them. But as a pragmatic thing, if there are not physicians who are trained or willing to do the procedure, other options have to be considered." Those options include physicians' assistants, nurse-practitioners and nurse-midwives.

While physicians' assistants already perform abortions in Montana and Vermont, forty-three states and the District of Columbia currently have laws on the books specifically barring anyone but physicians from doing abortions. So ACOG's recommendation is unlikely to make abortion more available in the near future.

ACOG's abdication seems at least partly driven by its members' fears of harassment and threats. "There's a deterrent effect on physicians," says Ann Allen, ACOG's legal counsel. "A young doctor looking at the evening news is going to say, 'Forget it.'" But passing the buck to another group of professionals doesn't exactly look good. As columnist Anna Quindlen wrote, "No one wants to be seen as saying, 'They're shooting doctors! Quick! Send in the nurses!'"

Considering how territorial gynecologists are about most aspects of their practice—opposing nurse-midwives handling routine pregnancies, and nurse-practitioners performing Pap smears—it seems obvious that if abortion were more lucrative, conferred a higher status, and involved no personal risk, organizations such as ACOG would be insisting that only physicians could provide the service safely.

Besides providing abortions, another way physicians could show their support for women would be to get involved in lobbying for the availability of RU-486, a medical alternative to surgical abortion. Because no special training would be needed to prescribe RU-486, any physician would be able to give the drug to women needing an early abortion. If the drug's use was not limited to family planning clinics, there would be no locus of attack for anti-abortion groups. Even though RU-486 is not the perfect answer for women who wish to end a pregnancy—it requires several trips to the doctor and must be taken early in a pregnancy—it would provide a nonsurgical alternative for women. Yet the medical profession still seems reluctant to endorse this option. Wrote a disgusted Quindlen, "The big medical organizations . . . were more fired up about our right to choose breast implants than they have ever been about our right to choose abortion."

■ REPRODUCTIVE TECHNOLOGIES: BREEDING FALSE HOPE?

In contrast to doctors who perform abortions for little money and no prestige, high-tech infertility specialists have taken an opposite course: They've decided to concentrate on achieving pregnancies for relatively few women who have a lot of money to spend. These physicians, while seemingly altruistic, may be doing many women a grave disservice.

At a Chicago fertility clinic, however, the decor doesn't obviously echo that conclusion. The wall leading to the suite of examining rooms is plastered with Polaroids of babies: scrawny babies, plump babies, rosy-cheeked babies, red-haired and black-haired babies, white, African-American, and Asian babies—all testimonials to the miracles of high technology.

For more than five years Connie walked past this "hall of wonder babies," back to the inner sanctum where her doctor removed close to a dozen ripe eggs from her aching, drug-stimulated ovaries and placed several of them, along with her husband's sperm, in her fallopian tubes. If fertilization occurred, the hope was that at least one embryo would make the fantastic voyage to her uterus, where it would implant.

Two weeks later Connie would return to the Chicago fertility clinic for a blood test—another walk down that hall—to learn whether she was carrying her very own wonder baby. Month after month, year after year, the answer was always negative. Like the majority of infertile women who turn to technology to fulfill their procreative urges, Connie was not to become pregnant. There would be no Polaroid to contribute to the great wall of babies.

"I feel like it was a racket," she now says about the dozens of invasive fertility procedures she endured. "They hold out just enough hope to tantalize you and keep you signing those nine-hundred-dollar checks before you walk out the door." She figures she and her husband dropped close to thirty thousand dollars before finally calling it quits.

Assisted reproductive technologies such as in vitro fertilization (IVF) and gamete intrafallopian transfer (GIFT), the procedure Connie underwent, are billed as the great success stories of modern medicine, a view reinforced by the media. A 1991 cover story in *Time* typifies the press's seduction by this biomedical technology. "More than a million couples seek treatment for infertility each year," the story began. "Now some remarkable insights into the mating dance of sperm and egg are bringing answers to their prayers." The article went on to discuss the "infertility epidemic" and the cutting-edge technology enabling couples to take home high-priced designer babies.

In article after article the message is always the same: Persevere and you'll eventually hit the jackpot, you'll win the thirty-, fifty- or hundred-thousand-dollar baby. Such a noble—albeit risky—quest is culturally sanctioned. That it's normal and natural to desire a baby is an unspoken assumption underlying almost every encounter with a fertility specialist. "The urge to have children is a basic, primeval, biological drive," says Zev Rosenwaks, M.D., director of the Center for Reproductive Medicine at New York Hospital–Cornell University Medical Center. "It can be devastating for a couple to have this problem. The couples we see are desperate to have children."

In a culture that views motherhood as instinctual, as the essence of what it means to be a woman, the more subtle message is that worshiping at the altar of technology is a small price to pay to carry on one's genetic heritage, achieve immortality, and, particularly for women, fulfill one's obligation to society. But is it truly?

When the technology works—and even when it doesn't—the answer is often an unqualified yes. "No one has the right to say what's too much for one person and what's not enough," says Terry Stoller, who attempted to conceive for seven years before finally giving birth to a healthy baby girl through IVF in 1992. "I do feel it was all worth it and I think I would have said that whether I got pregnant or not. I needed to know I did all I could. If it hadn't worked, though, I could have accepted a child-free lifestyle."

The flip side of the story, the side that's frequently omitted, is that the success rates of some of these procedures are remarkably low. Most women do not get to smile for the camera and show off a miracle baby. In fact the take-home-baby rate for IVF averages 15.2 percent per retrieval. Zygote intrafallopian transfer (ZIFT), in which the egg is fertilized in a test tube and the zygote transferred to the fallopian tube, is slightly better—at 19.7 percent, similar to the chance a fertile couple has of conceiving in any given cycle. Gamete intrafallopian transfer (GIFT), because it more closely simulates the act of conception—and even improves upon it—has a more respectable 26.6 percent success rate. Attempting these procedures more than once betters a couple's odds, but for some unknown reason effectiveness diminishes after three to four treatments.

The problem with these statistics is that they can't be taken at face value. For one thing the industry is almost entirely unregulated. Specialists may set up shop on the strength of a forty-eight-hour training program.

There's nothing to stop clinics from including in their statistics babies who die within a month of birth. What's more, most clinics' tallies do not include the 30 to 40 percent of women who drop out of programs because they can't produce eggs or their eggs can't be fertilized. In fact the best epidemiological data suggest that IVF yields fewer than ten live births per one hundred treatment cycles.

Says one woman who unsuccessfully ran the techno-baby chase, "That's why they scrutinize you so carefully beforehand. They don't want people who are dead in the water because they don't want to screw up their statistics. It's like the stock market. They want their stock to go up."

On the other hand reputable fertility specialists who know the score are loath to give false hope. "If a couple said to me, 'We have twenty thousand dollars, should we spend it on IVF or adopt?' I'd say, 'No question, adopt,' " says Patricia M. McShane, M.D., vice president of medical affairs at IVF America. "None of these techniques is a sure thing, a guarantee. Adoption is."

Still, it's understandable that women, desperate for a child and offered an increasingly vast array of options, might feel compelled to try them all. With ever more maverick technologies, it becomes difficult to decide when enough is enough. Despite the toll each failed attempt takes on a woman's emotional life, and often on her relationship with her partner, she can easily become addicted to each spin of the infertility wheel of fortune.

But every high—for instance the day a woman learns she's produced twenty eggs—has a corresponding low: None of the embryos implant in her uterus. Soon the treatments become beads of indignity strung one against the other, from men ejaculating into tiny plastic cups to women lying spread-eagle on an examining table holding a catheter in their uterus so that the millions of squeaky-clean sperm have a chance to do their thing. The early, relatively benign procedures—endometrial biopsies and hysterosalpingograms (an X-ray examination of the reproductive tract)—are often followed by laparoscopy, a procedure performed under general anesthesia in which a scope inserted into the naval is used to view the reproductive organs. Then it might be on to oral doses of the fertility drug Clomid and, later, injections of Pergonal and HCG (human chorionic gonadotropin). With these drugs come blood tests and ultrasounds to both monitor egg development and make sure the ovaries aren't becoming hyperstimulated.

If Pergonal combined with intrauterine insemination doesn't work, it's on to IVF, GIFT, or ZIFT. This next step involves more shots and procedures, continual trips to the doctor, and hours spent in overcrowded hospital waiting rooms. Ellen, a New York City art director who attended New York Hospital's fertility clinic, summed up her feelings this way: "They treated you like cattle. You were just a name and a number. There would be forty women sitting in the waiting room in the morning. I'd go in at seven in the morning so I wouldn't have to wait an hour.

"You couldn't ask questions when the doctor was doing the ultrasound. If the cycle failed, you couldn't just go to the doctor and ask what happened. You'd have to make an appointment and wait four weeks. They'd say, 'The doctors will meet and discuss your case and we'll report back to you.'"

After a while the poking and prodding, the needle pricks and surgical procedures, become the center of a woman's life. "My second IVF attempt was emotionally and physically getting too draining for me," admits Terry Stoller. "I started worrying that this was becoming a lifestyle for me, rearranging my personal life so that my husband could give me a shot every night at eight o'clock. I reached a point where, if this hadn't worked, I knew I couldn't go right back to it.

"The drugs affect you emotionally too," she says. One day in the middle of a Pergonal cycle, Stoller had to shop for a baby gift for a co-worker. As she and her husband approached the cash register, Terry bolted for the door in tears. "Seeing pregnant women was unbearable," she says. "I couldn't control myself."

Given that the majority of procedures take place in women's bodies, it's not surprising that they are more distressed than their male partners by infertility. In one study 57 percent of the women but only 12 percent of the men thought that infertility was the worst thing they ever had to face in life.

Few studies, however, examine the emotional toll that infertility takes on single women and lesbian couples. Indeed programs seem to be consciously pushing nuclear family building: until recently many IVF clinics accepted only married couples. Most also refuse to treat women over the age of forty-five or fifty—even though they have a chance of conceiving using donor eggs. The major issue is "whether the child will have living parents," says Patricia McShane of IVF America. "We feel very strongly about this, unlike some of our colleagues, who say if IVF isn't medically risky, then go ahead with it."

Applying the same logic as McShane, doctors in Britain recently refused to treat a childless woman who decided, at age fifty-nine, that she wanted to become a mother. Their grounds for refusal: She was too old to face the stress of child rearing. "There are deep ethical considerations," said the British secretary of health. "A child has a right to a suitable home." Yet there's no ethical debate when a man in his sixties or seventies becomes a father. As Margaret Carlson wrote in a 1994 article in *Time*, "When it is a man having the baby, few seem to question whether the stress will be too much for the old geezer. One could contend that the assertion that a child is worse off with a mother who may die before the child is grown than a father who might is an argument for more equal parenting."

So far only a handful of postmenopausal women over the age of fifty have given birth through assisted reproductive technologies. Whether they face the same psychological fallout as younger women undergoing fertility treatment is not known. Studies do show that after the failure of a first try at IVF, 25 percent of women experience depression, versus 10 percent of men. For women who have nurtured successful careers, infertility may be their first major disappointment. It doesn't help when a couple's sex life flies out the window, as it invariably does when couples must time sex to correspond with ovulation. Nor does it help when well-meaning friends and family tell women that, if they would only relax, they would become pregnant, a scenario totally unsupported by research. As their lives spin out of control, women can't help but feel as if they're damaged goods. "Intellectually you know it's a medical problem," said Pamela Loew, who eventually conceived through GIFT. "But emotionally you can't get it out of your mind that you're not like a normal woman."

If a woman has finally had enough and decides to get off the fertility merry-go-round, her infertility doctor may scarcely notice. After all, there are plenty more names and numbers waiting to take her place. "When I left the program," says Ellen, "no one ever called me to say, 'We haven't seen you in six months, what's happening?' They didn't care. It was brutal. It was inhuman."

In her book *Women as Wombs: Reproductive Technologies and the Battle Over Women's Freedom*, feminist scholar Janice Raymond calls these technologies "publicly sanctioned violence against women." She writes, "Reproductive technologies are the next step enhancing male access to women and the increasing abuse of women's bodies under the guise of scientific advancement. Women are required to spread their legs too frequently for medical probing and penetration."

In an interview Raymond said, "The wider ethical and political question for me is why, at this point in history, are women being encouraged to go through these invasive and interventionist procedures when there's very little chance of taking home a baby? A lot of women who want children will go through almost anything to get them.

"Adventure and adventurism are a big part of this. Many biologists claim that IVF has been developed not to help infertile women but to advance biology. That point has been made very much invisible in this whole debate. There's a hype of altruism surrounding this."

The real kicker is that in 40 to 50 percent of the cases infertility is related to a male factor; that is, the man is having difficulties. While there's been a real move to examine and deal with men's problems—more and more men are undergoing varicocelectomies to remove varicose veins that cause abnormal blood flow to the testicles—reproductive technology is still almost exclusively applied to women's bodies. Even though both partners are now routinely examined, assisted reproduction represents one of the few medical procedures in which the person with the medical condition frequently is not the one who is being treated.

▪ FERTILITY DRUGS:
SETTING THE STAGE FOR A CANCER EPIDEMIC?

Women who have deferred childbearing often find themselves in a panic when they finally decide to start a family and then don't immediately conceive. They've read about the infertility epidemic and, certain they're one of the statistics, may prematurely rush to treatment. Yet contrary to what many believe, there is no infertility epidemic in this country. An estimated 4.9 million women—or 10 to 15 percent of couples—are infertile, a statistic that has remained unchanged for more than twenty years. The tendency to postpone childbirth has resulted in an increase in the number of infertile women between the ages of thirty-five and forty-four (from 454,000 in 1982 to 620,000 in 1988), but a corresponding jump in the population has held the infertility rate steady among older women.

What *has* changed is the number of people seeking treatment—primarily a response to the explosion in new reproductive technologies. In 1988, the last year for which data are available, there were 1.35 million medical visits for infertility services, up from 600,000 in 1968. Couples spend some $1 billion a year on their quest for a child, and the industry is rapidly expanding to meet the demand. The number of fertility clinics has increased from twelve in 1985, to some three hundred today.

And the U.S. experience is only the tip of the iceberg. France boasts more IVF centers per capita than any other country in the world, and

Australia has had such success with its IVF technology that it has exported it to the United States. As Janice Raymond writes, "Rarely has a technology that has had such dismal success rates been so quickly accepted." Indeed, noted a 1990 World Health Organization report on IVF, "The rapid proliferation of IVF services in nearly all industrialized countries is driven by the interests of providers, industry and other special interest groups, rather than by rational planning based on the needs of the population."

If women's needs were a priority, countries would require fertility specialists to be board certified and licensed, and there would be a mechanism for reporting clinical data. As things stand, anyone can hang out a shingle and start a practice. Even though there are laboratory guidelines specifying which tests and equipment to use, there is no way to assess a practitioner's expertise, nor is there a set fertility work-up. In the absence of any regulations, the technology is being driven by market rather than scientific forces. "The bulk of the research on IVF," said the WHO report, "has focused on perfecting clinical protocols and finding new and expanded uses for the technology."

Some blame the male domination of the field. Only twenty-eight of the IVF program directors in the United States are women. If women were in charge, says Dr. Florence Haseltine, director of the Center for Population Research at the National Institute of Child Health and Human Development, the technology would be more advanced and, it should follow, more successful. Haseltine says research is desperately needed on such things as egg development and the cell cycling of eggs and sperm, areas women have been interested in pursuing. "We don't know much about the mechanisms of these things," she says. "We're stuck in how to manipulate the female cycle when the issue should be how to make eggs and sperm more viable."

The real holdup has been the male specialists' focus on the business of IVF. "Men are more involved in making money," says Haseltine. "The men who started in this field are more like entrepreneurs. Because the whole infertility area is not regulated, we didn't get scientists who were making a career out of this to carry out research. We got good brains, but not the best. Things were done really amateurishly."

And women, as usual, end up paying the price. Yet how many women are aware that the procedures they're eager to undergo have never been studied in randomized controlled trials and that no one is certain of the long-term health consequences—for them or for their offspring?

For one thing women who use fertility drugs have a greater chance of having a multiple pregnancy, which puts their babies at risk for premature birth and low birth weight. Birth defects occur at a rate comparable to that in the general population, but public health experts know from experience that this may not ensure a lack of problems down the road. As a chilling reminder of this, "DES-exposed women appeared normal at birth," writes Michael Steinkampf, M.D., of the University of Alabama at Birmingham. So far there have been no long-term follow-up studies of children who were conceived with the help of fertility drugs.

The high-octane drugs used in the fertility process may be damaging to women as well. Up to 60 percent of women undergoing ovulation induction with such drugs as Pergonal and HCG (human chorionic gonadotropin), an integral part of most assisted reproduction, will experience a mild ovarian hyperstimulation syndrome. In the severe form of the syndrome, which occurs in up to one percent of cycles, blood clots can form in a woman's lungs and kidneys, and her ovaries can literally burst.

The biggest worry is whether these drugs will end up increasing a woman's chances of getting cancer. Women who never bear children already have a higher risk of developing cancers of the breasts, ovaries, and endometrial lining. But women who are infertile as a result of ovulatory dysfunction have an incidence of endometrial cancer four times that of women without a history of infertility. Ovarian cancer, too, may be related to an inability to conceive.

There are also suggestions that the potent hormonal cocktails used to stimulate ovulation may, in and of themselves, lead to ovarian cancer, a disease that kills almost half its victims within five years. Compiling data from three case-control studies, Alice Whittemore, Ph.D., of Stanford, found that white women who used fertility drugs were three times more likely to develop ovarian cancer than women without a history of infertility. Women who had used fertility drugs and never borne children had twenty-seven times the risk of an ovarian malignancy.

When news of the ovarian-cancer study broke in 1993, many women felt betrayed. Ellen, the New York City art director, had taken fertility drugs every other month for three years. When she'd asked her doctor if there were any long-term risks, he'd told her, "These drugs have been around for twenty years and no one has had problems."

Ellen proceeded to take Clomid and then Pergonal and the drug Metrodin, at doses so high, she guesses she produced hundreds of eggs over the three-year period. Her eight IVF attempts—four of which were with frozen embryos—all failed. "In my heart of hearts I knew there had to be incredible side effects from these powerful drugs," she says. "But it seems particularly cruel that it was the people who had not conceived who faced the risk of cancer. Talk about adding insult to injury. We were all guinea pigs."

As fertility clinics fielded calls from frightened, angry women, the American Fertility Society attempted spin control, pointing out that Whittemore's study was not able to identify what fertility drugs the women had used or for how long they had used them. "It was a limited study, not very well done," adds New York Hospital's Zev Rosenwaks. "The study had nothing to do with IVF or with Pergonal, for all we know—we don't know what these women were treated with."

Whittemore openly acknowledges the study's shortcomings. Nevertheless independent researchers say her research was beautifully designed and executed. "Most clinicians haven't been trained to understand epidemiology's purposes, uses, and limitations," says Carolyn Westhoff, M.D., associate professor of clinical obstetrics, gynecology, and public health at Columbia University.

What's more, a link with ovarian cancer is biologically plausible. According to the so-called incessant-ovulation theory, anything that promotes ovulation—for instance, stimulation of the ovaries by fertility drugs—can increase the risk of malignancy. Another theory holds that carcinogenesis might be related to elevated levels of circulating pituitary gonadotropins. The fertility drug Clomid, in particular, increases the production of these hormones.

Whittemore's results are further bolstered by eight published case reports of ovarian cancer in women treated with fertility drugs. Two additional cases have been submitted for publication, and five others have been reported to the FDA. In France there are reports of twelve ovarian tumors following ovulation induction. The FDA is taking the data seriously. In 1993 it began requiring the makers of fertility drugs to include a warning in their package inserts about the possible risk of ovarian cancer.

Around the same time, the National Institute of Child Health and Human Development announced plans to launch a study into the drugs' safety. "On the most fundamental level, we don't know what's going on," says Westhoff, who hopes to be an investigator on the study. "The puzzle pieces don't add up. It's not weird to suspect that drugs that deliberately alter the ovaries may change risk. Also, do fertility drugs increase breast cancer risk? No study has been big enough or sufficiently targeted enough to give precise answers."

All of which worries Terry Stoller, who took Clomid as well as Pergonal. Breast cancer runs in her family, and a cousin has ovarian cancer. "I'm scared to death," she says.

Additionally there are worries about health risks to egg donors who get involved in IVF—and take fertility drugs—for money or altruism. "There is no medical benefit to them to get pregnant, but there is a concern about the potential for an increased risk for ovarian cancer," says Maria Bustillo, M.D., director of the Division of Reproductive Endocrinology in the department of ob-gyn at Mount Sinai School of Medicine in New York City. "It could be that these women are at low risk anyway for ovarian cancer, since they're not part of an infertile subgroup."

But no one really knows what risks both fertile and infertile women may be subjecting themselves to by taking these powerhouse drugs. Given so many unknowns, it's reasonable to worry about a future cancer epidemic among women unwittingly partaking in what the World Health Organization has dubbed an "experimental" treatment.

The WHO considers IVF unproven because it has not yet been rigorously tested. Women may be surprised to learn that the National Institute of Child Health and Human Development, which is responsible for research on infertility, has never funded a major prospective study on the safety of IVF in humans. (Because they follow subjects forward over time, prospective studies are considered the gold standard in research.)

The institute has had its hands tied by a series of bureaucratic missteps dating back to 1975. That was the year the then-Department of Health, Education and Welfare issued regulations requiring that an Ethics Advisory Board advise HEW's secretary on the ethical acceptability of research that involved the fertilization of human sperm and eggs. In 1979, after meeting for a year, the board declared IVF research ethically acceptable.

But through a misunderstanding the board was mistakenly dissolved. With no entity to review and approve proposals, research into the efficacy and risks of infertility treatments would not be eligible for federal funding. A 1989 congressional report, "Infertility in America: Why Is the Federal Government Ignoring a Major Health Problem?," noted that, in the time since the board has been disbanded, "IVF has gone from a rarely used technique to an established medical procedure. Research is needed to improve the efficacy of IVF, to improve the success of freezing and thawing of embryos, and to develop techniques for successfully freezing and thawing human eggs that are not yet fertilized."

Despite fifteen years of entreaties by scientists and major medical associations, the Ethics Advisory Board has not been reconstituted. The ban on human fetal tissue transplantation research during the Reagan and Bush administrations further prevented basic research involving fertilized human eggs. In 1993, President Clinton lifted the ban on fetal tissue research and the NIH Revitalization Act established ethical guidelines for carrying out such research, eliminating the need for the Ethics Advisory Board. But the years wasted in bureaucratic wrangling have delayed research findings important to women. Florence Haseltine, of the National Institute of Child Health and Human Development, estimates that one hundred IVF-related grant proposals would have been submitted to NIH every year if such research had been fundable.

The lack of federal funds for research on assisted reproductive technologies has resulted in treatments that are both ineffective and costly. IVF averages $6,000 to $7,000 per attempt and can easily go as high as $10,000. In many cases patients must pay out of pocket, since private insurance often does not cover these procedures. Infertile couples, whether they know it or not, are actually helping to support biomedical research. At some clinics a proportion of patients' medical fees are used to fund studies.

The bulk of funding, however, comes from private industry—for instance, from Serono Laboratories, Inc., which makes the fertility drugs that are the lifeblood of the technology and which is a major sponsor of continuing medical education courses on the treatment of infertility. Serono's domination of the field has shaped the direction of both research and treatment and is the reason the discussion has not gone in a much more important, albeit low-tech, direction: the prevention of infertility.

■ SEXUALLY TRANSMITTED DISEASES AND INFERTILITY: A NEGLECTED PUBLIC HEALTH ISSUE

If prevention of infertility were a priority, we'd be hearing a lot more about sexually transmitted diseases. There would be a particular emphasis on chlamydia, which, if left untreated, can lead to pelvic inflammatory disease. PID in turn can damage a woman's fallopian tubes, causing an ectopic pregnancy and rendering a woman infertile.

The twelve million STD infections that occur annually take their harshest toll on women and teenage girls—both because they are more easily transmitted to women and more difficult to diagnose. Even so, one national survey found that women were in denial about their risk of getting an STD, and the federal government is partly to blame. The bulk of federal funds to diagnose and treat sexually transmitted infections is directed toward public health clinics, which primarily serve men. While women are welcome, they rarely feel comfortable in such a setting. At one overburdened clinic in Prince George's County, outside Washington, D.C., for instance, men begin lining up for services at seven-thirty in the morning. As Lisa Kaeser, of the nonprofit Alan Guttmacher Institute, facetiously says, "Women just love to be seen standing outside an STD clinic in their own community for all the world to see."

Women who rely on family-planning clinics or private doctors for STD care should fare better, but many primary care physicians do not perceive their patients to be at risk. Only one-third of women who sought family-planning services from a private doctor were screened for STDs, compared with more than half of those who went to a family-planning clinic. Perhaps this should come as no surprise. Medical schools and residency programs offer little instruction in STD diagnosis and treatment.

A strong effort by the federal government to fight STDs would make a difference. But in 1994 the Centers for Disease Control and Prevention spent a paltry $90 million on STD prevention services. Most of these funds were directed toward secondary prevention—that is, testing and treating people. There are concerns, even at the CDC, that the money is not being well spent. A Guttmacher report questioned why 70 percent of federal funds were allocated toward syphilis and gonorrhea, which account for only 10 percent of all STD infections, while chlamydia, which is ninety times more common than syphilis, gets less than one-third of the federal budget.

As far back as 1986, James Mason, then director of the CDC, testified at a congressional hearing that the federal government would need to spend $50 million to $60 million each year to prevent and treat chlamydia. The CDC has spent only about $4.5 million a year.

The irony is that the people in the trenches—the health care providers who work in the clinics—are aware of the need for universal chlamydia screening but lack the funds to provide it. When Planned Parenthood's Southern Indiana region received a grant from Abbott Laboratories to do universal screening at eighteen clinics, 13 percent of the women turned up positive for chlamydia, an extremely high rate for that part of the country. When the money ran out, the screening came to an abrupt halt. "Medical directors of most clinics know chlamydia is out there, but they can't do anything about it," Lisa Kaeser says in frustration.

This is ludicrous, especially given evidence that universal screening is cost-effective. A 1986 California study found that offering all women chlamydia screening and treatment—including treatment for their infected partners—would save $6 million in the first year alone. Thereafter the program would save $13 million a year in medical costs associated with the prevention of chlamydia-related PID, ectopic pregnancy, and tubal infertility. Considering that the United States has some of the highest STD rates in the industrialized world—in some cities rates approach those of developing countries—neglecting prevention amounts to medical malpractice.

The message about STDs may finally be getting out, however. The Centers for Disease Control and Prevention has awarded grants of about $150,000 each to twelve state and local health departments to stimulate innovative approaches to STD prevention. And the American Medical Women's Association is developing a model curriculum on reproductive health, to be introduced to medical schools across the country, that will cover such topics as STDs and abortion training.

While there is a lot more to women's health than reproductive medicine, there's no question that the way women's gynecological and obstetric health concerns are treated goes to the very heart of the way medicine mistreats women. As the twentieth century draws to a close, women still face limited and unsatisfactory contraceptive choices, difficulty obtaining abortions, missed diagnoses of sexually transmitted diseases, pregnancies treated as illnesses, and infertility treatments in which the means—no matter how torturous—seem to justify the end. Women must realize that they have the clout to demand humane and complete reproductive care.

9

FROM MIDLIFE
TO THE MATURE YEARS
The Medicalization of Aging

To many women the menopause marks the end of their useful life. They see
it as the onset of old age, the beginning of the end. They may be right. Having
outlived their ovaries, they may have outlived their usefulness as human
beings. The remaining years may be just marking time until they follow
their glands into oblivion.

—David R. Reuben, M.D., 1969

Since the mid-nineteenth century, when the term *menopause* was first coined, the medical profession has been quick to blame a middle-aged woman's depression, anger, irritability—you name it—on her womb. Or, more precisely, on the betrayal by her womb. If, according to the medical perspective, a woman's body is useful only when it is capable of making babies, "by extension menopause implies failed production, breakdown of the ovaries, waste and decay," writes Kathleen MacPherson, R.N., Ph.D.

Along the same lines, the end of childbearing capacity would certainly herald a woman's loss of femininity, sexuality, and beauty. As Dr. David Reuben wrote, when "estrogen is shut off, a woman comes as close as she can to being a man. Increased facial hair, deepened voice, obesity, and the decline of breasts and female genitalia all contribute to a masculine appearance. Coarsened features, enlargement of the clitoris, and gradual baldness complete the tragic picture. Not really a man but no longer a functional woman, these individuals live in the world of intersex."

The view of menopause as a deficiency disease—the decline in the production of estrogen was said to be at the root of all women's emotional and physical problems—has had plenty of takers in the last several decades. In 1978 one researcher described the middle-aged woman as "red-faced, emo-

216

tionally labile, in need of some sort of medication, whether tranquilizers or estrogen." In contrast a middle-aged man was "a rugged outdoorsman, virile, dignified, who projects the image of success, self-satisfaction and sexual potency."

Even today some doctors and biomedical researchers still characterize the menopause as a kind of death, as if subconsciously to validate the turn-of-the-century view that a woman was nothing more than "a pair of ovaries with a human being attached; whereas man is a human being furnished with a pair of testes." And when these ovaries cease pumping out hormones, as they certainly must, the doctor stands ready to "fix" what is broken using a grab bag of medical interventions, from D&Cs to hysterectomies to hormone replacement therapy (HRT). Indeed the story of modern menopause has become virtually synonymous with the story of HRT.

The deficiency-disease model—against which the women's health movement of the 1970s fought vigorously—is very much alive and well today. "There's been a focus on menopause as a disease," says Dr. Diana Taylor, director of the Women's Health Program in the School of Nursing at the University of California, San Francisco. "There's a paternalistic view that medicine knows what's best for women." Underlying this perspective is the belief that middle-aged women are a deviation from the norm, in this case not only from the bodies of men but from the bodies of women of reproductive age as well. Whether discussing bone mass or cardiovascular function, "the chemistry of women of reproductive age is . . . taken as the standard measure for what is normal and healthy, and the aging body is designated as abnormal," says Margaret Lock of McGill University.

Rarely do researchers start with the assumption that the transition into menopause might be normal and healthy. All too often clinical trials examine the pathologies associated with menopause, most notably heart disease and osteoporosis. But by zeroing in on these diseases, the medical community is missing the bigger picture. It's missing a larger passage known as midlife, which encompasses but is not limited to menopause.

"Menopause is only one of many transitions a woman goes through," says Diana Taylor. "It's the end of menstrual life. To focus on just one aspect of reproductive health diminishes other aspects of women's health."

In March 1993, against this backdrop, the National Institutes of Health convened its first national conference to assess the current knowledge on menopause and make recommendations for research. "Menopause is a universal phenomenon experienced by all women, yet very little is known about the biological, behavioral, and psychosocial aspects associated with the menopausal process," noted a press release issued by the National Institute on Aging, one of the conference sponsors. Considering that in the next two decades approximately 40 million American women will pass through menopause and that, by the year 2012, women over fifty will comprise about half of the patients visiting ob-gyns, this statement would seem an embarrassing admission. As one researcher said, "Medicine's sudden interest in the treatment of problems associated with the postmenopausal period of life is at least twenty years late."

■ THE MISGUIDED CAMPAIGN
TO ELIMINATE MENOPAUSE: THE BIRTH OF HRT

At the NIH meeting battle lines were drawn, not along the usual basic versus clinical science, but along gender lines. In a breakout session in which a group of reproductive endocrinologists, ob-gyns, pathologists, neuroscientists, molecular and cellular biologists and nurse-researchers met to discuss the female ovary, the men all said what a good idea it would be to prevent or—at the very least—delay menopause. After all, they argued, humans are the only animals that go through a menopause. It must be an aberration. And with all these fortysomething women trying to have babies, wouldn't it be better to keep all women menstruating as long as possible, just in case?

To which the women researchers replied, "Absolutely not. There are many reasons we want to go through menopause. We want to stop breeding, we want to stop worrying about contraception, we want to stop bleeding every damn month. We want to experience this passage. We want research dollars to focus not on how to eliminate menopause but on how women can better get through it."

"When women are told by their doctors, 'You don't have to have menopause. You don't have to age,' feminists hear it as a gender put-down," says Brenda Weiss, a New York City psychotherapist specializing in midlife women's issues. "Menopause is a part of who we are. And who we are is, we're getting older. What's wrong with that?"

The campaign to eliminate menopause is nothing new. It was initiated by men, most notably male gynecologists, who, like some twentieth-century Pygmalions, believed they could create a class of middle-aged Wonder Women, women with firm breasts and skin, whose rich vaginal tissue ensured they would remain forever sexually appealing.

The way to accomplish this miracle of modern medicine? Through the ingestion of hormones. The medical community's love affair with estrogen began in the early 1960s with Brooklyn gynecologist Robert Wilson, who, like the legions of male doctors before him, considered menopause a deficiency disease. Much as diabetics needed insulin, he reasoned, menopausal women needed estrogen to prevent "being condemned to witness the death of their own womanhood."

Wilson, who viewed estrogen as a panacea, administered it to five thousand patients over a period of forty years. In 1963 he began prescribing it to premenopausal women as a means of preventing menopause. Wilson based his practice on flimsy science: a nonrandomized study of eighty-two women between the ages of thirty-two and fifty-seven, to whom he gave an estrogen-progestin oral contraceptive. Twenty-six of the twenty-seven premenopausal women taking the pill never experienced the usual menopausal symptoms, including hot flashes, thinning of the vaginal walls, and dry skin. Fifty-one of the fifty-five postmenopausal women taking estrogen got symptom relief.

In 1966, armed with these questionable data, Wilson published *Feminine Forever*, a book expounding his theories on estrogen. In it he described his Femininity Index, a means of measuring the amount of estrogen present in vaginal tissue. The more estrogen, he believed, the more feminine the woman. Wilson had become estrogen's biggest advocate. No one seemed to question the fact that his "study" was funded by Ayerst Laboratories, a maker of ERT, and G. D. Searle, a marketer of birth control pills.

In his book Wilson bemoaned the bone loss and metabolic disturbances estrogen-depleted women were certain to suffer, a deficiency that put them "in mortal danger," he wrote. "What impressed me most tragically is the destruction of personality. Some women, when they realize that they are no longer women, subside into a stupor of indifference."

Women who took estrogen could remain forever young. Wrote Wilson, "The outward signs of this age-defying youthfulness are a straight-backed posture, supple breast contours, taut, smooth skin on face and neck, firm muscle tone, and that particular vigor and grace typical of a healthy female. At fifty such women still look attractive in tennis shorts or sleeveless dresses."

Wilson made a convincing case for estrogen replacement. By 1975 six million women (one-third of those over age fifty) were taking Premarin, the Wyeth-Ayerst product, making it one of the top five prescription drugs sold in the United States. Yet the FDA had not cleared these birth control pills for the treatment of menopausal symptoms, nor had any research shown that estrogens were safe.

Then the bubble burst. Between 1975 and 1976 the *New England*

Journal of Medicine published four papers linking estrogen use with endometrial cancer. Two weeks after the first articles appeared, Wyeth-Ayerst
sent out a letter deriding the new research findings. But when the threat
of cancer enters the picture—no matter how remote—emotions rule. Estrogen prescriptions dropped 40 percent, and pharmaceutical companies
rushed in to do damage control.

The intensive campaign to rehabilitate ERT began with the collection
of data to demonstrate that the risks of endometrial cancer could be reduced by adding progestin to the ERT regimen. The theory was that progesterone would block the accumulation of estrogen in the uterine lining
and prevent the overstimulation of the endometrium, a process that was
thought to lead to the development of first hyperplasia and then cancer.

Soon all women who still had their uteruses were being told that they
must take progesterone with estrogen. Given the known dangers of unopposed estrogen, "it's almost malpractice to use estrogen without progestin
in a woman with a uterus," noted Isaac Schiff, M.D., a gynecologist at
Massachusetts General Hospital.

But progesterone is not without side effects either. Ninety percent of
the women who take it have menstruallike bleeding. Other side effects include depression, bloating, and fluid retention—in other words, good old
PMS. For a small group of women the adverse effects are even more troublesome. At the First Annual Congress on Women's Health in June 1993,
Karen Johnson, M.D., a San Francisco psychiatrist, stood up after a talk by
Isaac Schiff and told the group of three-hundred-plus physicians and nurses
that some of her menopausal patients came close to killing themselves
when taking HRT. "I have nine clinical cases of women who had no history of affective disorders but who developed major depression on hormone therapy," she said. "I almost lost people and I think it's secondary to
progestin."

During a break at the convention, Ruth Merkatz, Ph.D., the FDA's
special assistant for women's health issues, rushed over to Johnson. "You
need to report these adverse events. The FDA wants to hear about this."
For one thing the agency has not approved progestins for the treatment of
postmenopausal women and in fact has insisted on including the following
warning in every package of Premarin:

> Morphological and biochemical studies of endometrium suggested that
> 10 to 13 days of progestin are needed to provide maximal maturation of
> the endometrium and to eliminate hyperplastic changes. Whether this
> will provide protection from endometrial carcinoma has not been clearly

established. There are possible risks which may be associated with the inclusion of progestin in estrogen replacement regimens.

While the risk associated with unopposed estrogen is real and accepted by most public health experts, odds ratios are statistically small—about five per one thousand women taking unopposed estrogen will develop endometrial cancer, versus one in one thousand nonusers—indicating low to moderate associations, which are difficult to even confirm epidemiologically. What's more, studies didn't bother to screen out women who had preexisting disease, so the estrogen may simply have accelerated the growth of tumors that were already there.

The American College of Obstetricians and Gynecologists urges doctors to counsel women about the need for protection against endometrial cancer, and says that if estrogen-only therapy is used, a "biopsy should be performed prior to the initiation of therapy and annually thereafter." But because biopsies are painful, some physicians recommend them only if a woman experiences unexplained bleeding. Still others are prescribing small amounts of progesterone intermittently, which may be just as effective at sloughing off the endometrial lining as taking the drug for either twelve to fifteen days every cycle or on a daily basis.

What these varying practices point out is that no one knows at what doses, how often, or indeed whether progesterone even needs to be taken. Should all women take it or only the relatively few who are at an increased risk of developing endometrial cancer? How can these women be identified? No one knows. Once again women are unwitting participants in a massive, uncontrolled experiment.

■ OSTEOPOROSIS AND HRT

One of the few confirmed health-related benefits of HRT is its positive effect on women's bones. For the one-third or so of postmenopausal women who will develop osteoporosis, the consequences can be severe. The bone-thinning disorder is responsible for 1.3 million fractures and thirty thousand deaths annually as well as painful spinal deformities and disability.

In fact all women—and men—lose bone as they age. In the first five years after menopause a woman's bone density declines by about 2 percent a year. Although the rate slows to 1 percent a year and then remains constant, it can add up to a hefty 30 percent drop in bone mass by age eighty, the point at which women are more susceptible to fractures.

If osteoporosis is billed as the nemesis of aging women, then estrogen is their White Knight—studies have found that the use of postmenopausal estrogen can prevent bone loss and reduce the risk of a future hip fracture by more than 50 percent. Taking calcium seems to add to estrogen's effects.

It had been thought that estrogen was required for a minimum of five years to obtain a long-term effect on bone, but a 1993 Boston study suggested that at least seven years was necessary to preserve bone through age seventy-five. Women seventy-five and older, according to the study, were not protected by early ERT use.

Unfortunately these data are at odds with the way estrogen is actually used. Women tend to take it soon after menopause for short-term relief of such symptoms as hot flashes—the way pharmaceutical companies originally marketed it—and then discontinue it as they reach their sixties. When estrogen is stopped, however, bone density declines at a rate similar to that just after menopause. So by the time a woman reaches her eighties, when she's most likely to experience a hip fracture, she's also lost the protective effect of her early ERT use.

One option, posed in an editorial accompanying the Boston study, is to start estrogen at menopause and never stop. But most healthy women do not relish the idea of taking a drug for the rest of their lives. Then there is this question: Should all women be prescribed the hormone replacement regimen or only those known to be at risk for osteoporosis?

To further complicate the picture, even the agreed-upon risk factors—small bone structure, smoking, alcohol abuse, Caucasian race—may be red herrings, since they're based on studies of populations, not true predictors. Because these studies have tended to focus on upper income white women, they're not representative of the general population of middle-aged women. The studies don't differentiate women according to whether they've had a surgical or a natural menopause. And they don't include reliable assessments of potential risk factors.

While researchers have recently discovered the gene responsible for osteoporosis, until there is a way to screen women for this genetic propensity, the best way to gauge who will benefit from estrogen is to test bone mass at menopause. Such techniques as dual-photon absorptiometry (DPA) and dual-energy X-ray absorptiometry (DEXA) are 90 to 96 percent accurate at detecting bone loss in the hip and spine. What's more, bone densitometry tests are fast, painless, and safe.

But despite the fact that bone densitometry has been around for ten to fifteen years, Medicare considers some types of bone mass measurements experimental and will not reimburse their $150 to $200 cost. One reason for Medicare's resistance is that there have been no randomized clinical trials to determine whether a national program of bone mass measurement would lead to a reduction of fractures. Given the twenty- to thirty-year lag time between the start of bone loss and the occurrence of hip fractures, such trials will probably never take place.

Nevertheless the National Osteoporosis Foundation (NOF) believes the use of bone tests for women at high risk will reduce the rate of fractures. A 1989 study by the NOF found that the cost of providing bone mass measurement tests and therapeutic interventions for women at high risk produced a twentyfold savings to Medicare in terms of fracture reduction, says Sandra C. Raymond, NOF executive director. "The medical system becomes the benefactor of earlier measurement, because it won't have to pay the back-end cost of the hip or spinal fractures. It's so ridiculous that Medicare is not putting its imprimatur on this. They haven't focused on prevention."

The fact that Medicare doesn't reimburse means that other insurers don't either. So, says Ethel Siris, M.D., professor of clinical medicine at Columbia-Presbyterian Medical Center, "If you're a fifty-year-old woman trying to decide, 'Should I take estrogen? Maybe I'll do it if my bone mass is low,' your insurance company won't pay for the test.

"Not to reimburse when we have good ways to prevent osteoporosis is outrageous. This technique is so well standardized, it's not experimental. However, the message hasn't gotten through to the bureaucracy in Washington."

Indeed the only message that seems to have gotten out—courtesy of estrogen makers—is that all women should consider taking hormones if they want to avoid osteoporosis. A magazine ad for the Estraderm patch fairly shouts, "HOW TO KEEP THE CHANGE OF LIFE FROM CHANGING YOUR BONES." The copy explains that "you could lose up to 50 percent of all the bone mass you'll ever lose in just the first seven years after menopause begins." And doctors unfortunately play along.

■ HEART DISEASE AND HRT:
THE GREAT UNKNOWNS

In contrast to the marketing campaign waged around osteoporosis, drug companies have wisely kept away from discussions of HRT and heart disease, despite a raft of studies suggesting a decreased risk of heart problems in women taking estrogen. The 1991 Nurses' Health Study, for instance, found that women who used estrogen had a 50 percent reduction in the incidence of heart disease. It's telling, however, that the FDA has not found enough evidence to list cardiovascular protection as an indication for postmenopausal estrogen. Still, that hasn't stopped doctors from touting estrogen's supposed heart-healthy benefits, much to the chagrin of some women.

"I tried to find a gynecologist when I moved from Long Island to Manhattan," says Jane Porcino, the 71-year-old editor of *Hot Flash*, a newsletter for midlife and older women. "A friend recommended a doctor very highly. I went to her, and within five minutes she was talking to me about estrogen. I was not interested in estrogen. It was clear she didn't want me as a patient. She said, 'Don't call me in the middle of the night if you're having heart pain and you won't take estrogen.'"

She failed to mention to Porcino that women who take estrogen are probably healthier to begin with than those who don't. Estrogen takers tend to be slim, educated, upper-middle-class white women, factors that, by themselves, lower their risk of heart disease. These demographics alone may account for some or most of the apparent reduced mortality rates of estrogen therapy. Although, says William Harlan, M.D., of the Women's Health Initiative, "most of us believe the benefit [of estrogen on heart disease] is so striking that it goes beyond the self-selection of women who take estrogen."

Nevertheless, there is a concern that "we're dealing with epidemiologic data that essentially reflect what happened 10 years ago," says Wulf Utian, M.D., Ph.D., professor and chair of the department of ob/gyn at Case Western Reserve University. "The data cannot tell us what is happening now. A decade ago, because of the suspected association between heart disease and birth control pills, women with a history of heart disease were discouraged from taking estrogen [i.e., going on ERT]. How much of the reduced incidence of heart disease among women on estrogen replacement therapy is attributable to this pre-selection?"

Even with a large body of literature looking at cardiovascular risk, the mechanism by which estrogen supposedly prevents heart disease is still unknown. Some studies suggest that estrogen may directly affect the arterial walls by inhibiting the formation of plaque and improving the ability of blood vessels to expand as needed. Estrogen has already been shown to increase the "good" HDL cholesterol and lower the "bad" LDL cholesterol, but whether this action is responsible for the reduction in heart attacks is unknown.

Once again the uncertainties are mind-boggling, among them whether progestin will negate the apparent beneficial effects of estrogen on the heart. Of sixteen prospective trials on estrogen replacement and heart disease, almost none looked at the effect of progestins, even though they're known to increase LDL and decrease HDL, a worrisome side effect.

"To think of estrogen therapy as prevention for cardiovascular disease is really frightening," says Diana Taylor. "We don't have enough data. There's been no prospective randomized clinical trial of HRT until now [the Postmenopausal Estrogen/Progestin Interventions trial], and we won't have data for years."

Even William Harlan admits, "We've been distributing these drugs for decades without doing any randomized clinical trials. It's a black mark against the profession."

■ BREAST CANCER AND HRT: A TROUBLESOME CONNECTION

Perhaps the biggest worry about HRT—at least in the minds of women—is whether it causes breast cancer. A review of the studies on estrogen replacement without an added progestin suggests that there is no increased risk of breast cancer if a woman uses it for five years. After fifteen years, however, risk increases by 30 percent. Although this is a small statistical risk, for an individual woman, who already has a one-in-eight chance of getting breast cancer in her lifetime, it's an understandable cause of concern.

But because most of the breast cancer data come from women who used estrogen twenty or more years ago, when the average dose was 50 percent higher than what is currently prescribed, it's unknown whether the risk applies to today's lower-dose regimens. What is more, most studies have examined estrogen alone, not in conjunction with progestin. Of six studies that looked at combined estrogen-progestin therapy, two showed a protective effect, two showed an increased risk of breast cancer, and two showed no change.

All of which means that when it comes to HRT and breast cancer, the most the research community can offer is one big question mark. "Despite more than 50 epidemiologic and clinical studies and several meta-analyses that have considered the effect of estrogen replacement therapy on breast cancer risk, there is still no consensus on which women should not take supplementary estrogen because of a suspected increased risk of breast cancer," noted an article in the *Journal of the American Medical Association.*

Even Trudy Bush, Ph.D., an epidemiologist at the Johns Hopkins School of Public Health, admits, "I honestly don't know whether it's estrogen or menopause that increases the risk of breast cancer. When you look at the literature, you can see what you want to. It's an emotionally charged issue.

"My perspective is that if menopausal hormonal therapy does increase the risk of breast cancer, it is too small for us to be able to detect at this time. We're not going to have the answer to this question until we follow a cohort of women to see if the lifetime risk of breast cancer is increased with hormone use. That's because there is a very real reason to suspect that estrogens may promote the growth of in situ tumors [those that haven't invaded neighboring tissue], permitting them to be diagnosed at an earlier stage and looking like there is an apparent increase." In other words, perhaps estrogen does not cause new breast cancer but stimulates the growth of existing tumors.

The lack of knowledge is particularly frustrating for women who have had breast cancer, many of whom enter premature menopause as a result of their treatment and desperately want to go on estrogen not only to preserve their bones but to relieve bothersome menopausal symptoms. The package insert for estrogen advises against its use by women who have had a malignancy, but Bush is not convinced these women should be steered away from replacement hormones. She explains, "If you go back and read the literature of twenty or thirty years ago, the major hormonal therapeutic agent used to treat postmenopausal breast cancer was estrogen, and you got a 35 to 40 percent remission rate, which looked very good. Somehow, in the interim, we've lost that information. I think we can be somewhat reassured that we probably would not be doing harm by giving women with breast cancer hormone therapy."

Of course the fear is that in a cancer patient malignant cells will travel through the bloodstream to another part of the body, where they'll cause a recurrence. "There aren't any data that say estrogen makes breast cancer worse," says Peter Hickox, M.D., a gynecologist specializing in reproductive endocrinology at the Cleveland Clinic in Fort Lauderdale, Florida. "The question is, 'Is estrogen a carcinogen? Does estrogen have some cancer-promoting effect?'"

In a climate of uncertainty, he says, "there is physician fear and patient fear of taking estrogen—and rightly so." But perhaps the biggest barrier to prescribing estrogen to women with a history of breast cancer is the fear of a medical malpractice suit. "You don't want to be the physician who has their signature on an estrogen prescription when the breast cancer patient has a recurrence."

■ HRT: OTHER POTENTIAL DANGERS

Few women are aware of some less publicized concerns about estrogen: for instance, the facts that it might be both habit-forming and adversely affect the immune system. Estrogen is known to suppress T cells, the disease-fighting white blood cells. "Many women are getting estrogen supplementation after menopause, and we have absolutely no idea how these estrogens will affect the immune system," says Deborah Anderson, Ph.D., an associate professor at the Harvard Medical School. "We know that natural estrogens promote some effects of aging, including a decline in immune function. In some studies synthetic estrogens are even stronger in that effect, so they could presumably make autoimmunity worse."

Another rarely discussed issue is that of estrogen addiction. In an editorial in the British journal *Lancet*, Susan Bewley, M.D., an ob-gyn at the University College Hospital in London, suggests that HRT injections (or implants as they're called in Great Britain) promote feelings of well-being. "Drugs that rapidly promote a feeling of well-being are more likely than other types of drugs to induce dependence, and those taken by injection can produce dependence faster and more powerfully than substances taken orally," she wrote. "Those taking HRT might be investigated for DSM-III-R criteria of dependence."

Howard Judd, M.D., a reproductive endocrinologist at UCLA, dittos Bewley's theory. "I believe there is a drug dependence with estrogen," he says. "We and others have shown that when you administer estrogens to postmenopausal women, opioids within the hypothalamus go up. So that's a clear way that an individual has the potential to become dependent." Even if a fraction of the 9 percent of postmenopausal women taking estrogen in the United Kingdom, and the 15 percent in America, are dependent, it adds up to a worrisome number. Despite Bewley's legitimate concerns, she has not been able to get funding to administer a simple questionnaire to investigate estrogen dependence.

■ THE MARKETING OF HRT

A large body of evidence suggests a cautious approach to the use of hormone replacement therapy, but this is not the message the makers of the drug want to convey. Indeed, they have worked hard to co-opt the discussion of menopause and, in doing so, have helped to reinforce the image of "the change" as a disease in search of a cure. In 1992 Wyeth-Ayerst spent

$9.2 million advertising Premarin in women's magazines, while Ciba-Geigy forked out $4.7 million on ads for its Estraderm patch. Besides ads in national magazines and top medical journals, companies also put their marketing dollars into sponsoring medical conferences, where they preach to the converted and try to convert the undecided. Ciba-Geigy has been sponsoring menopause seminars around the country since 1988. Led by local doctors and nurses, the meetings have drawn as many as one thousand women eager for information. While the programs do not push estrogen nor the patch, women leave with brochures on HRT, courtesy of Ciba. The message is clear: Estrogen, like the Pill—which has been shown to reduce a woman's risk of ovarian cancer—is good for you.

Ciba-Geigy has also sent out direct-mail solicitations promoting its patch. Cynthia Pearson, program director of the National Women's Health Network, told a congressional hearing that her organization was "outraged that a potentially risky drug is being promoted with the same techniques used by Publishers Clearinghouse Sweepstakes."

In 1993 Wyeth-Ayerst established the Women's Health Research Institute which, among other endeavors, will attempt to develop new therapies to treat menopausal symptoms. Wyeth-Ayerst also donated 100 million tablets of Premarin for use in the Women's Health Initiative. "They realize the potential to treat the postmenopausal women in the baby boom," says Nancy Reame, R.N., Ph.D., a menopause researcher at the University of Michigan.

By most accounts the campaign to market hormone therapy has been a success. In 1990 U.S. sales of estrogen were estimated at $460 million and in 1992 Premarin, the top-selling estrogen, became the most prescribed drug in the country.

■ HRT IN THE REAL WORLD:
A DISQUIETING LACK OF INFORMATION

To a large degree, however, drug companies have succeeded only in persuading doctors to prescribe HRT. For the majority of women, though, estrogen has been a hard pill to swallow. Consider that only 15 percent of the postmenopausal women in the United States take estrogen, and the majority of them stay on it for an average of only nine months, hardly a resounding endorsement.

The medical profession has a word for this situation—noncompliance—and it's trotted out at every meeting in which the subject of menopause is discussed. Doctors' jobs are to treat disease, usually with medication. When they prescribe a drug, they expect their patients to use it for as long as the doctor thinks it's necessary. That they can't achieve compliance with HRT utterly discombobulates them. Why, they want to know, aren't women eager to take a drug with so many wonderful fringe benefits? How, they ask, can we change women's irrational behavior?

"The problem is, women don't know if [estrogen is] of any benefit," says Lewis Kuller, M.D., an epidemiologist at the University of Pittsburgh. "I don't blame them. We have forty years of the largest uncontrolled experiment ever perpetuated on the human population. Now, after forty years, we're trying to get basic answers."

As one sixty-six-year-old HRT user lamented, "I'd love to stop taking it, but I'm afraid to stop taking it, and I'm afraid to keep going on. It's a dilemma because there's no one place to get definitive advice. It's gotten to be a very confused issue."

Just how confusing became apparent to Marilyn Rothert, Ph.D., R.N., a professor of nursing at Michigan State University. Rothert and her colleagues handed out three pages of information about the trade-offs of HRT, which they asked women to read as part of a study. "The women were so hungry for information, they stole the information sheets," she says.

The National Institute on Aging's Sheryl Sherman sees the same hunger on the Washington social circuit. "I can't go to a cocktail party and tell people what I do professionally and not have them want information on menopause. Women don't understand what is normal, and physicians don't understand what is normal and can't answer questions about hormone therapy when they would like to, because they don't have information on the estrogen issue."

Even health spas are answering the call of the menopausal woman. Brenda Weiss remembers arriving at Tucson's Canyon Ranch one February to find a menopause roundtable on the schedule. To her surprise, Weiss, who was on the cusp of the change, "found a room filled to capacity. It was jammed, standing room only. People were sitting on the floor and tables. You could have cut the anxiety with a knife. It suddenly became clear to me, these were affluent, sophisticated, educated women. They had access to the top physicians in the country, but they felt that their needs weren't being addressed. They had little but old wives' tales to draw on. Many had bad-doctor stories. Others felt betrayed."

Women doctors live with the same sense of betrayal. Karen Johnson, the San Francisco psychiatrist, gets together regularly with a group of women physicians involved in women's health issues. "We're all in our forties and fifties. At some point in the evening the conversation turns to, 'What are you going to do about hormone replacement?' We're all in the field and none of us knows what to do. This is nuts. We're women. We're physicians. We're scientists. We're medical educators. And we're saying we cannot provide the kind of quality care to women that we want to because we don't have information."

Of course this doesn't stop most doctors. All too often, women say, hormone therapy is pushed on them, or they are excluded entirely from the decision-making process. Says Wulf Utian, "We can't expect women to comply with a medication regimen when they may not completely understand the reasons for doing so, or when they may not be receiving the best treatment option for their particular situation. The onus is on physicians to initiate discussions about menopause and tailor treatment to the individual."

Individualizing treatment is time-consuming but necessary. If a woman notices an untoward side effect on one form of estrogen, her doctor has to be willing to try another product or delivery system. If the pill isn't suitable, perhaps the patch will be. Doses, too, often have to be adjusted upward or downward. Some women return to their doctors half a dozen times until they get it right.

"A physician can't say, 'This is what you take, period,' " says UCLA's Howard Judd. "These are very powerful chemicals. They have very different effects from one patient to the next. You've got to be very flexible."

Yet studies show widely inconsistent prescribing practices. In one San Diego clinic, more than half of the postmenopausal women with intact uteruses were taking estrogen without progestin, as prescribed by their doctors. Another survey, of 330 gynecologists in Los Angeles, found that 47 percent had prescribed progestins to women *without* uteruses. This lack of uniformity may explain Congresswoman Patricia Schroeder's stinging comment: "If you get six menopausal women together, you'll find that their doctors are doing six different things. Our joke is that you might as well go to a veterinarian."

Women want an unbiased presentation of facts. They want true informed consent. Here the medical profession has fallen woefully short. When Phyllis Kernoff Mansfield, a health education researcher at Pennsylvania State University, and Ann Voda, a nursing professor at the University of Utah, surveyed 505 middle-aged women about menopause, they found that these women's doctors were amazingly uninformative. Only 16 percent of the women surveyed said health professionals were the major source of advice. When one woman asked what changes to expect during menopause, her physician told her to ask her mother.

In terms of symptom relief, physicians are incredibly myopic. A 1993 Gallup survey found that 67 percent of the physicians had discussed treatments with their patients for such symptoms as hot flashes and night sweats, and 84 percent of these discussions centered on HRT. Interestingly, in another study, female doctors were more likely than male doctors to prescribe HRT, perhaps because they had more empathy with their female patients' complaints.

The Gallup survey also found that fewer than 2 percent of physicians discussed such nonhormonal therapies as diet, exercise, stress reduction techniques, and smoking cessation. "What women want to know is not what doctors want to tell them," says Ruth Jacobowitz, whose own traumatic menopause led her to write two books on the subject. "It's outrageous that 51 percent of the population goes through this period in life and the medical profession doesn't know what it's doing. You'd think they'd be more embarrassed than they are."

Women want to know more about the role of calcium and exercise in preventing osteoporosis, and about alternative therapies for hot flashes, urinary incontinence, and vaginal dryness. Studies by Robert Freedman, Ph.D., at Wayne State University, have shown that a combination of progressive muscle relaxation and slow, deep breathing reduced women's hot flashes by about 50 percent. Other women are getting symptom relief with such natural remedies as Chinese herbs, vitamins, and minerals. Further research in this area would be welcomed by women.

■ EMOTIONAL CHANGES OF MIDLIFE

Menopause is often thought to be the only event of midlife. But there are other issues that concern women—incontinence, cognitive function, depression, and sexuality—during this important period of their lives. An examination of these issues might not make money for drug companies but would have far-reaching effects for women.

Women's sexuality at midlife is poorly understood. While both men and women lose some sexual function with age, women may suffer needlessly from decreased libido. Studies suggest that adding the male hormone testosterone, an androgen, to postmenopausal estrogen therapy increases well-being, sexuality, and libido in surgically menopausal women. Morrie Gelfand, M.D., a Canadian researcher who has been studying and prescribing androgens for twenty-five years, says the estrogen-androgen combination is the fourth top-selling drug in Canada.

But doctors, particularly in the United States, are loath even to mention it to their middle-aged patients. "Of the women who finally find their way to our clinic," says Gelfand, "four out of five have been told to see psychologists about their sexual problems. Women really are treated like second-class citizens, and doctors are the culprits. They don't think about the quality of life in older women. They think they're just lucky to be alive, so why should they be worrying about their sexuality. If they had the same hormones for men, they'd be lining up all the way from Washington to L.A. to get them."

Yet questions remain about the regimen's safety. In studies at McGill University in Montreal, androgens appear to be antiestrogenic in terms of the breast, which means they may reduce the risk of breast cancer, but no one knows for sure. The FDA's Jean Fourcroy has been hearing sporadic reports of a disturbing adverse effect: decreased liver function. "The FDA is uncomfortable with the use of testosterone hormone replacement," she says. "We have little data on its safety or efficacy."

Much more also needs to be known about the emotional changes during midlife. Some women complain about moodiness, depression, anxiety, and irritability, yet there are no data linking these disturbing symptoms to the hormonal changes of menopause. Several studies that followed women forward through time have found that depressive symptoms do increase with age but not with menopausal status. The most depressed women are not older women but mothers in their thirties raising young children. "Menopause does not cause depression," one researcher states flatly.

Women troubled by depressive feelings at menopause consider this attitude dismissive. Why, they want to know, are their subjective experiences of their own menopause being discounted?

Maybe they should be thanking doctors for refusing to saddle them with that nineteenth-century construct, climacteric insanity, which eventually made its way into the American Psychiatric Association's diagnostic manual as "involutional melancholia." While the mental disorder originally applied to both women and men, it quickly became a menopausal disease, characterized by restlessness, motor agitation, anxiety, hypochondriasis, insomnia, and feelings of guilt and worthlessness.

With the APA's stamp of approval, psychiatrists could achieve the heady thrill that comes from researching a "cure." Small, uncontrolled studies, usually conducted on institutionalized women, led to treatment with ovarian extracts in the 1920s, estrogen in the 1930s, and electroshock therapy in the 1940s. In 1979, when it had been determined that depression did not peak at menopause, involutional melancholia was stricken from the psychiatric manual. If a woman became depressed during menopause, she usually had a prior history of major depression.

Still, the debate over menopausal mood changes rages on. Research confirms that the brain, like a woman's uterus and breasts, contains estrogen receptors, sites through which hormones enter cells. Studies suggest that a drop in estrogen may cause a corresponding drop in the brain chemical serotonin, a neurotransmitter related to mood, which could explain women's feelings of anxiety and irritability around the climacteric. Research at McGill University suggests that taking estrogen can improve memory as well as mood swings, irritability, and anxiety.

Some researchers go so far as to suggest that estrogen may act as an antidepressant, a point on which many doctors are not well versed. "Typically women go to the doctor and they are told there is nothing wrong with them," says Gillian Ford, a PMS and menopause educator in Auburn, California. "Their doctors imply that they're neurotic and say, 'You need to go see a psychiatrist and go on antidepressants.' And many times these problems can be solved very easily by giving them low doses of natural hormones. The side effects are far less dangerous than a drug like Prozac."

There are hints that a drop in progesterone may also affect one's emotional state, but even if this association proves correct, there are important nonhormonal reasons why a woman may get the blues. If night sweats are waking her ten times a night and she floats through the next day sleep deprived, is it any wonder she feels irritable and out of sorts? All she really needs is a good night's sleep, not a prescription for Prozac.

■ CULTURAL EXPECTATIONS AT MIDLIFE

A more rational and less medicalized view of menopause begins with the understanding that it is not a single event and it does not occur in a vacuum. Rather menopause is a transition during which many women choose to reexamine their lives, a time when a variety of major life changes converge. Adult children may be leaving—or moving back—home. A woman may be contending with divorce, the death of a spouse or partner, or caring for her aging parents. Menopause, when seen in this context, is not just a transition from reproductive to nonreproductive status, but from youth to midlife.

It doesn't help that the climacteric has become synonymous with aging. "The culture has managed to make women fearful that mid-life marks the fall into aging, and menopause means you wake up overnight an alarmingly diminished person," wrote Margaret Morganroth Gullette in *Ms.* "The fear of the sudden loss of self begins long before a woman nears the likely age of her menopause."

Indeed it's young women who dread it the most. In a youth-oriented society that brands a woman old at the first sign of a wrinkle, in which the fears of aging are reinforced in the mass media, it's no surprise that women spend their forties dreading their impending disintegration. Gullette contends that menopause "is on its way to becoming a psychosomatic disease for women who haven't had it yet, who are being made hyperconscious of the ailments of old-old age and of 'female' causes of death. The last half of adulthood is collapsed into itself, mercilessly shortened. This is a form of cultural terrorism."

Difficulties with menopause are greatest in patriarchal cultures that offer older women few significant social roles. In castes in India, in contrast, women have few hot flashes and other symptoms. "Menopause, for them, is a time of positive changes," says physical anthropologist Marcha Flint, a professor at Montclair State University. "Until then they had to remain veiled and secluded. But after menopause they could leave seclusion and interact with men."

In some Muslim cultures a woman is thought to be holier after menopause because she's stopped menstruating. In Indonesia a woman partakes of a celebratory ceremony when she crosses the great divide into midlife. "The woman is regarded as a source of wisdom, an asset to the community," says Flint. "In America we write women off after menopause."

■ OLD AGE: THE INVISIBLE WOMAN

If our culture writes women off after menopause, it renders them downright invisible when they traverse midlife into old age. Nothing throws the gender gap in women's health into sharper relief than the issue of aging. Women currently constitute more than two-thirds of those eighty-five and older. By the year 2020 there will be sixty-nine men for every one hundred women aged sixty-five, and thirty-six men per one hundred women aged eighty-five. Yet along with women's survival advantage comes more chronic conditions and disabilities, making them more likely than men to spend the last years of their lives in a nursing home.

Much of the age-related decline in women is not due to the natural aging process but to a complex interaction between disease, lifestyle, nutrition, psychological status, and social support. Concluded a report by the Office of Research on Women's Health, "Women survive through the decades that claim their male peers from cardiovascular disease and cancer. They provide care and succor, but when they become ill, they have neither social support nor caregivers. If they survive the common diseases, they live long enough to develop the devastating illnesses that are unique to the very old: geriatric malignancies, osteoporosis, incontinence, and neurological degenerative diseases."

Yet, the report noted, research on the gender-specific biological and psychological processes that lead to disease and frailty in older women has been conspicuously absent. It's difficult to separate out how much of this neglect is due to ageism, how much to sexism. Because there are more elderly women than men, ageism, in a strange sleight of hand, becomes sexism, which is compounded by the medical profession's proclivity toward turning aging—like midlife—into a disease.

Because there are more elderly women than men, aging—and, by extension, geriatric medicine—is primarily concerned with women's health. Unfortunately, as in other areas of primary care, new physicians are not flocking into the field. In 1992, 270 fellowship positions were available in geriatrics programs within internal medicine, and only 181 were filled. A paltry eight of this country's 126 medical schools require separate courses in geriatric medicine. And only one medical school, Mount Sinai in New York City, has a department of geriatrics through which all medical students are required to rotate.

"Physicians don't understand what old age is," says Mildred Seltzer, Ph.D., a researcher at Scripps Gerontology Center at Miami University in Ohio. "They associate it with illness and don't differentiate between the two. The result is a lot of discriminatory behavior, both conscious and unconscious. For example, if an old woman has a disorder, it's not diagnosed as quickly as it would be if it were in a younger woman, because her complaints are assumed to be simply a matter of age."

Elderly women are less apt to be screened for breast and cervical cancers. They get less aggressive treatment compared with both men and younger women and are less likely to be included in clinical trials. Many studies of the elderly are conducted in Veterans Administration hospitals, virtually ensuring that older women will be excluded. When women are interested in participating in research, they often find there are criteria that specifically exclude all people over the age of sixty-five.

Women past the menopause no longer have troublesome hormonal fluctuations to confound study results, so it could be safely assumed that researchers would be eager to study them. No such luck. "They enter the netherworld of the elderly, where researchers begin to worry about the in-

creased risks of side effects," says Myrna Lewis, M.S.W., a gerontologist
and assistant professor at the Mount Sinai School of Medicine. "This, too,
was a complication that until recently was avoided by limiting research to
middle-aged and young-old men." As a result little is known about normal
aging in women.

The Baltimore Longitudinal Study on Aging (BLSA) is a case in
point. One of the largest and most important studies of its type, it included no women for its first twenty years—because the ward at the
city hospital in which the study was being conducted had only one toilet. It took until 1968—ten years into the study—to improve the facilities, but still no women were enrolled. The excuse this time: funding
and staff shortages.

Myrna Lewis was amazed at how deeply ingrained the anti-female bias
was. Strolling the corridors of the Gerontological Research Center at the
National Institute on Aging, the site of the BLSA, she saw a research assistant rush by with a box of young mice.

"Are they headed for a research lab?" she asked.

"No, they're headed for the incinerator."

Why? Because they were females.

The assistant explained that the little mice's estrous cycles would complicate the research and confound the results.

It was the same old party line. Rather than presenting a unique
research opportunity, female hormones were a source of annoyance.

One accomplishment of the Baltimore Longitudinal Study was its November 1984 report "Normal Human Aging," which summarized the major published findings from the study's first twenty-three years. It included
important data from men in their twenties all the way to their eighties. But
the report had no longitudinal data on aging in women because they had
not been in the study long enough. Due to this glaring omission, "years of
information on how women age has been lost," says Anne Colston Wentz,
M.D., of Northwestern University Medical School. Physicians who had
hoped to use these data to counsel and treat their elderly female patients
were out of luck.

Despite the eventual inclusion of women in the BLSA, there were not
always a sufficient number in the various age groups to yield useful data.
Testifying before Congress in 1990, the General Accounting Office's Mark
Nadel admitted to hearing "of a case in which there were not enough
BLSA women in the 45 to 60 year age group to perform certain studies re-
lating to menopause."

"Considering that the majority of older people are women, it's quite a shock that all the data you've got on normal aging is based on men," says Mildred Seltzer.

HEALTH PROBLEMS OF OLD AGE

Only in the last few years have there been good data on the barriers to successful aging in women. One of them—caring for an ill or disabled spouse—is an example of a social issue that has become an important women's health issue. When men become infirm, they're more apt to have their wives around to care for them. Yet numerous studies are finding that caretaking exacts a harsh toll both physically and psychically. Work by Janice Kiecolt-Glaser, Ph.D., and her husband, Ronald Glaser, Ph.D., of the department of psychiatry at Ohio State University College of Medicine, suggests that elderly caregivers who lack social support have higher systolic blood pressure compared with their younger counterparts. In other studies caregivers reported more days of infectious illness, and there are hints that the stress of caregiving has an adverse effect on the immune system. Caregiving also places older women at an increased risk of depression. At least one-third of the caregiving spouses of demented older adults are thought to suffer from a diagnosable depressive disorder.

Frailty—impaired physical functioning and susceptibility to injuries and acute illness—is especially problematic for elderly women and is the major reason they require long-term care. "It turns out that women, at a given level of dysfunction, are more frail and disabled than men," says William Hazzard, M.D., director of the J. Paul Stricht Center on Aging at Wake Forest University's Bowman Gray School of Medicine. "You take an eighty-two-year-old woman with osteoarthritis and an eighty-two-year-old man with osteoarthritis and the woman is functionally more disabled than the man. Most people think that because she's weaker in her muscles, there's less strength in her bones, but it may well be a hormonal or genetic issue. The bottom line is: women are disabled and tend to have to live longer with their disability."

As these women outlive their spouses—and if they don't succumb to heart disease or cancer—they are often afflicted with nonfatal age-dependent diseases. Things like arthritis, incontinence, visual and hearing impairments, dementia, and Alzheimer's. "These illnesses haven't attracted nearly the amount of scientific interest and research support as fatal diseases," says Christine Cassel, M.D., director of the Center of Aging, Health and Society at the University of Chicago. "Alzheimer's is our single biggest fear about aging, yet we spend one-two-hundredth the amount on Alzheimer's research that we do on heart disease or cancer."

Incontinence has received even less research attention. Although some 37 percent of women over age sixty who reside in the general population and half of nursing-home residents suffer from the condition, its causes are still not known. The age-related decline in estrogen is thought to be a major factor. Indeed estrogen is often used to manage urinary incontinence during and after menopause. But studies supporting this practice are scarce.

After reviewing data from twenty-three clinical trials on estrogen and urinary incontinence conducted between 1969 and 1992, the most genitourinary specialist J. Andrew Fantl, M.D., could say is, "There seems to be an effect [with estrogen]. It's subjective. People say they're better, but we can't quantify it objectively."

Incontinence is not a life-threatening disease, but it can severely impair a woman's quality of life. Fantl tells stories about patients who stop socializing and give up their favorite activities to accommodate their bladders, or resign themselves to wearing adult diapers, not aware there are treatments.

Many women never even tell their doctors they're having problems, and their doctors usually don't ask. In a study conducted by Fantl, professor of obstetrics and gynecology at the Medical College of Virginia, the mean time between a person's initial symptoms to when they showed up at his office was ten years. When urogynecologist Peggy Norton of the University of Utah School of Medicine asked women why they waited so long before seeking help, 50 percent said they were too embarrassed to discuss the subject with their doctors.

"Incontinence is not an inevitable part of the aging process," says Fantl. But doctors often behave as if it is. Fantl shakes his head as he describes the "pats on the back given to women with incontinence. The prevailing attitude is: 'You had three babies, what do you expect?' " Such an attitude is not surprising given that incontinence is not appropriately covered in medical school nor in residency training. Why? "It isn't considered a real disease," says Norton.

That female urinary incontinence is a low priority was driven home when Fantl participated in a committee convened by the Agency for Health Care Policy and Research to develop guidelines for treating the condition. As he set about analyzing the data, he was floored by the lack of good studies. "There are six controlled trials in the world's literature and seventeen uncontrolled trials. The study design is totally erratic. There's no standardization in patient selection, and quality of life is rarely included in outcomes of clinical trials in women. It's not enough to say we treated women and decreased their incontinence 64 percent. What does that mean to a woman, that instead of playing three sets of tennis, she can play one?"

If incontinence is what one researcher calls the last taboo subject, sexuality may be a close second. Painful intercourse is the most common sexual complaint of older women, but unless a physician asks, a woman rarely tells. Unfortunately physicians are often just as uncomfortable bringing the subject up. It's probably not surprising given that few medical school training programs emphasize sexuality, particularly among the elderly.

When the subject is raised, doctors are often repelled by the thought of an elderly woman having sex. June LaValleur, M.D., an ob-gyn and director of the Mature Women's Center at the University of Minnesota, recalls a course in human sexuality that she took as a medical student in the late 1980s. "We had to look at films of people having sex with animals. We saw young heterosexual couples, young homosexual couples, and old couples having sex. What turned people off was not the sex with animals, it was a couple in their eighties making love. All around me young men were saying, 'Oh my God, what does he see in her?' "

What would happen if an elderly woman were to consult one of these doctors today? Would he raise the subject of sexuality with her? Would he be able to empathize with her if she brought up a sexual problem? In all likelihood, no.

Cultural biases die hard. The nation isn't ready to accept an elderly woman as sexually attractive. "Elderly women are not supposed to have sexual desires," says LaValleur. "They're supposed to be frail and unable to make love even if they wanted to. They're considered physically unattractive. The whole notion of older people having sex is considered shameful and perverse."

For these reasons there are very little data on the sexual practices of the elderly, let alone older women. Only three of the 1,700 pages in the two Kinsey reports are devoted to people over sixty. A mere one-half page focuses on elderly women. Fewer than 5 percent of the men and women studied by Masters and Johnson in the 1960s and 1970s were over sixty-five.

Yet studies suggest that two-thirds of women between the ages of sixty and seventy remain sexually active. Some elderly women notice an improved body image, despite their gray hair, drooping skin, and chronic illnesses. "Older women can begin to accept themselves," says Sheryl Kingsberg, Ph.D., a Case Western Reserve psychologist who trains medical students and residents in sexual history taking. "They've matured, come into their own. They've stopped striving to meet an unrealistic ideal."

When a woman's sexual activity does decline, notes the Kinsey report, it is usually "controlled by the male's desires, and it is primarily his aging rather than the female's loss of interest or capacity which is reflected in the decline."

OLDER WOMEN, DISMISSIVE HEALTH CARE

Just as doctors characterize menopause as a deficiency disease, aging, too, is seen as a disorder in need of a cure. While some elderly women do suffer from ailments and disabilities, aging per se is a normal transition. "Aging is not a disease," says Wake Forest University's William Hazzard. "It's a backdrop against which disease develops. But as the population ages and as the problems of older people are highlighted, the problems of women emerge as more important than previously thought because they are surviving."

Women's survival is bringing other social and economic issues to the forefront. When elderly women lose their spouses, they often lose their main source of financial support. And since in the United States, as of this writing, health is a function of socioeconomic status because one's finances determine access to medical care, it only follows that more women than men will be locked out of the health care system.

Between the ages of forty-five and sixty-four, women comprise 84 percent of the widowed population and 87 percent of the uninsured. Relative to their numbers in the population, women are overrepresented on the Medicaid rolls, the health insurance program for the poor. In 1993, there were more than 19 million women enrolled in Medicare—the federal insurance program for people sixty-five and older—versus 13 million men.

With chronic health problems, and no one to care for them, elderly women are more likely than men to become institutionalized. Women make up three-fourths of the two million nursing-home residents. Because most women do not have private long-term care insurance, they or their families end up paying more than half of their nursing-home costs out-of-pocket.

The one-two punch of ageism followed by sexism knocks many women out of the health care ring entirely. And when they're fortunate enough to be able to afford medical care, that care is often shoddy at best. Says Mary Harding (a pseudonym), a seventy-five-year-old retired office manager in New York City, "When you talk about your aches and pains, doctors tell you, 'Well, you're getting older.' But every ache and pain doesn't have to do with getting older. There can still be some kind of help for you."

On numerous occasions, however, there was no help for Harding. When she saw an internist about a condition known as reflux, a backup of stomach acid into the esophagus, he dismissed the problem and instead lectured her about the pneumonia and phlebitis from which he was sure she would suffer in the near future. More than five years later none of his dire predictions have come true. Her reflux, meanwhile, went away on its own, no thanks to her doctor.

On another occasion a female gynecologist who had come highly recommended did a pelvic exam on Harding without sufficiently lubricating the speculum. Harding screamed in pain. "It was like a rape with an instrument," she says. The gynecologist should have been aware that older women who are not on estrogen are more likely to experience vaginal dryness; she should have taken precautions. (To prevent mishaps like this, more doctors are beginning to specialize in geriatric gynecology.)

As Nena O'Neill, a seventy-year-old New York City widow, laments, "We've become invisible. After a while we accept it as a part of life. It's hard to distinguish if our poor care is because of gender or age, or both. The tricky thing with bias is that it's hidden, so there are always other possible explanations for it."

Whether it stems from ageism or sexism, the paternalistic treatment of elderly women comes off as a gender put-down. How else to explain what happened to Hazel Johnson? When the seventy-six-year-old Baltimore woman began having fainting spells, her family took her to a respected internist, who proceeded to schedule every high-tech test in the book.

"Hop up on the examining table," he said, his back to Johnson.

A short, petite women, Johnson's hopping days were long over. She stayed put.

"I thought I said, 'Get up on the examining table,'" the doctor barked.

Johnson was stunned. "Goddammit, I can't get up," she shot back.

Appalled by the doctor's lack of sensitivity, Johnson's family promptly got her to a geriatrician, who was the first physician to deal practically with her functional difficulties. First he got her on blood pressure medication, which alleviated her fainting spells. Then, with the whole family present, he talked to Johnson and genuinely seemed to care. He asked her what she felt her everyday problems were, whether she could get dressed by herself, whether she still drove. He asked to watch her walk. "It was like coming out of a tunnel into lightness," her daughter, Sylvia Eggleston-Wehr, says.

If elderly women subjectively feel that their health concerns are being minimized by the medical profession, studies bear this out. Marjorie

Pearson, Ph.D., of the Rand Health Sciences Program, wanted to know whether older women were in fact being treated differently than men. In examining hospital records of 11,242 men and women sixty-five and older who had been treated for congestive heart failure, acute myocardial infarction, pneumonia, and cerebrovascular accidents, she found that women received slightly worse care than men, regardless of their age. Although the difference was small, the fact that there was any difference at all disturbed Pearson.

The medical profession's track record with preventive services isn't much better. If a woman is seeing a young physician, she's less likely to get rectal and pelvic exams. If she seeks care from an ob-gyn, she has a decent chance of receiving Pap smears and breast cancer screening, but few older women see ob-gyns for regular care. After their childbearing years are over, women often mistakenly believe that they no longer need gynecological care, so they shift to internists, who tend not to perform pelvics and Paps. In one study, 15 percent of women over age sixty-five reported never having had a Pap smear and another 25 percent said it had been more than five years since their last Pap. In general, internists are not trained in gynecological care, but even so, they should at least refer their elderly female patients to ob-gyns. Often they don't.

"The most famous line on many charts is 'pelvic deferred,' " says Robert Butler, M.D., chairman of the Department of Geriatrics at Mount Sinai School of Medicine in New York City. "This means that instead of doing the pelvic examination, the doctor simply avoided it."

An Atlanta woman recalls poring through her seventy-four-year-old mother's three-quarter-inch stack of medical records, only to find the ubiquitous "pelvic deferred." "It pissed me off," she says. "The gerontology clinic where she went for a full work-up hadn't even done a pelvic on her. She hadn't had a Pap in twenty-four years."

Some doctors wrongly believe that older women don't need to be screened for cervical cancer. But women sixty-five and over develop one-quarter of the new cases of cervical cancer each year and account for 41 percent of the deaths from the disease. In order to reduce mortality, therefore, screening programs need to target elderly women.

Unfortunately, official screening guidelines are confusing and inconsistent. The National Cancer Institute no longer sets screening policy. The American Cancer Society and the American College of Obstetricians and Gynecologists, meanwhile, recommend screening throughout a woman's lifetime, with no upper-age limit. And the Canadian Preventive Services Task Force recommends that screening stop at age seventy, assuming a woman has had two recent normal smears and has had no abnormal Paps within the previous nine years.

"Women develop cervical cancer in their sixties because of a lack of screening, not because of new disease," argues Anthony Miller, M.D., of the University of Toronto. "Providing you can be certain a woman has been well-screened previously, then screening at an older age is not required."

The United States Preventive Services Task Force apparently agrees, recommending that screening stop at age sixty-five, provided a physician can document that a woman's previous smears have been consistently normal.

As some of the major public health agencies backed away from screening the old, in the late 1980s Medicare announced plans to cover screening every three years with no upper age limit. Marianne Fahs, Ph.D., of Mount Sinai's Department of Community Medicine, and Jeanne Mandelblatt, M.D., were recruited to the Medicare project. A fellow in preventive medicine at Mount Sinai at the time, Mandelblatt knew firsthand that elderly women were not being adequately screened: they were showing up at the public hospital where she worked with invasive cervical cancer—one of the most preventable malignancies.

As they began work on the Medicare guidelines, says Fahs, "we realized that the data on older women was almost nonexistent. We don't know the natural progression of the disease in older women. We just don't have the studies. Older women have been ignored, and we've falsely assumed that they were fine."

Medicare's new guidelines went into effect in 1990. A subsequent analysis by Fahs, Mandelblatt (now at Memorial Sloan-Kettering Cancer Center), and others showed that screening elderly women for cervical cancer is indeed cost-effective. "Early detection of cervical neoplasia extends life for elderly women of all ages," their report notes. "Universal screening would result in a 74 percent reduction in cervical cancer-related deaths in the elderly. The cost-effectiveness ratio of $2,254 per year of life gained after triennial Pap smear screening is similar to expenditures for other preventive services for the elderly."

However cost-effective, preventive services, including mammography, are sorely underused in older women. As discussed in chapter 5, older women are less likely to get mammograms, even though they're at the greatest risk of developing a breast malignancy. And they receive fewer diagnostic evaluations—including lymph node dissections—which are considered essential for determining the stage of a tumor.

Kathleen Brenneman, M.D., a Washington, D.C., geriatrician, recalls a 72-year-old woman who came to her office after a year-and-a-half absence. "She had been going around the city . . . to health-fair screenings for senior citizens. She brought to me a stack of papers: cholesterol levels, blood pressure readings, hearing tests, eye exams, blood sugars. Not once did anyone mention a mammography to her.

"On exam, I found a large breast tumor that had already spread to her axilla. The woman now has a modified radical mastectomy and is undergoing radiation therapy. If a mammogram had been recommended at one of the health fairs . . . maybe the disease could have been caught much earlier and she could have avoided . . . this mutilating surgery."

In general, older women are less likely than younger women to undergo breast-conserving surgery, even when lumpectomy is appropriate. Whether or not they get a lumpectomy seems to depend on where they live. In 1986, for instance, the percentage of women sixty-five and older with early-stage breast cancer who underwent breast-conserving surgery varied from 3.5 percent in Kentucky to more than 20 percent in Massachusetts, New York, Pennsylvania, and Vermont.

Such variations in care are hard to explain, but they may partially be due to lifestyle considerations. "There are many older women for whom mastectomy may be preferable because they don't want six weeks of radiation therapy and they may not have a way to get to the appointments," says Rebecca Silliman, M.D., Ph.D., a geriatrician at the New England Medical Center in Boston. "The critical issue is whether they are offered the choice."

Equally troubling, those elderly women who receive breast-conserving surgery are less likely to get follow-up radiation, yet lumpectomy alone is considered to be inadequate. So far, there are few data on whether less aggressive care results in poorer outcomes. It is known that older women are more likely to be diagnosed with advanced disease and, when they are, their mortality is considerably higher than that for younger women.

What accounts for older women's less vigorous care? Part of the problem is that physicians may base treatment decisions on their personal beliefs about the elderly. In many cases, doctors are not even aware of life expectancy data that should influence decision-making. For instance, a study of practicing physicians found that one-third estimated the average life expectancy of a 75-year-old woman to be four years or fewer. "Fewer than 10 percent of the doctors were within two years of the actual life expectancy of 12 years," writes Silliman.

Doctors may also take their cue from their older women patients, who tend to ask fewer questions and end up facilitating physicians' paternalistic behavior. "It is well recognized that physicians spend either the same amount or less time with their older patients than their younger patients and do not actively involve them in medical decision-making," notes Silliman.

PUSHING PILLS TO THE ELDERLY

Older women take drugs at two times the rate of older men and are more likely to be on multiple medications. With more women than men surviving into old age, it seems obvious that women should make up the bulk of the study population in trials of drugs for which they will later be the major consumers. But women's patchwork quilt of illnesses, their use of multiple medications, and the chance that there may be gender differences in drug metabolism—issues that should be examined in their own right—are seen as confounding factors and form the basis for shutting women out as research subjects. As a result, age-related gender differences in drug response are seldom investigated.

Although 64 percent of patients eighty-five and older who die of acute myocardial infarction are women, most clinical trials to test new therapies exclude women over seventy. A review of 214 trials of drug therapies for heart attack involving 150,920 people found that fewer than 20 percent of randomized subjects were women. More than 60 percent of the studies excluded persons over the age of seventy-five. Studies with exclusions based on age had a smaller percentage of women compared with those without such exclusions.

"While traditional explanations for excluding women from clinical studies have included risk of teratogenicity [congenital abnormalities in offspring], hormonal fluctuations, the protective cardiovascular effects of estrogens, and reduced statistical power due to the less frequent occurrence of measured outcomes, these reasons would have little relevance to the vast majority of female acute myocardial infarction patients," wrote principal investigator Jerry Gurwitz.

If anything, it's ethically and scientifically advantageous to include women. Because death or recurrence—the most commonly measured outcomes in heart attack studies—are more likely to occur in elderly women, their inclusion would increase the chances of detecting the positive effects of a treatment. From an epidemiological standpoint, a therapy that reduces the risk of death by 25 percent in elderly patients will result in a substantially larger number of lives saved than a greater reduction in risk among younger patients, says Gurwitz. No matter how you look at it, studying older women is good science.

Excluding them means the insights gained from research cannot be extrapolated to older women with any kind of assurance. Indeed, physician confusion about how to apply data derived primarily from research on middle-aged men may explain the pervasive underuse of such drugs as clot-busters, beta-blockers, and antihypertensive therapy in elderly women.

It is known that older women have a higher fat-to-muscle ratio compared with men. This suggests that fat-soluble drugs—including such tranquilizing agents as benzodiazepines—have a longer half-life in women; that is, the same dose remains in a woman's bloodstream longer than it does in a man's.

Do most clinicians take such sex differences into account? "No," says Bruce Pollock, M.D., Ph.D., a geriatric psychopharmacologist at the University of Pittsburgh.

What's the practical effect of this neglect? "Women's dosages may be excessive," says Pollock, "which could, depending on what drug we're talking about, result in more impairment."

Antipsychotics, for instance, have greater efficacy in women compared with men. It's possible that unnecessarily high doses in women may put them at a greater risk for chronic side effects such as tardive dyskinesia, a neurological disorder that results in abnormal movement of the mouth and tongue. One study suggested that the incidence of tardive dyskinesia is far greater in women over age sixty-seven. "At best the disorder is unpleasant to look at," says Pollock. "At worst it can occur in the trunk and interfere with respiration."

Antidepressants also have varying effects depending on gender. Dextroamphetamine tends to sedate postmenopausal women, while inducing euphoria and increased alertness in young men. If one bought into the cultural stereotype—that elderly women have outlived their usefulness—then it wouldn't matter if they sat at home in a drug-induced stupor. In reality many older women have careers, travel, and lead active social lives. Not only can they not afford to be slowed down by a drug, the sedation can trigger a domino effect of negative health consequences.

One of those negative consequences is hip fractures, which can occur as a result of falls while on mood-altering drugs. Research conducted in 1987 in a Medicaid population suggests that up to 14 percent of hip fractures are directly attributable to psychotropic drug use. If this estimate can be generalized to all the elderly, it means that the use of these drugs may result in some thirty thousand excess hip features each year, most of which will occur in women. "Among these patients," wrote the study's authors, "there will be a 10-to-15 percent excess mortality rate in the year following the fracture, 50 percent will lose the capacity to walk independently, and up to one-third of those formerly dwelling in the community will require long-term nursing home care. The annual direct medical care cost associated with these 30,000 cases is approximately $1 billion."

Drug interactions present additional problems for elderly women. A 1989 study in the *Journal of Clinical Psychiatry* discussed case reports of four women who were taking an MAO inhibitor for depression in conjunction with over-the-counter cold and cough preparations. All of the women developed severe hypertensive reactions, but one of the women, who took an MAO inhibitor with an Alka-Seltzer Plus cold medication, died from the reaction. Said Philip Hansten, Ph.D., a professor at the University of Washington School of Pharmacy, "If this is from one center—I suspect . . . this is happening elsewhere, where it is not reaching the medical literature."

Elderly women taking multiple drugs are at an even greater risk of dangerous drug interactions. Since it will never be feasible to examine all the various drug combinations and their potential complications, clinicians must be scrupulous about filing adverse effect reports with the FDA. Although these data are after the fact, they may at least provide a body of evidence on which health care providers can base rational treatment decisions. Women's health advocates are eagerly awaiting the FDA's new guidelines for the inclusion of the elderly in clinical trials, due in 1994.

■ NEW HOPE

Despite the gloomy reports about the treatment of older women, new studies are focusing on successful aging and finding that there's much to celebrate. "One of the things we learned early on is that aging isn't as bad as we thought," says E. Jeffrey Metter, medical director of the Baltimore Longitudinal Study on Aging. "Many parts of the body continue to function quite well as one gets into older ages."

Other major longitudinal studies—Duke University, National Institute of Mental Health, and Swedish studies—have found that physical and mental decline is not an inevitable part of aging. Researchers at the Yale Health and Aging Project are drawing the same conclusion. The project, which has been surveying close to three thousand men and women over age sixty-five annually since 1982, is examining the psychosocial and biomedical factors that predict successful aging.

"A lot of people in their seventies are functioning like people in their fifties and sixties," says Lisa F. Berkman, Ph.D., codirector of the project. "We've also found that people improve in functioning." Self-efficacy— maintaining one's activities, using cognitive skills, and exercising choice— appears to be a more important predictor of functioning than age itself.

These data should help plot a course for future research. If aging is indeed normal, if we are not genetically programmed to decline, age, as Betty Friedan says, can "offer the opportunity to develop values and abilities, for each of us and for society, that are not visible or fully realized in youth."

One can only hope that the middle-aged women of today will march gloriously into old age, proudly paving the way for the next generation of women. "There's a massive group of women who have grown up in the women's movement," says Mount Sinai's Myrna Lewis. "These women simply don't accept the status quo. I'm fifty-five. Many women of my generation are still somewhat intimidated by physicians, but the next generation has a different mind-set. In their childbearing years they completely turned obstetrics and gynecology around. Now you're seeing what they're doing to the menopause, and they will be doing the same thing to old age."

10

"IT'S ALL IN YOUR HEAD"
Misunderstanding Women's Complaints

Just as the physical diseases of women are poorly understood, so, too, are a panoply of psychosomatic disorders, extremely controversial diagnoses in which emotional distresses are transferred into physical symptoms for which people then seek treatment. Somatization, as this process is known, has existed for centuries and is, to this day, remarkably common: Some 80 percent of healthy adults are believed to have psychogenic symptoms in any given week—for instance a stomachache that coincides with an important deadline or a headache that comes on after a fight with the boss.

On a more extreme scale are such disorders as chronic fatigue syndrome (CFS); fibromyalgia, a musculoskeletal condition characterized by diffuse aches and pains; and twentieth-century disease, a total-allergy syndrome. The mere mention of these disorders in a chapter on psychosomatic disease is bound to raise the ire of some readers, so it's important to state up front that these illnesses are not imaginary. Although a woman's pain or grinding fatigue may be psychogenic in origin—and even this contention is not settled—the disorders they cause are very real. A woman can't be expected to simply pull herself up by the bootstraps and get over her symptoms any more than a person can will herself to grow an extra four inches in height.

But it's equally important to note that despite intensive research efforts, these disorders have no known organic causes—no virus or other pathogen has yet to be identified. In terms of chronic fatigue, the hottest of the new diseases, a 1993 study by Alison Mawle, Ph.D., of the Centers for Disease Control and Prevention, concluded that "none of the abnormalities seen in CFS are unique to the disease and therefore cannot be used as a marker for diagnosis. . . . The epidemiological evidence for an infectious agent is weak at best."

Given the long history of psychosomatic disease, the more likely explanation is that symptoms are a result of the workings of the unconscious mind; that is, the symptoms are ascribed "to an underlying organic disease for which the patient could not possibly be blamed," writes Edward Shorter, Ph.D., in his book *From Paralysis to Fatigue: A History of Psychosomatic Illness in the Modern Era.*

"The unconscious mind desires to be taken seriously and not be ridiculed," explains Shorter.

> It will therefore strive to present symptoms that always seem, to the surrounding culture, legitimate evidence of organic disease. . . . As the culture changes its mind about what is legitimate disease and what is not, the pattern of psychosomatic illness changes. For example, a sudden increase in the number of young women who are unable to get out of bed because their legs are 'paralyzed' may tell us something about how the surrounding culture views women and how it expects them to perform their roles.

As might be expected, illnesses vary from country to country, again reflecting the strong cultural influences on what is an acceptable symptom to take to a doctor's office. The French, for instance, have embraced spasmophilia, an abnormal tendency toward convulsions, while in Germany people seek treatment for low blood pressure, a condition that is generally ignored in North America and Britain. The British and Europeans meanwhile have their own version of chronic fatigue, called myalgic encephalomyelitis, or muscle pain accompanied by inflammation of the brain and spinal cord.

To what can these strange disease phenomena be attributed? Advances in biomedical technology seem to be playing a prime role. People in Western industrialized societies now expect to be in top form every day, notes Donna Stewart, M.D., a Canadian psychiatrist who is an expert in psychosomatic diseases. The result is "that they believe that most of life's infirmities are preventable or medically treatable. North Americans, in particular, have become increasingly preoccupied with their health."

The culture of somatization requires doctors who are sympathetic to the ever-changing symptom pool. "Patients want to please doctors, in the sense that they do not want the doctor to laugh at them and dismiss their plight as imaginary," writes Shorter. "Thus they strive to produce the symptoms the doctor will recognize. As doctors' own ideas about what constitutes 'real' disease change from time to time due to theory and practice, the symptoms that patients present will change as well. These medical changes give the story of psychosomatic illness its dynamic: the medical 'shaping' of symptoms."

Such a dynamic has a great bearing on women: they make up the majority of people suffering from such psychosomatic disorders as chronic fatigue syndrome, fibromyalgia, irritable bowel syndrome, and chronic pelvic pain (which can also be the result of an organic disorder such as endometriosis). The hidden scandal is that there is no shortage of doctors who will treat women's psychogenic complaints as if they're organic in origin, often leading to a chamber of medical horrors, including an array of unnecessary surgeries instead of the treatment women may really need: help in understanding the emotional reasons for their disease.

Of course women are willing participants in their mistreatment. Resisting psychological consultation, they embark on a medical odyssey, dragging their strange array of symptoms from specialist to specialist until they find someone who will give them the one thing they desperately need: a diagnosis. "These are very beleaguered patients," says Nortin Hadler, M.D., a North Carolina rheumatologist with a particular interest in somatization. "The worst thing to happen to any patient is not to be believed. You can't get better if you can't prove you're ill."

The corollary is that, because women suffer from psychosomatic illness disproportionately and express their medical problems in a more open and emotional style compared with men, their complaints frequently *aren't* listened to—even when they're directly related to an organic disease. "The perception among many physicians is that women tend to complain a lot, so you shouldn't pay too much attention to them," says Donna Stewart, head of women's health at Toronto Hospital, a teaching hospital affiliated with the University of Toronto. As a result, many of women's *legitimate* physical ailments are not attended to, sometimes with serious consequences.

■ DISEASE-OF-THE-MONTH CLUB

Just as bustle dresses and miniskirts are hallmarks of particular eras, so, too, is the parade of psychosomatic disorders. For instance, neurasthenia, nerve weakness for which women and men took to their beds, was popular in the nineteenth century. While the diagnosis gradually lost currency in the early part of the twentieth century, it managed to reemerge in the 1950s as neuromyasthenia, muscle weakness supposedly caused by an infectious agent. By the late fifties this new "disease" was epidemic.

A decade later Michael Epstein and Y. M. Barr discovered the virus that caused infectious mononucleosis. Mono, however, wasn't adopted by large numbers of somatizers because doctors could test for the white blood cell abnormality that characterized the disease. But Epstein–Barr, or EBV, although a true infectious agent, also had the makings of "a disease of fashion, because the vast majority of the population bears EBV antibodies in the blood," writes Shorter. "Disproof was impossible. Finally 'Evidence' was at hand that sufferers were 'really ill': Their blood tests (and everybody else's) showed antibodies."

It was only a matter of time before Epstein-Barr became a socially sanctioned disease. In 1984 there was an outbreak of an illness of undetermined cause at Lake Tahoe. It turned out that some of the victims had EBV antibodies in their blood. Like clockwork Epstein-Barr became the putative cause of a full-fledged disease, and soon transformed itself into the "yuppie flu," to which fast-tracking upwardly mobile professionals were especially prone. Symptoms included debilitating fatigue, fever, malaise, headaches, muscle and joint aches, sore throat and lymph glands, confusion, and decreased memory.

At the same time that EBV was hitting its peak, an older psychosomatic disorder was also in vogue. Fibrositis, more commonly called fibromyalgia, emerged from the ranks of rheumatologists, who used the terms to describe patients who had generalized muscular aches and pains or stiffness, fatigue, sleep disturbance, and bowel irregularity. Patients with fibromyalgia often suffered from Epstein-Barr as well. And so fatigue became the disease of the late twentieth century.

But there was a major problem with Epstein-Barr: The virus couldn't actually be linked to the symptoms. So in 1988, much to the dismay of patient-advocates, the Centers for Disease Control renamed the condition chronic fatigue syndrome. The objective was to emphasize fatigue as the major symptom and to avoid making unproven assumptions about its origin. A working research definition released that year included persistent or relapsing fatigue or easy fatigability that does not resolve with bed rest and that is severe enough to reduce a person's average daily activity by 50 percent. It also included a list of eleven possible symptoms that must have persisted or recurred over a period of six months: such things as mild fever, sore throat, lymph node pain, unexplained muscle weakness and discomfort, headaches, forgetfulness, and depression.

Women suffering from psychosomatic disorders have one thing in common: a willingness to switch back and forth among the currently popular diseases. People with CFS, for instance, have been quick to embrace twentieth-century disease, also called environmental hypersensitivity disorder or multiple chemical sensitivity, characterized by allergies to food, water, clothing, environmental chemicals, furniture, and sometimes even the air. Any exposure to the environment is said to trigger such symptoms as fatigue, nausea, dizziness, bowel disturbances, respiratory distress, depression, menstrual disturbances, headaches, and irritability. Some women claim to have total body yeast infections, or candida; temporomandibular joint syndrome; or mercury poisoning from the fillings in their teeth.

A study by Donna Stewart demonstrated how these "diseases of the month" overlap. Stewart asked fifty patients suffering from twentieth-century disease to list other conditions from which they'd suffered in the preceding ten years. Ninety percent said they'd had at least "one other media-popularized condition." In 1985, at the start of the study, most believed their symptoms were caused by allergies to environmental agents. By 1986 most had shifted to candida albicans, and by 1987 chronic infection with Epstein-Barr was the disease of choice.

Interestingly women suffering from these disorders often suffer simultaneously from severe premenstrual syndrome, an established condition that nevertheless has a psychosomatic component.

In an attempt to establish a relationship between PMS symptoms and the hormone changes during the premenstrual period, one important study took three groups of women with prospectively confirmed PMS and administered agents to manipulate their progesterone levels. Peter Schmidt, M.D., of the National Institute of Mental Health, created one group in which menstruation occurred at mid-cycle; a second group that had bleeding at the expected time; and a third group in which the cycle remained unaltered. Neither blocking the action of progesterone nor altering the luteal, or postovulatory, phase changed the course or severity of the women's PMS symptoms as one might have expected. While these findings are open to interpretation, they suggest subjectivity in women's perceptions of their condition.

Other research has drawn similar conclusions. A study by psychologist Sheryle Gallant found no large differences in reports of symptoms among four groups of people: women with severe premenstrual symptoms, women without symptoms, women on oral contraceptives, and men who were assigned a random cycle and had their hormone levels tested. After reviewing one-month symptom diaries for all four groups, Gallant found that many women who said they had severe symptoms reported daily ratings that didn't meet the most liberal standard for confirmation of the diagnosis. It's particularly telling that when both men and women fill out checklists of symptoms, men report as many "PMS" symptoms as women.

"There are very few other diagnoses where more people claim to have something than actually do have it," says Nada Stotland, M.D., associate professor of clinical psychiatry and obstetrics and gynecology at the University of Chicago. "I mean, if I hang out a sign that says 'Schizophrenia Clinic,' only a few people would show up. Not true with a sign that reads 'PMS.' So a whole culture is driving it."

In fact the interpretation of premenstrual symptoms varies widely from culture to culture, even though women's bodies function the same worldwide. In the Middle East, for instance, premenstrual changes are not considered cause for medical intervention. In contrast, in the United States studies show that both women and men expect women to experience negative changes in mood and behavior associated with the menstrual cycle.

"It's part of our cultural belief system that the menstrual cycle will produce debilitating hormonal changes and inevitable negative symptoms," says Stotland. "When you think about it, though, women's lives in society today, their condition en masse, would lead many reasonable people to be irritable and angry. These allocations of blame often come from the woman herself. Yet this could be a way of being crabby, and maybe she should legitimately feel crabby more often."

■ "TREATING" THE BODY

Women who can't admit their underlying anger or pain are more likely to obsess on physical symptoms, which may successfully divert their attention away from unsatisfactory life conditions. Once they've taken this route—which they often do unconsciously—they are compelled to follow a well-worn course. First they need a diagnosis, a label on which to pin their symptoms and, finally, treatment to ease their suffering. Their exhaustive searches for sympathetic doctors are chronicled on numerous electronic online services. During these meetings in cyberspace women tell harrowing tales.

"The weight of never really knowing what is going on with your body and not being able to function in any normal fashion is not something that can be understood except by someone who has been there," a woman wrote to her fellow sufferers on Prodigy's medical support bulletin board.

Unless her doctor recognizes chronic fatigue, she continued, she can go years without being diagnosed. This particular woman made the rounds of specialists for eight years before having her chronic fatigue syndrome confirmed. She told others that once they recognize that "having 20 symptoms is normal [they] will actually feel less fear and frustration."

People prone to somatization, like the woman above, are oblivious to the fact that having twenty symptoms is not "normal." After all, these people want so much to be taken seriously. They want their pain eased. Because their symptoms change and expand over time, they also demand a great deal of attention, a commodity in short supply in most medical practices. As a result their physician encounters are almost always unsatisfactory. "If the perfunctory examinations get done and they're not positive, the woman gets shunted off and told nothing is wrong," says Donna Stewart. But just because there's nothing physically wrong doesn't mean the woman is not ill.

Those who persevere will eventually find someone to proffer treatment, which, depending on the symptom and condition, may include antihistamines; antifungal, antiviral, and anti-inflammatory drugs; immune modifiers; steroids; surgery; wheat-free diets; vitamin B^{12} injections; and megadoses of zinc—few of which have been tested in controlled clinical trials. When these don't work, women beg for the latest experimental treatments. One woman suffering from chronic fatigue, fevers, sore throats, irritability, and memory loss exploded at her doctor: "I want the cure. I don't care what you have to inject into my body. Just fix it now."

Stewart has seen women with low-back pain who have had disks inappropriately removed and young women with chronic pelvic pain who have had unnecessary hysterectomies—a chilling callback to the legions of nineteenth-century women who underwent the same surgery to relieve their "hysteria."

Hysterectomy is often the treatment of choice for irritable bowel syndrome (IBS) as well, even though women's debilitating bowel irregularities, including diarrhea, constipation, abdominal pain, and gas, rarely abate with the surgical removal of their uteruses. In her job as research coordinator at the Women's Mental Health Program at Toronto's Clark Institute, Alisha Ali interviews women with IBS for entry into studies. She's amazed at the "astoundingly large percentage of women in their twenties who have had hysterectomies in the hope that it would get rid of their symptoms."

Not surprisingly, one study found that women with somatization disorder, a psychiatric illness characterized by chronic sexual, neurological, and gastrointestinal complaints, had three times as many hospitalizations and operations—including abdominal and pelvic surgery—as women with major depression. "Even though somatization disorder has been well described in the medical literature for thirty years," concluded the researchers, "somatizers still receive excess medical care."

Gerald Weissmann, M.D., a rheumatologist at New York University, describes these "treatments" as "a series of major assaults by authoritarian physicians on women and their genitals."

Fibromyalgia, which falls under his bailiwick, is also mishandled, he asserts. At an NYU rheumatology conference that he moderated, Weissmann asked the audience, "How many of you have treated a patient with fibromyalgia in the last year?" The majority of the several hundred doctors raised their hands.

"How many have used tricyclics?" he asked, referring to a kind of antidepressant. Most hands went up.

"Steroids?" The majority again.

Weissmann didn't attempt to hide his contempt. "You've seen a roomful of physicians who are giving their patients drugs with serious side effects to treat a disease I don't believe exists," he chided his peers. "I think we're poisoning our patients."

When told of Weissmann's outburst about steroids, Stewart replied, "Good for him. Rheumatologists tend to think fibromyalgia is totally neuromuscular. I'm surprised they didn't lynch him. However, the use of antidepressants is often effective for fibromyalgia and is possibly underutilized."

In the same vein doctors frequently prescribe "aggressive rest therapy" for women with chronic fatigue syndrome, despite the lack of scientific evidence that it alleviates the condition. Indeed there is evidence that exercise and cognitive therapy may do a better job of alleviating symptoms. The same holds true for women with environmental hypersensitivity, who are often encouraged to eat severely restricted diets, drink triply distilled water, and undertake costly environmental renovations of their homes. Writes Stewart, "Some ecologic treatment programs are harmful; they impose isolation, reinforce invalidism, cause nutritional compromise, and prevent patients from obtaining treatments proven to be effective."

These women patients clearly view themselves as chronically unwell. In one of Stewart's studies only 38 percent of patients expected to ever recover their health, despite the fact that their physical examinations and lab tests were all normal.

■ TREATING THE MIND

This isn't to say that women should shut up and live with their pain. Far from it. But rather than targeting symptoms, a better approach may be to get at the underlying emotional causes of the disorder. Donna Stewart has found that women who are willing to examine their lives often remember that a disturbing or traumatic event directly preceded their illness.

"These people have often had very sad, difficult experiences," she says. "A woman may be married to a man who mistreats her, or she may have a terrible job that she can't leave because she needs the money. When a woman looks back, she may realize, 'That was the year I had my miscarriage,' or 'That was the year my husband left with his secretary.' That's when we begin to talk about what sort of things might help her manage this in a different way."

One of Stewart's patients was so felled by fatigue, she dropped out of work for a couple of years. During her therapy sessions with Stewart, she revealed that she was romantically involved with a married man, which was causing her a great deal of emotional distress. "When she was finally able to work that out and leave him, she began to feel much more in control of her life and her symptoms gradually abated," says Stewart. She's now back at work.

Psychotherapy, however, doesn't help everyone, and even if it could, it would be difficult to get women to sign on to this approach. No one wants to believe her disease is in her mind—though the majority of women suffering from psychosomatic disorders appear to have underlying anxiety and depression. For instance, one study of twenty-eight patients who met the criteria for chronic fatigue syndrome found that 75 percent had had a lifetime prevalence of psychiatric disorders including anxiety or affective disorders, substance abuse, or somatization disorder. The mental disorder was more likely to have preceded the chronic fatigue than the other way around. Another study found that 66 percent of one hundred patients complaining of chronic fatigue had mood and other psychiatric disorders that triggered their fatigue.

For a woman to accept a diagnosis of depression, however, she must acknowledge she has a psychological disorder. "Having a physical symptom is a more socially accepted venue into a doctor's office," explains Stewart. "It's seen as being beyond a person's control. These women see a physical cause as legitimizing their distress. If you tell them a big part of their illness is emotional, they see it as stigmatizing and trivializing, as blame."

That these women need to believe their pain and disappointment are out of their control fits the description of somatization as "the language of the powerless." To follow this argument farther, it's understandable how a woman with a history of physical and sexual abuse might develop gastro-intestinal pain or chronic pelvic pain. As a survival mechanism, the mind refuses to face what the body has been forced to endure. "If you really feel trapped in a situation and unable to act, as many women do," says Stewart, "then sometimes this is the only socially acceptable expression of your distress."

One of Stewart's case histories illustrates the degree to which women with psychosomatic diseases cling to their diagnoses. A 41-year-old woman who was "allergic to the world" complained of feeling dizzy and faint, had insomnia, chronic vaginal itching, premenstrual tension, disorientation, muscle twitching, recurrent upper respiratory tract infections and depression. After being diagnosed with twentieth century disease, she moved to the country and isolated herself in an "ecologically safe oasis."

Writes Stewart, "She forbade cigarette smoking or the use of synthetic materials, sprays, shampoos or perfumes in her home, and she installed an oxygen line into her room. The few people who were allowed to visit had to wear natural fiber clothing that had been washed only with Ivory Snow soap and had never been dry cleaned. These visitors had to wear surgical caps, masks and gowns over their regular clothing. She 'went into a coma' when there was any 'ecological insult' to her."

Her medical records revealed a troubled past. She'd suffered postpartum depression after the birth of both of her children, and her relationship with her husband was strained. By age thirty she had ninety complaints involving fifteen organ systems, without any sign of organic disease. One year she'd consulted nineteen specialists and several general practitioners.

During a consultation Stewart raised the possibility that psychiatric treatment might enable the woman to live a less restricted life. Her response: "Why should I do that? I'm better than I've been for years. Discovering that I have twentieth-century disease has made my life so much happier."

And in fact there was evidence that the diagnosis had improved her life. "The isolation imposed by her illness had solved many of her problems with her husband, as he no longer made sexual requests of her and now undertook most of the housekeeping and child-care tasks," wrote Stewart. "She was relieved of any conflict about not working outside the home, and she exerted considerable control over her environment and the people who visited her."

For some women, apparently, social isolation is not too high a price to pay to relieve their psychic pain. Such a solution, while extreme, nevertheless works. In sharing "success" stories such as these, women have managed to rally support from the clinical and research communities. Certainly it's reasonable to study these diseases and search for an offending pathogen. But by overlooking the mind's effect on the body, the medical profession is facilitating women's denial. The practical effect of this neglect is that it keeps women in their places, which begs the question: How far must a woman in our society go to express her rage and helplessness? To answer this question is to get at the heart—and soul—of women's health.

■ MISSING REAL DISEASE

If, as we've seen, the traditional medical approach to psychosomatic disease is misguided, so, too, is the propensity to write off women's real organic disorders as psychogenic. Unfortunately women's complaints are dismissed by doctors far too often—and much more readily than men's. One study found that primary care physicians judged 65 percent of women's symptoms, versus 51 percent of the men's, to be influenced by emotional factors. Perhaps not surprisingly women's complaints were more than twice as likely as men's to be identified as psychosomatic. Misdiagnosing a woman is bad enough, but misdiagnosing her as a result of a sexist bias is unforgivable. At the very least it can delay appropriate care; at worst it can threaten her life.

Shortly after the birth of her first child, Patricia Niemin began experiencing a light fluttering sensation in her chest. Her doctor, a family practitioner, assured her that it was normal, that this happened to women all the time. During her second pregnancy the palpitations disappeared, only to return less than a year after her son was born. Over the next five years, instead of having palpitations one to two times a day for a few seconds each, she had them almost constantly.

Then one day Niemin looked up at the large clock in the Walgreen's where she worked as a cosmetologist and realized she couldn't read the numbers.

Am I having a heart attack? she wondered. *What's wrong with me?*

By 1980, almost ten years after the palpitations began, Niemin's resting heart rate had increased from a worrisome canter to a fast-and-furious gallop. Without running any tests, her doctor put her on digitalis. Although it slowed her racing heart, her family was not sold on the treatment. After all, she hadn't ever gotten a diagnostic workup.

Niemin consulted an internist, who immediately took her off the digitalis and hospitalized her for tests. *Finally,* she thought, *I'll get answers. I'll find out what's wrong with me.*

But all the tests came back negative. With nothing organically wrong, the hospital cardiologist questioned her about her home life. When Niemin said that she was in the middle of a divorce, she could almost see the light bulb go off above her doctor's head.

"Honey," he said, patting the back of her hand, "go home and take some stress out of your life."

"Wait a minute," Niemin said. "I don't operate badly under stress. I enjoy certain kinds of stress."

What's more, now that her husband was out of the house and, most important, out of her life, Niemin was happier than she'd been in more than ten years. She was under less—not more—stress.

She'd been reading medical books and she had her own theories about what was wrong with her. "It's got to be my thyroid," she told her doctors. "Everything points to my thyroid."

"No," she heard over and over again, "that's not possible."

Over the next decade Niemin had accumulated a grab bag of strange symptoms: hives when she showered, occasional hair loss, and more intense palpitations. By January 1993, at the age of forty, she had lost thirty pounds, her cheeks were hollow, and her skin had taken on a grayish, deathlike pall. Hot all the time and extremely fatigued, she couldn't walk from one room to another without gasping for breath.

Niemin stared at herself in the mirror and thought, *I look just like my brother did a few months before he died of cancer.* She was scared.

The endocrinologist she consulted took one look at her and said, "I can tell you what's wrong with you. You've got a thyroid problem." Finally, some twenty years after her initial symptoms appeared, Niemin's condition had a name. She had Graves' disease, a thyroid disorder that affects three women for every man. The chilling part of her story is that, had she gone much longer without treatment, she could have been courting a fatal heart attack.

Feeling angry and betrayed, Niemin worked Prodigy's electronic bulletin boards and found dozens of others like herself. It had taken all of them years and numerous medical consultations to get their thyroid conditions diagnosed. And they'd all heard the same tired lines from the people who should have been trying to heal them: "You're not handling stress well" or "A lot of women go through this."

Niemin wanted to scream. "A lot of women are going through it because no one is doing anything about it." She's convinced that "they didn't look thoroughly enough because I'm a woman."

That Patricia Niemin suffered needlessly for almost two decades, that her doctors had no qualms about blaming her symptoms on stress, on her emotions, is unforgivable. But when it comes to medical care, as we have seen, women are often subjected to such outrageous practices over and over again. If there is no obvious cause for a woman's medical complaint, her condition must be all in her head.

In twentieth-century medicine there's a long legacy of writing women's organic diseases off as emotional disorders. Menstrual cramps, morning sickness, and endometriosis—all of which occur exclusively in women—top an extensive list of real medical conditions that were once considered nothing more than physical expressions of some inner angst.

"When women have problems it's always due to hormones or their psyches. People look inward," says psychiatrist Ann Turkel, of the Columbia-Presbyterian Medical Center. "Women's pain is more misunderstood and overlooked. Since men are stoic, their complaints of pain are more believable. Women are more often dismissed as hypochondriacs."

Researchers maintain that such sex biases exist because women are more often diagnosed as suffering from emotional and psychogenic illnesses than men. For instance women are more likely than men to seek medical care for such symptoms as headaches, nervousness, insomnia, and palpitations. And overall they're more communicative about their problems.

"The open and emotional behavioral style used by women in reporting their illnesses may prompt physicians to react to women's complaints as though they were expressions of emotional problems, whereas the more stoic style found in men reporting a similar complaint does not elicit a psychosomatic diagnosis from the physician," write Barbara Bernstein, M.D., and Robert Kane, M.D.

Interestingly, nonexpressive women in a study by Bernstein and Kane were still more likely than nonexpressive men to receive a psychosomatic diagnosis. "Physicians do have preconceptions about women patients, and some of these judgments resemble the biases described in popular literature."

The tendency to dismiss women's health concerns stems not only from the belief that women are more emotional but that they are more emotionally unstable than men. Doctors know that women are more often diagnosed as suffering from depression and other mental illnesses and are twice as likely as men to receive prescriptions for psychotropic medications. As a whole, women receive more health care services than men, are more concerned about their health, and are more vocal about their medical problems, all of which lead physicians to unfairly stereotype them as overanxious, perhaps even hysterical.

This view is reinforced in medical education. In conversations with medical students, physicians and patients in the early 1970s, Harvard doctor Mary Howell found a pervasive pattern of discrimination against women patients. Howell noted that in most medical-school lectures patients are referred to by the male pronoun *he*. The notable exception, she says: "In discussing a hypothetical patient whose disease is of psychogenic origin, the lecturer often automatically uses 'she.' For it is widely taught, both explicitly and implicitly, that women patients (when they receive notice at all) have uninteresting illnesses, are unreliable historians, and are beset by such emotionality that their symptoms are unlikely to reflect 'real' disease."

A decade later a British study drew similar conclusions. In surveying the attitudes of second-year medical students at the London Hospital Medical College, the researchers wrote, "It is disturbing to find that 12 percent of the male students agreed that women were less creative, and one-third that they were less logical because of their hormones. . . .

"This attitude might well explain the feeling that women express that their complaints are not taken seriously and the doctor often prescribes a tranquilizer when what they would like is an explanation of their symptoms."

When doctors assume that women are more emotionally unstable than men, it can't help but affect the kind of care they give. Overexaggerating psychological disturbances among women patients can result in more prescriptions for psychoactive drugs in lieu of treatment.

Reaching in a knee-jerk fashion for the emotional explanation can also result in a failure to detect and treat real illness. As mentioned in chapter 4, men have cardiac catheterizations ordered at a disproportionately higher rate than women. One study found that 4 percent of the women with abnormal radiological tests were referred for catheterization, compared with 40 percent of the men. Although the women tended to be more symptomatic than the men, cardiologists attributed almost 33 percent of the women's problems—but only 16 percent of the men's—to somatic and other noncardiac causes.

Concerned about this problem, in 1991 the American Medical Association's Council on Ethical and Judicial Affairs issued a report, "Gender Disparities in Clinical Decision Making." "Society and medicine have addressed and are working to remedy sex stereotypes and biases," the report said. "Yet, many social and cultural attitudes that endorse sex-stereotyped roles for men and women remain in our society. The medical community cannot tolerate any discrepancy in the provision of care that is not based on appropriate biological or medical indications."

But such inequities still exist. Not only do sex-role stereotypes adversely affect the care women receive, they also affect the kind of research being conducted. Beth Meyerowitz, Ph.D., of the University of Southern California, suspected she'd find just such a sex bias in cancer research. Indeed, when she examined 139 articles on the psychosocial aspects of cancer, she found that women comprised 77 percent of the subjects in studies of emotional and social support but only 45 percent of those in studies of functional capacity. Even in cancer research there's an unconscious bias that women are more concerned with emotional issues and less with the practical effects of their illness on their lives. "There's a lot we don't know about women's ability to return to work after being treated for cancer," says Meyerowitz. "Even with cancers that men and women both get, studies about work are limited to samples of men."

As the AMA report noted, the research and medical communities cannot afford to operate under such misconceptions. They cannot justify interpreting women's demonstrative patient styles as signs of mental weakness any more than they can justify interpreting men's stoic styles as signs of strength. As Bernstein and Kane write, "A physician's reaction to a female patient may point him in the direction of treating a physical ailment as an emotional one." Meanwhile "his response to a male patient may cause him to treat an emotional problem as a physical ailment and may deny emotional support or psychiatric help to a patient who cannot be open about his needs."

Any good clinician knows that prejudging patients according to cultural stereotypes means that everyone—women as well as men—misses out.

11

WOMEN'S MENTAL HEALTH
A Cruel Double Standard

Pick up any women's magazine and you'll learn that women eat too much, eat too little, are food obsessed, worry too much about their appearance, have low self-esteem, try too hard to please, don't handle stress well, make the mistake of trying to have it all—and that these "neuroses" exact a harsh toll on women's mental health.

The reality is women are twice as likely as men to suffer from panic disorder, manic-depressive disorder, phobias, and major depression, a statistic that holds true across cultures and continents. Close to 25 percent of women will experience major depression in their lifetimes, versus 12 percent of men. Why?

Studies suggest that depression may be related to a drop in the brain chemicals serotonin, norepinephrine, and dopamine, neurotransmitters that regulate mood. Other studies report that depression runs in families, suggesting a genetic component. Still other researchers have linked depression to the hormonal changes brought on by menstruation, pregnancy, and menopause, although this theory hasn't been proven.

Ultimately the truth about depression and other mental illnesses may lie in a combination of biological and sociocultural factors, the most important of which may be women's life conditions. Feminists argue that women's disadvantaged position in society puts them at a higher risk for mental illness. Incest, rape, and domestic violence—to which two to four million women a year fall victim—are known to increase susceptibility to mental illness. One study found that up to 35 percent of the difference between male and female depression rates is attributable to the childhood sexual abuse of women.

Frequently, women who work face salary inequities and sexual harassment. Full-time homemakers often contend with work that is frustrating, thankless and low in prestige. As a consequence, full-time mothers with young children at home have the highest rates of depression. Working mothers, on the other hand, may have the best—and worst—of these two worlds. While the data tell women that having a variety of roles should be reducing their stress, women know all too well the push-pull effect of endless juggling.

No one needs to tell women that feeling powerless and alienated and being economically deprived can impair their mental health. Noted *Washington Post* columnist Judy Mann, "You don't have to be a psychologist to figure out that a class of people who are underpaid in the workplace, beaten up at home and raped almost routinely on college campuses are going to suffer much more from depression than people who aren't victimized."

Still, the mystery of depression is far from solved. For instance, recent analyses of epidemiological data suggest there may be no true gender difference in the prevalence of major depression. Perhaps the mood disorder is merely underrecognized in men, who, unlike women, may express their pain and inner angst through violence and aggression or by abusing alcohol or drugs. If this is the case, any discussion of depression—and of other mental disorders—must examine possible gender bias in diagnosis, a major focus of this chapter.

■ GENDER BIAS IN DIAGNOSIS

If it's folly to try to separate women's mental states from their lot in life, it's equally foolish to ignore the overt biases that are built into the way psychiatric disorders are detected in the first place. Among the widely used diagnostic tools is the American Psychiatric Association's (APA) Diagnostic and Statistical Manual, the DSM. The psychiatric bible, the DSM influences the practice of both psychiatry and psychology all over the world. In its pages, one can find hundreds of mental illnesses and their symptoms, all referred to by code numbers. Not only do these codes enforce uniformity among clinicians and researchers, they're used by insurance companies to determine coverage for treatment.

The newly published fourth edition of the DSM, the DSM-IV is a reassuringly scholarly book, but its purview seems almost limitless. It has grown from a mere 106 disorders in its 1952 edition to some 300 in 1994. The DSM's expanded scope has raised questions about exactly what constitutes a mental disorder. Certainly no one would argue over whether depression, schizophrenia, or bipolar disorder (manic depression) belong in such a tome, but it's not obvious why such things as sexual dysfunction and marital difficulties are listed as mental disorders. The problem in including such commonplace situations in the DSM, notes psychologist Carol Tavris in *The Mismeasure of Woman*, is that "if a label is there, many users of the manual assume, it must be valid."

Yet this is not necessarily true. Sex-role stereotypes have already been found in a number of diagnostic criteria, leading to some heated debates about the legitimacy of some of the established mental disorders and raising concerns that women are ill served by the mental health profession. Even the results of an early seminal study on sex-role stereotypes by Inge Broverman confirmed that clinicians were "significantly less likely to attribute traits which characterize healthy adults to a woman" than they were to a man.

For a woman to be healthy "she must adjust to and accept the behavioral norms for her sex," Broverman found. This means she has to be more submissive and dependent, less aggressive and competitive, more excitable in minor crises, more emotional, and more conceited about her appearance. Trying to adhere to these "norms" places women in the "conflictual position of having to decide whether to exhibit those positive characteristics considered desirable for men and adults, and thus have their 'femininity' questioned, that is, be deviant in terms of being a woman; or to behave in the prescribed feminine manner, accept second-class adult status, and possibly live a lie to boot."

To be sure, both genders are penalized for failing to live up to their sex-role expectations. For instance, because depression is considered more congruent with the female experience, when men are depressed they're believed to be more disturbed than their female counterparts. Even so, women are likely to be diagnosed for both overconforming and underconforming to sex-role stereotypes.

As psychologist Marcie Kaplan describes it, "To be considered an unhealthy adult, women must act as women are supposed to act (conform too much to the female sex role stereotype); to be considered an unhealthy woman, women must act as men are supposed to act (not conform enough to the female sex role stereotype). Not only does this catch-22 predict that women are bound to be labeled unhealthy one way or another, but also the double bind itself could drive a woman crazy."

A case in point is Histrionic Personality Disorder—formerly Hysterical Personality—which can be found in the DSM. To be diagnosed with this disorder, an individual must satisfy four of the following eight criteria:

1) constantly seeks or demands reassurance, approval, or praise
2) is inappropriately sexually seductive in appearance or behavior
3) is overly concerned with physical attractiveness
4) expresses emotion with inappropriate exaggeration, e.g., embraces casual acquaintances with excessive ardor, uncontrollable sobbing on minor sentimental occasions, has temper tantrums
5) is uncomfortable in situations in which he or she is not the center of attention
6) displays rapidly shifting and shallow expression of emotions
7) is self-centered, actions being directed toward obtaining immediate satisfaction; has no tolerance for the frustration of delayed gratification
8) has a style of speech that is excessively impressionistic and lacking in detail, e.g., when asked to describe mother, can be no more specific than, "She was a beautiful person."

Most of these characteristics are amazingly similar to the way the mental health professionals in the Broverman study described a healthy woman. Remember: "more excitable in minor crises," "more emotional," "more conceited" about her appearance, "cries very easily." Not surprisingly, women are diagnosed with Histrionic Personality Disorder far more often than men, suggesting that biases are indeed codified in the DSM. In this and other disorders, the APA officially sanctions labeling women who overconform to what society expects of them as nuts. (Although the diagnostic criteria for Histrionic Personality Disorder have been revised for the DSM-IV, only time will tell whether they will be used judiciously.)

"Is it possible," asked a National Institute of Mental Health report, "that normal processes in women are sometimes viewed as pathological because the baseline for normality was established on or by males?"

Good question. When it comes to Self-Defeating Personality Disorder the answer is an unequivocal yes. The criteria for this disorder—originally called Masochistic Personality Disorder—began to take shape in the mid-1980s when the DSM-III was under revision. After objections from the committees on women of both the American Psychiatric Association and the American Psychological Association, the name was eventually changed to Self-Defeating Personality Disorder (SDPD), which appeared in the appendix of the DSM-III-R under "proposed diagnostic categories needing further study."

Feminists had managed to keep the disorder out of the main body of the DSM, but their goal was to have SDPD entirely stricken from the books on the basis that it was conceptually flawed and biased. In the

DSM-III-R the disorder is described as "a pervasive pattern of self-defeating behavior," with such criteria as: "chooses people and situations that lead to disappointment, failure or mistreatment," "rejects or renders ineffective attempts of others to help him or her," "engages in excessive self-sacrifice," "fails to accomplish tasks crucial to his or her personal objectives despite demonstrated ability to do so."

The fear among feminists was that, as was the case with Histrionic Personality Disorder, women would be unfairly penalized for doing what they have been socialized to do. SDPD, they argued, pathologizes the culturally accepted behavior of women.

To point out the bias inherent in this diagnosis, Paula Caplan, a psychologist at the University of Toronto, proposed criteria for a new disorder—Delusional Dominating Personality Disorder—and suggested that sufferers were unable to "establish and maintain close relationships," "identify and express their feelings," and "respond appropriately to the feelings and needs of others." They also used "power, silence, withdrawal, or avoidance rather than negotiation in coping with conflict."

Most psychiatrists took the proposed disorder as a joke, but Caplan was serious. She knew that if this were a real disorder, it would be applied disproportionately to men. Her point: It's just as biased to explain stereotypical male behavior as an abnormal personality disorder as it is to explain women's as such.

Although SDPD's criteria specifically noted that the disorder should not be applied to people who have been sexually or physically abused, there was no way to prevent it being used in this way. For one thing battered women often don't reveal their history of abuse to their therapists. And since most homicides of abused wives occur after they leave their husbands, it may be rational, not pathological, for a woman to remain in an abusive relationship if she fears that by leaving she'd be risking her life.

Despite the inherently stigmatizing nature of this diagnosis, many psychiatrists favored its inclusion in the DSM. But critics pointed out that no matter how you looked at it, the diagnosis was methodologically flawed. In fact a study to test its validity found a great deal of overlap with other personality disorders and some mood disorders as well.

Psychiatrist Margaret Jensvold had long argued that SDPD was conceptually flawed. She had both a professional and a personal interest in the debate's outcome. The disorder was invoked against her after she charged her supervisors at NIMH with sexual harassment and sexual discrimination. In essence the defense in the case was labeling Jensvold crazy, saying that as a self-defeating person she'd gotten what she deserved. Using the diagnosis against Jensvold, who was a victim of abuse—during a brief marriage she had been beaten twice by her husband—was everyone's worst nightmare, and now it had come to pass.

At the same time that SDPD was making its way into the DSM, a second worrisome diagnosis was slipping in the back door. Despite contentious debate, in 1987 Late Luteal Phase Dysphoric Disorder (LLPDD) joined SDPD in the appendix of the DSM-III-R. It was also included in the main body of the text in a list of "unspecified mental disorders," signaling its ambiguous status.

This gobbledygook of a term—and its newer, less cumbersome incarnation, Premenstrual Dysphoric Disorder, or PMDD—refers to severe premenstrual symptoms, such things as persistent and marked anger or irritability, anxiety and tension, depressed mood, a decreased interest in one's usual activities, easy fatigability, and a marked change in appetite. Thanks to the psychiatric powers that be, a disabling form of PMS was on its way to becoming a full-fledged mental disorder.

It was easy to view this move with suspicion. PMS had already had a long and checkered past. In 1931 gynecologist Robert Frank declared that "premenstrual tension" made women a liability in the workforce. Interestingly, writes psychologist Carol Tavris, Frank made these claims at a time when women were losing the gains they had made in the workplace during World War I. At the beginning of World War II, when women were again needed to replace men in the workforce, studies curiously found that premenstrual tension was no longer a problem.

There was another backlash after the war. At about the same time that women were once again forced out of their jobs, British physician Katharina Dalton published widely on the dangers of menstruation, which she linked to crime, accidents, and acute mental illness. In 1953 she coined the term *premenstrual syndrome*, which she saw as a pathological condition that made women unfit for the rigors of professional life. In the preface to her 1969 book, her husband, Tom E. Dalton, wrote, "The reader will begin to realize that there is a biological basis for much that has been written, or said, about the whims and vagaries of women.

"The old cliché 'It's a woman's privilege to change her mind' calls for an even greater tolerance than before now that it is realized that every woman is at the mercy of the constantly recurring ebb and flow of her hormones."

One cannot even take comfort in the thought that Dalton's beliefs are hopelessly out-of-date—articles based on her theories continue to appear in the medical literature. As we've pointed out throughout this book, there's a long history of medicalizing women's natural reproductive events, from pregnancy to menopause. Why should menstruation be an exception?

Apparently it's not enough that women's monthly cycles are pathological; now they're associated with a mental disease. Exactly what kind of mental disease no one is quite certain. In fact, although PMDD is ostensibly a dysphoric, or depressive, disorder, the nation's top mental health professionals cannot agree on whether it is in fact a true depression. It's telling that the six-member work group charged with reviewing hundreds of studies in the literature and making recommendations on whether PMDD should be moved to the main body of the DSM-IV could not reach a consensus.

Work-group member Jean Endicott, Ph.D., argued that PMDD was a depression. Endicott has studied more than two thousand women at her PMS clinic at Columbia-Presbyterian Medical Center and is convinced that some of them have "quite severe premenstrual depression and anxiety" and that they are "worthy of treatment. I was seeing women with very clear premenstrual problems. I was seeing the difficulties they were having. They were usually told, 'It's all in your head. There's nothing wrong. You're just neurotic.' It became very clear to us there was a biological component." (This, however, does not rule out a psychogenic component.)

Research by LLPDD work-group member Barbara Parry, M.D., also suggested a biological base. Her studies have found a consistent decrease in the levels of the brain chemical melatonin in PMS patients versus controls. Other studies have found a decrease in serotonin, a neurotransmitter related to mood.

While such evidence is intriguing, it's far from conclusive. And even if PMDD is a depression, it may have nothing to do with a woman's cycle. The literature review conducted by the LLPDD work group found that women who seek treatment for premenstrual problems often have mental or other medical conditions "that may account for many, if not all, of their 'premenstrual' complaints." Such things as major mood disorders, dysthymia (a mild depression), bulimia and anxiety, substance abuse and personality disorders.

Some women appear to have major depression that worsens premenstrually. If this is the case, argues Paula Caplan, why not simply treat women's depression and leave their menstrual cycles out of it?

Then, too, "why are women's hormonal cycles regularly characterized as negative?" asks Nada Stotland, M.D., associate professor of clinical psychiatry and obstetrics and gynecology at the University of Chicago. Is it possible that women might experience positive changes during their menstrual cycles? Studies going as far back as the 1950s noted such positive attributes as increased energy and sex drive and feelings of well-being and excitement during the premenstrual period. In 1980 psychologist Mary Brown Parlee went so far as to suggest naming a "premenstrual elation syndrome."

Intrigued with these earlier positive data, psychiatrist Donna Stewart surveyed one hundred women making routine visits to a gynecologist and found that two-thirds of them had at least one positive change during the premenstrual week, including an increase in sexual enjoyment, energy, and creative ideas. Twenty percent of women reported five positive changes. "I've heard terrible anecdotal stories of women who have had their whole lives wrecked because of menstrual cycle mood changes," says Stewart, "but I've never seen them in my clinical practice."

That still leaves the question, Is PMDD a real disorder? The debate, much like the one over its predecessor, PMS, seems to be as much about science as it is about feminist ideology. As Margaret Jensvold explains it, "In the fifties and earlier, biological differences between men and women were readily acknowledged and used to justify keeping women out of the workforce. In the sixties you had the women's movement and the downplaying of biological differences. The hope was that women would have more access to power. In the late eighties and early nineties, well-intentioned research was done on men and extrapolated to women. Suddenly people said, 'Oh, there are biological differences.'"

In light of this, she says, "we know that a small proportion of women do have severe symptoms premenstrually that have a negative impact on their personal and professional lives. We need to acknowledge it, study it, and come up with treatments."

In a perfect world this might be the perfect solution. But PMDD is an imperfect diagnosis whose very existence raises serious questions about scientific integrity and gender equity. For example:

- *Why is there no corresponding category for men?* There's plenty of evidence of significant cyclical variability in men's psychological states and functions. "There's clear data that men get into more car accidents and are more daring and reckless and this is hormonally related," says Nada Stotland. "This is a social and biological circumstance that causes measurable damage and yet we have no category for this, like Testosterone-related Syndrome."

• *Is it discriminatory to require women to keep symptom diaries prior to giving them a diagnosis?* In order to get the label PMDD, women must experience at least a 30 percent change in the intensity of their symptoms six days prior to menstruation, and they must document it through two months of daily ratings. Researchers argue that the only way to identify women with true PMS is through such prospectively confirmed ratings. As it is, there's some subjectivity involved in using self-rating scales, although they are perhaps more reliable than asking women to recall their symptoms over time.

Jensvold disagrees. "If your symptoms are too severe," she argues, "you won't make it through the two months of daily ratings. If you're not willing to do the daily ratings for two months or you can't do them because you're suicidal, you can't get the diagnosis of PMDD.

"This is the part I find discriminating. Major depression requires being depressed every day for two weeks, but you don't make people fill out daily rating forms and have them come back in two weeks to find out if they have major depression. Dysthymic disorder requires depression most days for two years, but you don't make people fill out ratings for two years and come back.

"It's only in this condition that they don't believe a patient's words. Part of the PMS dogma is that women have to do daily ratings because they're not good reporters of their own experience. I really object to that. Just because a woman's self-report and the daily ratings are discrepant doesn't mean that the daily ratings should be the gold standard."

• *Can carrying a diagnosis of PMDD harm a woman?* Stotland is convinced that "the official labeling of symptoms related to menstruation, pregnancy, and menopause as mental illness threatens to stigmatize women as unstable, unreliable, and inferior." Such a category may also pose social and political dangers for women. Paula Caplan, one of the most vocal opponents of PMDD, worries that "at Senate confirmation hearings, job interviews, custody proceedings, and mental competence hearings, women could be asked, 'Have you been diagnosed as having Premenstrual Dysphoric Disorder?' " (While the use of PMS as a legal defense has succeeded in Canada and England, it has been generally unsuccessful in the United States.)

• *Is there a financial incentive in making this a mental disorder?* As the psychiatric community focuses increasingly on biological medicine, practitioners are more apt to turn to medication over therapy in treating PMDD. "It's clear it's the drug-company money that's behind a lot of this," says Caplan, who points to the fact that psychiatrists fail to prescribe such benign treatments as diet, support groups, and exercise and instead prescribe medication.

PMDD proponent Robert Spitzer, M.D., claims that the inclusion of PMDD in the DSM-IV will encourage research into the condition. "You can't do research unless you have accepted criteria," he asserts.

To which Caplan responds, "Nonsense, I've gotten grants. It's just harder to get drug-company money."

• *Is PMDD an accurate name?* Not only was Late Luteal Phase Dysphoric Disorder cumbersome to use, it was also misleading, given increasing evidence that its symptoms may not have been exclusively linked to the hormonal milieu during the late luteal phase of the cycle. But PMDD has its own shortcomings. For one thing it excludes women who no longer menstruate because of hysterectomy but who still have cyclical changes. What's more, research using the criteria for LLPDD was just starting to come into the literature when the LLPDD work group met. "Changing the name would only serve to confuse things even more," argued work-group member Sally Severino, M.D.

In the end, with impassioned arguments from feminists on both sides of the issue, the work group stood hopelessly divided. Ultimately the American Psychiatric Association's Assembly recommended that PMDD replace LLPDD in the appendix of the DSM-IV and be listed in the main body of the text under "depressive disorders not otherwise specified," a compromise that didn't please anyone. On the one hand it meant that PMDD wasn't accorded full status, but it also meant that the disorder was one step closer to being labeled a depression. Now it was up to the APA's board of trustees to make the final decision.

With only months to go before the official vote, opponents got in gear. The American Psychological Association believed the research base was too weak to warrant creating a new disorder and said so in a letter to work-group chairperson Judith Gold. Raymond Fowler, the psychological association's chief executive officer, also voiced "the APA's concerns about the potential for misdiagnosis, abuse and pathologizing of women inherent in the inclusion of this diagnostic category."

Gail Erlick Robinson, M.D., chair of the American Psychiatric Association's Committee on Women, expressed her group's concerns in a letter to Allen Frances, chair of the APA's Task Force for the DSM-IV. She wrote that the "suggestion to move this diagnosis into the main body of the DSM-IV . . . is premature."

As the psychiatric association's board of trustees met in San Francisco in July 1993 to vote, members of the National Organization for Women protested outside. Said Deborah Glenn, vice president of NOW's San Francisco chapter, "When a woman feels angry, the response of the medical establishment has always been to say there's something wrong with her, that she has a psychiatric problem."

And indeed, that's exactly what happened with PMDD. While Self-Defeating Personality Disorder was finally expunged from the books, PMDD was retained. It didn't matter that the data had not proven it to be a form of depression. Now severe premenstrual symptoms were officially declared a sign of mental pathology.

"The DSM-IV is a document of disempowerment, an attempt to sell psychiatry and drugs to the American public," says Peter Breggin, M.D., a psychiatrist and author of *Toxic Psychiatry*. "It takes ordinary human problems and redefines them as medical problems. PMDD itself is a continuation of the chronic tendency in psychiatry to take a patriarchal stance toward women."

■ TOO MANY PILLS, TOO LITTLE PROGRESS

The same biases that affect diagnostic categories in the DSM are also apparent when psychiatric drugs are studied. Consider the case of the Burroughs Wellcome antidepressant buproprion (Wellbutrin). In 1986, while testing the drug among female bulimics, Burroughs researchers got a rude surprise. The drug caused seizures in four of fifty-five patients, an alarmingly high rate and one that was far above the three seizures per one thousand patients seen when the medication was tested for depression.

Despite almost ten years of clinical testing, both Wellcome and the FDA had discounted the factors that could have contributed to the high seizure rate in women—women's lower body weight compared to men, and their greater sensitivity to the stimulant effects of Wellbutrin.

What makes this story truly disturbing is that, by the time this increased seizure rate showed up, Wellbutrin had already been approved as safe and effective by the FDA and had been shipped to pharmacies. Approved in 1985, Wellbutrin's labeling carried a warning that seizure rates appeared slightly above those seen with most other antidepressants and that it should not be used by patients either prone to seizure or using other drugs associated with seizure risk. However, there was no mention of a greater seizure risk in female patients compared to males, which would have alerted physicians to be more cautious in prescribing it.

When the elevated seizure rate showed up in bulimic women, Wellcome voluntarily withdrew Wellbutrin from the market, hoping that the drug could be relabeled to exclude bulimics and quickly rereleased. The FDA's Psychopharmacologic Drugs Advisory Committee called a meeting on April 25, 1986, to examine the company's seizure data and determine whether further testing was required on Wellbutrin and, possibly, on other antidepressants.

Amazingly, the company had no depression data broken down by gender; Wellcome scientists simply assumed there were no gender differences in seizure rates. However, in a reanalysis of Wellbutrin seizure data already published, James Goldberg, Ph.D., who conducts investigatory drug trials at Vista Hill Hospital in San Diego, found that women had three times the seizure rate of men. Goldberg said that the initial recommended dose of Wellbutrin—450 mg per day—had been too high for most of the women.

Other side effects of Wellbutrin had also been ignored, despite the fact that they appeared more probable in women. For instance, rather than diminishing libido, as is the case for most antidepressants, Wellbutrin might boost sexuality and increase physical genital sensation in some women. Additionally, in contrast to other antidepressants which often cause weakness and fatigue, Wellbutrin had stimulant-like qualities, or as the FDA's Paul Leber, M.D., has said, "you get on a jag with it." While such a stimulant action might be acceptable to women, it could also lead to a feeling of being "wired" or to a breakthrough of latent psychotic tendencies, says Goldberg.

Why were these special features of Wellbutrin and their particular relevance to female patients ignored by some of the sharpest medical minds in the country? While Wellbutrin was tested equally in women and men, the data on women were not analyzed separately and compared to the data on men, making it impossible to discover gender-related complications. Unfortunately, the problems in the evaluation of Wellbutrin are typical of psychiatric drug testing and review: doses are not tailored to women despite clear weight and metabolic differences; women's greater sensitivity to these drugs' adverse effects is not considered; and there is a conspicuous lack of involvement of women doctors in the testing, review, and approval processes.

And here's the cruel irony. Although women make just over half of all visits to physicians' offices, they receive 73 percent of all prescriptions written for psychotropic medication—and an incredible 90 percent when the prescribing physician is not a psychiatrist. Women receive up to 83 percent of prescriptions for antidepressants, well in excess of the 66 percent that would be expected based on the two-to-one female-to-male ratio for depression. (Numerous studies conducted over the last twenty years have shown that when men and women present themselves to doctors with the same physical or emotional complaints, women are significantly more likely than men to receive prescriptions for antidepressants, tranquilizers, and other psychotropic drugs, suggesting a pervasive physician bias in diagnosing and prescribing.)

Overall, women have twice as many fatal drug reactions as men. A 1992 article in the *Lancet* noted a seventeenfold increase in the risk of fatal myocardial infarction in young women taking psychotropic drugs, a troubling association that needs further study. Seventy percent more women than men visit emergency rooms to be treated for tranquilizer-related adverse consequences, and more than two times as many women as men enter ERs for adverse reactions to antidepressants.

While working at an NIMH neuropharmacology lab in 1980, Jean Hamilton, the researcher who settled a sexual discrimination case against the institute, was convinced there were sex differences in pharmacology. "With naive enthusiasm," she says, "I talked about this with my boss."

His reply: "There couldn't possibly be sex differences in response to drugs. If there were, we'd already know about it."

Undaunted, Hamilton continued to investigate whether the menstrual cycle or oral contraceptives affected drug response in women. "In animals," she says, "there was a clear sex difference in one of the antidepressants that our lab was studying in people. But when I tried to look at the data in our lab by age and sex, it turned out that the data were not even entered in the computer files by these variables."

After collecting an impressive body of research suggesting that men responded better to antidepressants than women, Hamilton went back to her lab chief. "I pointed out that the basic science work on antidepressants was done in male rats, partly in order to avoid the menstrual cycle, and that the early-stage testing of antidepressants was done only in men." It was possible, she reasoned, "that there was a sievelike effect, leading to the selection of drugs that worked better in men than women."

Hamilton's boss discouraged her from publishing her findings. Indeed, if she believed her male colleagues, what she was trying to study wasn't even pharmacology.

But Hamilton persisted, eventually demonstrating a menstrual-cycle effect on lithium levels, resulting in a premenstrual exacerbation of depression in some women. When she was finally able to get a breakdown of her lab's data by sex and age, "sure enough," she says, "there was evidence of a sex difference in responsivity to that antidepressant."

In 1983 Hamilton and Barbara Parry, M.D., then a staff psychiatrist at NIMH, published a review of sex-related differences in clinical drug response. They found that estrogens and oral contraceptives affected the therapeutic response of a wide variety of drugs, including antidepressants and antianxiety agents. For instance, antianxiety drugs and postmenopausal estrogen taken together increased seizures and reduced the effectiveness of estrogen in treating menopausal symptoms. Hormone replacement therapy and oral contraceptives decreased the liver's metabolism of tricyclic antidepressants, leading to a greater risk of toxicity in women. And, as mentioned in an earlier chapter, older women on antipsychotics were more likely than men to suffer from an irreversible abnormal movement disorder, tardive dyskinesia.

Although the Public Health Service has identified the study of sex differences in pharmacotherapy as an important research area, little effort has been made to find answers. In 1994, more than ten years after Jean Hamilton was dismissed from NIMH for working in low-priority areas, including psychopharmacology, not one study on gender differences in drug metabolism is being conducted by that institution.

The studies that form the state of the art in psychopharmacology have one major flaw: As was the case with Wellbutrin, even when women are included, researchers rarely analyze data by gender. At a November 1993 meeting convened by NIMH, Hamilton reported the results of a meta-analysis of 180 studies on the effect of the drug imipramine in treating depression. Only 35 studies—or 19 percent—had bothered to gather sex-relevant data. When taken as an aggregate, the studies revealed that men were 11 percent more likely than women to respond favorably to the drug.

Some twenty years after gender differences in drug response were first noted in the medical literature, researchers like Hamilton are still fighting to have the subject taken seriously. Meanwhile the body of evidence continues to grow. For instance it's now known from real-world experience that women often respond more slowly than men to antidepressants: four to six weeks versus two to three in men. In women over sixty-five, psychotropic drugs clear more slowly and have a longer half-life, meaning the medication remains in their systems longer. Hamilton says doses may need to be reduced by one-third in older women.

Some women whose depression is generally well controlled with medication get depressed premenstrually and need a higher dose of medication prior to menstruation. Doses of other drugs may need to be adjusted across the menstrual cycle as well.

Margaret Jensvold, the psychiatrist whose lawsuit against NIMH resulted in a jury finding sex discrimination and retaliation, is particularly interested in this question. She recalls working with a twenty-six-year-old woman hospitalized for the treatment of manic-depressive illness. Although the woman's mood stabilized when lithium was prescribed, she began to suffer from depression and mania premenstrually. Jensvold suspected that the birth control pills the patient had been taking since adolescence were contributing to her symptoms, but there was nothing in the literature to support her theory, since birth control pills in women with mood disorders had not been adequately studied. Jensvold tried an experiment. She had the young woman go off the Pill and found that, while the depression recurred, it became unrelated to her menstrual cycle. To curb the depression, Jensvold added a low dose of Prozac. Now the woman is doing fine.

"The moral is, we have very little understanding about the relationship between mood disorders and hormonal factors," says Jensvold. "This example points out that treatment needs to be individualized. Up until now people weren't even asking those questions, let alone studying them."

■ PATERNALISTIC TREATMENT

As we've seen, gender bias is rampant in both drug development and psychiatry's diagnostic categories, but it also rears its head in treatment regimens.

Judi Chamberlin knows this only too well. She'd fallen into a severe depression after suffering a miscarriage. When, over several months, she didn't respond to therapy or high doses of psychotropic drugs, she followed her psychiatrist's advice and committed herself to the psychiatric ward of a general hospital, which she describes as a "devastating" experience.

"You come in looking for help and you end up with a diagnosis that isn't helpful and you get prescribed a lot of drugs. Nobody wants to listen to your own assessment of what's going on in your life because once you get a diagnosis you're crazy, what you say doesn't matter."

Eventually Chamberlin was diagnosed as schizophrenic, a label she says many people get saddled with if they're in the system for any length of time. "You start out with a diagnosis that has something to do with what's going on with you—in my case, reactive depression. The longer you're there, the more they decide you must be seriously ill, and if you're seriously ill you must have a psychosis. What makes the mental health system different from any other is that people can be defined as patients and treated and confined against their will."

Like Chamberlin, Jeanne Dumont's hospitalizations are a litany of sexist and humiliating treatments. At one institution the doctor refused to talk with Dumont if she raised her voice. (Healthy women, as we saw earlier, are not supposed to be angry and aggressive.) Another time her psychiatrist suggested she put on lipstick and make herself more feminine. When she wore a skirt, he complimented her. As long as she adhered to her doctor's stereotypic view of how a woman should behave, she was declared on the road to recovery.

On another occasion Dumont became belligerent about being held against her will. The doctor ordered her into seclusion, which meant being locked in a small room devoid of all furniture except a mattress. The staff refused to tell her how long she could expect to remain in isolation, which set her off even more. Banging around the room, she screamed, "Let me out of here. Let me out of here." Soon she was strapped to a bed with four-point restraints.

Dumont and Chamberlin are the first to admit they've had difficulties. But they know they're not crazy. No matter. Once they pass from private citizen to "mental patient," no one cares if their anger is justified. If they don't submit to their doctor's will, play the good girl, give up the idea of self-empowerment—the tenets of traditional Freudian psychiatry—the punishment is severe.

Unlike many women, Dumont and Chamberlin were able to turn the tables. Both are now involved in patient advocacy work. Chamberlin is a member of the board of the nonprofit National Association of Psychiatric Survivors in Sioux Falls, South Dakota, while Dumont is working to create an alternative to psychiatric hospitalization that revolves around peer support.

But for most women, says psychiatrist Peter Breggin, the psychiatric profession is the worst kind of patriarchy, revolving around male doctors who subjugate female patients. It's particularly heinous in mental hospitals, Breggin says, where "patients are treated as helpless, dependent, sexless, unreasonable—as crazy."

Hospitalized women, who should be encouraged to become independent and assertive and to trust in their own internal resources, quickly "learn that being a mental patient is in many ways similar to being a wife," says Breggin. "This disillusionment often drives them to enact the helpless role with still more fervor."

This is especially problematic for women who, as previously discussed, are often depressed specifically because of their life conditions, what psychologist Phyllis Chesler describes as "a continual state of mourning—for what they never had—or had too briefly, and for what they can't have in the present, be it Prince Charming or direct worldly power." Madness, she says, "is a cry of powerlessness which is mercilessly punished."

Institutionalization is equally tough on men, but it's a particularly important women's health issue given that women comprise up to two-thirds of the patients in private mental health facilities, general hospital inpatient units, and outpatient psychiatric facilities. Once hospitalized, these women are strongly encouraged to embrace the culturally sanctioned roles they may be maddeningly trying to escape.

At the top of the hierarchy stands the psychiatrist, usually male, who rules autocratically. At the bottom is the woman, powerless, without an advocate. She's rarely consulted about her treatment plan, behavior few people would accept if it involved care for a physical problem. In fact psychiatrists—unlike other medical doctors—have almost unchecked power to diagnose and treat patients as they see fit. As Chamberlin says, "There's no blood test for what you have, no X ray. It's all a clinical impression."

A psychiatric nurse at Johns Hopkins Hospital was so upset at the way female inpatients were being treated, she eventually transferred out of the department. "Decisions about care would go on behind closed doors between the physician and the patient's husband," she says. "One woman was held against her will for a couple of months. The doctor was not assessing her so much as he was assessing her husband's readiness to have her back home. She felt controlled and thought nobody understood her. She was pretty enraged and objected in a histrionic manner. Of course when people are calm around you and you're hysterical, it's just more evidence against you."

Because women tend to be diagnosed with such "female" diseases as major depression, panic disorder, and a less severe form of depression known as dysthymia; when they stray from the norm, they're more readily labeled deviant and mentally ill. In a widely cited study, researcher Sarah Rosenfield analyzed data from 666 psychiatric emergency room patients in a large municipal hospital and found that women were much more likely than men to be hospitalized when they exhibited symptoms of antisocial personality disorder, aggression, or substance abuse. Says Rosenfield, "[W]hen women deviate in ways that are consistent with the masculine sex role and are more typical of men, the reaction to them is more severe than to men with the same behavior."

What's often missed is the true reason a woman is seeking help. Women are more likely to have multiple problems; for instance, depression plus a history of family violence and substance abuse. All too often, however, no one bothers to ask women what's really going on in their lives. There's an unwillingness to listen to women's stories, as if they have nothing of value to contribute to the therapeutic process. Sometimes doctors are aware of a history of abuse and choose to ignore it as if, following Freud's lead, they don't believe it's real. On several occasions, when the Johns Hopkins nurse consulted with anorexic patients who had been the victims of sexual abuse, the psychiatrists told the staff not to deal with that issue.

Vanessa Savage (a pseudonym), who was sexually and ritually abused by an uncle, had experiences similar to Chamberlin's in private mental institutions in Massachusetts. After being diagnosed with multiple personality disorder (MPD), she was hospitalized in 1992 for twenty-seven days, but her psychiatrist refused to address her abuse. "She didn't believe I had MPD. She said I had post-traumatic stress disorder and that I should forget about the incest because it wasn't real. But how could I have post-traumatic stress disorder without it being preceded by some kind of trauma? It didn't make sense."

Savage learned the rules of the game the hard way. During a group-therapy session one of her alternate personalities came out and started crying and speaking in Spanish. Savage was hauled out of the session screaming and told if she didn't shape up, she'd be transferred to another hospital. "The message was, 'This isn't stuff we do here. We do containment.' They didn't want my private therapist coming in and doing memory work with me. They wanted to contain me. There was no place you could go and scream or get a hug when you needed one. It does cause you to conform. It's such a scary atmosphere."

Savage was rarely offered individual therapy during her hospitalizations, but she was often doped up on tranquilizers and antidepressants. After several institutionalizations she knew enough to steer clear of Thorazine, a major tranquilizer and the one that causes "the Thorazine shuffle." "When you're on Thorazine, you feel like you're walking on the tops of your feet. You can't think. You can't do anything. It takes away all your feeling."

In fact drugs are often the mainstay of treatment. Writes Breggin, "Instead of understanding the woman's symptoms as an expression of frustration, outrage and despair over her place in society, the psychiatrist prescribes spirit-blunting medications that reinforce the status quo in her life."

Indeed, as the battle over the control of the nation's mental health care escalates, psychiatrists have sought to distinguish themselves from psychologists and other kinds of therapists by emphasizing the biological basis of mental disorders. With new knowledge about the chemical and genetic underpinnings of these illnesses, they have increasingly turned to psychotropic medication—which can only be prescribed by an M.D.—as a quick fix. Talk therapy is demanding and time-consuming. It's so much easier to give women a drug, shut them up, and send them on their way.

Ultimately, writes Breggin, "the woman's role in the family is reinforced by the hospital experience. She's not likely to be discharged feeling inspired with feminist fervor or brimming over with self-empowerment. Indeed, such attitudes would get labeled 'resistant' or 'oppositional' in the hospital and earn her more severe restrictions, a larger dose of medication or electroshock."

Shock therapy, an extremely controversial treatment, is of great concern to those in the consumer health movement because it is disproportionately applied to women, who comprise two-thirds of the more than 100,000 people who receive the treatment every year. Proponents of electroconvulsive therapy (ECT) say that this sex ratio should be expected since more women than men are diagnosed with depression.

But critics of the procedure—in which electrical pulses are transmitted to the brain through electrodes placed on one or both temples—say it is nowhere near benign. Although the American Psychiatric Association says that ECT is safe and effective in treating people with major depression, mania, and schizophrenia, it can have severe side effects, including some permanent memory loss. The myriad pros and cons of ECT are beyond the scope of this book. What is worrisome is that more women than men are getting a potentially damaging treatment, in many cases without full knowledge of what they're getting into.

Susan Witte was hospitalized in 1987 after suffering a nervous breakdown. A variety of medications hadn't curbed her severe depression, so she agreed to undergo three shock therapy treatments a week, for a total of twenty treatments. When she was discharged from the hospital two months later, Witte, then forty-one, didn't recognize the family car or her house on Long Island. She was amazed to see two grown children waiting for her at home. The last she recalled, they were ten and seven years old. Witte couldn't remember how to cook or how to operate the kitchen appliances or her washer and dryer. She didn't remember that she'd recently received her associate of arts degree at Nassau Community College. When she tried to read, she saw the words backward, as if she were suddenly dyslexic. When Witte complained about her memory problems, her psychiatrist said, "There's nothing wrong with you. This is all part of your depression."

No one told Witte or her husband that ECT could result in memory loss extending a year or two before and after treatment. Lee Coleman, M.D., a psychiatrist in private practice in Berkeley, California, and a critic of ECT, contends that the induction of amnesia is the whole point. "Traditionally, women have had less power and income to control their destiny," he says. "The doctor is far more likely to collaborate with the husband in making the decision to give the wife ECT. The assumption is that a housewife has nothing else to do. If she's a zombie for a month, she can usually still cook and clean and do the housework. It all has to do with power."

Especially vulnerable are elderly women, who, when judged mentally incompetent, are more likely than men the same age to have ECT forced on them. In December 1993 eighty-year-old Lucille Austwick refused to undergo the ECT her psychiatrists had prescribed to treat her major depression and dementia. Her public guardian filed an emergency petition to order her to have the procedure. One of her treating psychiatrists, Iradj Nabatian, M.D., of Rush Presbyterian Saint Luke's Hospital in Chicago, testified in court that psychotherapy had been ineffective in treating Austwick and that she'd had adverse reactions to certain antidepressants. Although she'd started on the antidepressant Zoloft five days prior to the hearing, he said it would take two to three weeks to see any benefits. Rather than wait, Nabatian said it would be better to get Austwick out of the hospital "rather than stay here and spend money and time." While he admitted under oath that the generally accepted treatment for both of her conditions was medication, he wanted to get on with ECT—three treatments a week for up to four weeks.

Austwick refused the treatments, saying, "I am wise enough to . . . make [the] decision for myself. I don't need anybody to make [the] decision for me."

Apparently Nabatian did not agree. In fact Austwick's physicians seemed unconcerned that serious medical complications are significantly more common in people over sixty-five years of age and that the elderly are at the greatest risk of cognitive impairment as a result of ECT.

Despite the risks, a trial court ordered Austwick to consent to the treatment. The State Guardianship and Advocacy Commission representing Austwick appealed the decision. Laurel Spahn, a lawyer for the guardianship, said, "I've explained the treatments to her several times, and each time she's said, 'That's ridiculous. If they want to do that, let them go shock themselves.'" As of early 1994, the new medication appeared to have worked, but Austwick's case was still pending in appellate court.

■ SUBSTANCE ABUSE: A WOMAN'S ISSUE

If women make up a disproportionate number of the mentally ill receiving electroshock therapy and psychotropic drugs, the reverse is true when it comes to research and treatment programs involving substance abuse. Here women are downright neglected, a result of deeply ingrained stereotypes about who uses drugs and alcohol.

Back in the early 1970s, when Sharon Wilsnack was a researcher at Harvard, a colleague published a book titled *The Drinking Man: Alcohol and Human Motivation.* Considered an important contribution to the field, the tome dealt exclusively with men. Wilsnack thought it was interesting that women were not included. Her curiosity piqued, she did a library search and found hundreds of articles on men and alcohol, but only six on women. "Even the animal studies involving alcohol at that time were conducted solely on males," she says. "There were experiments where they poured alcohol into goldfish tanks to gauge its effects on fish. Even the fish were male!"

It would be nice to think that things have changed, that in the last twenty years a large knowledge base has accrued on women and substance abuse. Granted, strides have been made, but when it comes to research and treatment, the seventy-kilogram male is still the norm. As we've seen in every other area of medicine, women's unique needs are just noise in the system. This is a shame given that women's addictions to alcohol and drugs constitute a major public health problem.

Women pay a heavy price, both physically and socially, for their addictions. Because drinking is still believed to lead to promiscuity, women who drink heavily are often branded "fallen women," making them acceptable targets of sexual aggression. A number of studies have documented the stigma attached to women who drink. In one such study, ninety-six male college students were asked to rate videotapes of a young woman drinking either beer or a soft drink. The students judged the woman drinking beer with a male companion highest in terms of sexual responsiveness and promiscuity. Furthermore, a woman's drunkenness is seen as an exploitable weakness. Research shows that women who are heavy drinkers are more likely than men to be the victims of physical or sexual assault.

Yet the belief that drinking makes women promiscuous is totally unsupported by research. In a survey of one thousand women who used alcohol, Sharon Wilsnack found that only 8 percent said they had become less selective about a potential sexual partner when they had been drinking. In contrast, 60 percent said that someone who was drinking had become sexually aggressive toward them. This held true whether the woman was a light, moderate, or heavy drinker. "Thus, the stereotype of women made promiscuous by alcohol is not merely inaccurate," writes Sheila Blume, M.D., medical director of the Alcoholism, Chemical Dependency, and Compulsive Gambling program at South Oaks Hospital in Amityville, New York. It promotes "the sexual victimization of drinking women."

THE RESEARCH GAP

The myth of the fallen woman, the belief that "nice girls" don't drink or do drugs, has rendered substance-abusing women invisible from all manner of scientific inquiry. They're conspicuously absent from epidemiological research and treatment studies, resulting in knowledge gaps as to how best to care for these women.

Concerned that women were being neglected, in the late 1970s the National Institute on Alcohol Abuse and Alcoholism (NIAAA) reviewed the literature to determine exactly what was known about women. Investigators found that in spite of plenty of evidence of gender differences in the effects of alcohol, "it was often impossible to tell from the title of an article, from the abstract, or even sometimes the article itself, whether or not women were included in the study at all."

A second look at the literature in the mid-1980s found an incredible lack of progress. In a review of thirty years of treatment outcome research Marsha Vannicelli found that of the 110,000 alcoholics included in the studies, only 8,000 were women. Data were analyzed separately for only three thousand women. Interestingly, women represented 13.4 percent of study participants when the first author was female but only 4.3 percent when the first author was male. Vannicelli concluded that "sex bias does appear to influence the ways in which women alcoholics have been studied."

Likewise a review of studies published since 1980 found a paucity of "large representative clinical data bases that would allow investigators to generalize to the overall population of women in treatment." As is the case in most areas of research, if it's too difficult to identify substance-abusing women and too time-consuming to analyze data by gender, researchers have no qualms about throwing all scientific integrity to the wind. Similar to women with AIDS, many substance-abusing women are African-American or Latina and live in poverty, making them easily disposable.

Women are overlooked as research subjects in part because much of the substance-abuse research is conducted in Veterans Administration hospitals, where most of the patients are men. Shorter hospital stays, a cost-cutting measure mandated by many insurance companies, may also undermine research in women. "If one is going to study the effects of different hormonal states throughout a menstrual cycle ..., one would require that the women in the study be hospitalized for a minimum of twenty-eight days, a period often longer than hospitalization plans allow," says substance-abuse researcher Beth Glover Reed, Ph.D., of the University of Michigan's School of Social Work.

Scientists have justified the exclusion of alcohol and drug-addicted women from research by pointing to the lower prevalence of these disorders in women. Thirty percent of alcoholics and nearly 50 percent of those who are chemically dependent are women. More than 4 percent of women meet the official diagnostic criteria for alcohol abuse or dependence, about half the rate of men.

But it's possible, as was the case with AIDS, that women are being vastly undercounted. When appropriate screening tests were used, studies found that 12 percent of women visiting a private gynecologist and an incredible 21 percent visiting a private PMS clinic met the DSM-III-R criteria for alcohol abuse. When women's centers screened patients for addictions, they found that 50 to 80 percent of the women either used alcohol or drugs, were spouses or partners of substance abusers, or were from families where there had been alcohol or other drug problems.

This suggests there are a lot more substance-abusing women than are officially counted. Unfortunately the stigma attached to being a woman addict keeps many of them in hiding, which explains why women are more apt to engage in these activities at home alone. Although a woman may seek medical help, it's usually for such complaints as nervousness and insomnia, and she'll be likely to leave with a prescription for tranquilizers rather than a referral to a treatment program.

Unless health care providers are really looking for drug- or alcohol-related problems, they're not going to find them, particularly among educated women with private insurance. "Women are misdiagnosed more often than men," says Sheila Blume. "If a woman is well dressed and doesn't look like she has a problem, the doctor will probably miss it." But it is relatively easy now for doctors to uncover alcohol abuse. A number of simple screening tools, such as the TWEAK and CAGE tests, ask several questions designed to get at drinking problems in a nonjudgmental way, and take only minutes to administer.

TREATMENT

If women are underdiagnosed and underresearched, they are underrepresented in treatment as well. Of more than 800,000 patients treated in drug and alcohol programs in 1991, only 27.5 percent were women.

No one consciously set out to refuse women treatment, but because more men than women abuse alcohol and drugs, there was more research on the effects these substances had on men. As a result, alcohol treatment programs from the 1950s through the early 1970s developed around white middle-aged men and were especially aware of their problems—that men generally use alcohol but not drugs, show up for treatment in the late stages of their disease, and have little psychiatric impairment outside of their alcoholism. The field defined the physiology of alcohol in the body, the causes and progression of the disease, and the state of the art in treatment based on the experiences of this largely homogeneous group of men. At the time it seemed like good science.

In the mid-seventies, when the National Institute on Alcohol Abuse and Alcoholism asked programs to be more responsive to special populations, it became obvious that women would bring a whole new dimension to the equation. To start, they were a much more heterogenous population. Women alcoholics start drinking later than men but have more dual diagnoses. Major depression, for instance, often precedes the development of problem drinking in women. How and when should antidepressants be used with these women? No one knows.

Not only are female substance abusers more likely to have coexisting mental disorders, they're more apt to have a history of physical and sexual abuse and to be using multiple drugs. In one survey almost half of female alcoholic patients were also using illegal drugs, in particular marijuana and cocaine. Another study found that about 70 percent of female alcoholics also abused sedatives and tranquilizers. Older women often combined alcohol with prescription drugs.

And there are these additional concerns:

- Women become physically addicted to alcohol more rapidly than do men.
- The phases of alcoholism are less distinct in women.
- Women reach higher peak blood alcohol levels than men when given a standard dose of alcohol, even when weight is controlled.
- Blood alcohol levels vary with the phase of the menstrual cycle.
- Women alcoholics tend to be more socially isolated than men. Men abandon their alcoholic wives at higher rates than women abandon their alcoholic husbands.
- Women develop liver disease after shorter periods of drinking and at lower levels of intake compared with men.
- As few as three to nine drinks a week may increase a woman's risk of developing breast cancer by up to 60 percent.
- Women alcoholics are at greater risk for osteoporosis, hypertension, and death due to heart disease.
- Women alcoholics are more likely than their male counterparts to attempt suicide.

The medical literature was reporting these gender differences as early as fifteen to twenty years ago. Back then "the attitude had been, train people in the ways in which women are different than men and services would change," says Beth Glover Reed. But the programs didn't change, and after a while most of the people working with women burned out and left the field. "Failures such as these probably are due in part to male-centered theories, assumptions and concepts," says Reed.

Whether being treated for alcohol or drug abuse, women are shoehorned into services developed solely for men. Programs have traditionally focused on what is known as ego-restructuring, a confrontational approach aimed at unmasking denial, which can be especially problematic for women. "Dealing with denial and responsibility is thought to be key in drug treatment programs and the approach is to challenge it, confront it, try and go through it, or let somebody bottom out so their denial defenses are broken down," says Beth Reed. "It was not unusual in earlier programs to make potential clients demonstrate their motivation for treatment by coming back multiple times before they would be allowed to come in and then to extend the intake process deliberately in order to be certain that, by the time somebody got into the program, they were motivated to work on their problem. By and large, such strategies aimed toward male denial do not work for women and are likely to increase depression and self-blame." The very fact that women who are substance abusers have so much depression and anxiety suggests that the psychological mechanism of denial isn't working. If it were, women wouldn't have these feelings.

Then there was that eighties buzzword *codependency*. Originally applied to women raised in families with alcoholic parents or living with alcoholic partners, the term expanded to include a pattern of behavior in which women took responsibility for the actions and well-being of those around them. Highly self-blaming, these women supposedly coped by trying to control themselves and everything else in their worlds. But by attempting to protect a dysfunctional spouse or other family member, the woman further "enabled" the abusive behavior. On the one hand the concept of codependency brought some real psychological issues in women's lives— dependency, low self-esteem, and women's habit of putting others first— into the treatment process. But by reinforcing a woman's expected gender role, programs may only serve to "perpetuate stereotypic perceptions of women," says Reed.

Jean Kirkpatrick, president and founder of the eighteen-year-old Women for Sobriety, one of the oldest treatment programs aimed squarely at women, is convinced that this male model of treatment disadvantages women. "Before 1976 all programs looked at alcoholics as a group, but men were getting well and women weren't," she says. "The basis of Alcoholics Anonymous and other twelve-step programs is that you are powerless to cure yourself, so you have to turn yourself over to a higher authority. We disagree. Women need to be empowered, not turn their power over to others."

Just being in a setting with men may prevent the underlying reasons for a woman's drug or alcohol use from surfacing. It's hard enough for women to talk about their incest, sexual molestation, or eating disorders with other women, let alone with a group of strange men, particularly when they're outnumbered three to one. Yet talking about and coming to terms with past abuse is a crucial part of the healing process and may be an important prerequisite to a woman getting off drugs or alcohol.

"There are a great many things that are difficult for women to talk about in groups with men," says LeClair Bissell, M.D., past president of the American Society on Alcoholism. "If a man says to the group, 'We got drunk and ended up in bed,' that's considered cool. Not so for women. And in fact treatment-center outpatient departments don't very tightly control social interactions among group members off the premises. Yet once a woman reveals to the group, 'We got drunk and ended up in bed,' almost invariably there's one male in the group who thinks she's available. It's harder for women to get good treatment because of this."

In most treatment programs there's a complete lack of gynecological, contraceptive, and prenatal care. Only 10 percent of women are treated in units providing child care, a major barrier to their participation in inpatient programs. Although vocational rehabilitation is sometimes offered, stereotypical attitudes toward what is appropriate for women discourage them from pursuing such "male" occupations as plumbing or construction work and push them into lower-paying "female" positions, such as clerical or service work.

In spite of these shortcomings it appears that women in coed programs do at least as well as men. Program administrators, however, feel they should be doing much better. An evaluation of 259 studies on substance abuse found twenty-three with enough data to evaluate treatment outcomes in women versus men. Eighteen studies found no significant gender differences, but four showed a better outcome for women than for men. When there were gender differences, women seemed to benefit from treatment more than men. Muses Sharon Wilsnack, "You have to wonder, if women are doing that well in nongender-specific programs, might they not do even better in more specialized programs?"

In an attempt to get answers, NIAAA has funded a large multicenter trial, "the first big study to ask whether certain types of alcoholics do best with certain treatments," says Frances Del Boca, Ph.D., an investigator in the Addiction and Substance Abuse Unit at the University of Connecticut School of Medicine. Of the 1,728 subjects, about 25 percent are women, a large enough sample to draw gender-related conclusions. "A lot of what we know or suspect about the subject of women and substance abuse is anecdotal," says Del Boca, whose center is coordinating the NIAAA trial. "There are not much good data because the right questions haven't been asked. We're still in the dark about what women think is important in treatment programs."

One thing is certain: Pregnant women want assurances that going for treatment will not result in criminal prosecution or the loss of their children to foster care. By all accounts they have good cause to worry. Between 1985 and 1992 more than 150 criminal cases had been brought against pregnant and postpartum women charging them with abusing their fetus or newborn through the use of alcohol or drugs. (For more on this, see chapter 13.) In a recent case in Connecticut an infant was taken from her mother at birth because the mother had used cocaine just prior to delivery. A lower court ruled to terminate the mother's rights, but on appeal Connecticut's highest court reversed the termination, saying that under the child-abuse-and-neglect laws of that state, the fetus was not a child and the pregnant woman was not a parent.

Until recently New York City hospitals had a policy of reporting positive urine drug tests on newborns, resulting in an automatic petition for a family-court neglect hearing. Some five thousand petitions were brought in 1989, and three-quarters resulted in a loss of parental custody. One woman, Ana R., had had a single positive drug test but three subsequent negative ones. Although she denied taking drugs, she lost custody of her child. In a 1990 lawsuit her lawyer argued that another woman with the same last name had delivered in the hospital that same day and that the urine reports may have been mixed up. New York State has since put an end to this fetal-protection policy.

In general, though, few of the criminal cases against women are successful. "There was a tremendous hue and cry from women working in this field, who said the focus was wrong, that this wasn't a way to fight drug abuse, because women became afraid to get treatment," says Paula Roth, a consultant to organizations on women and substance abuse. "In any case the focus shouldn't just be on the fetus."

Fetal rights took the spotlight in the late 1970s when public health officials discovered the "alcohol problem" in women. Fetal alcohol syndrome became headline news, and before anyone knew what was happening, "alcoholism was declared an epidemic among women," says Sharon Wilsnack. "All sorts of reporters, even the *National Enquirer*, called me about this topic. But the data found no epidemic at all."

Upon closer scrutiny Wilsnack realized that a host of health problems were being attributed to women who left the wife-mother role and entered the workforce, which at that time they were starting to do in greater numbers. "There were claims that women doing 'men's' jobs left them vulnerable to men's diseases, such as heart disease and alcoholism," she says. "Yet increases of heart disease among women were not being reported, and drinking levels were up only modestly."

Authorities had no qualms about punishing women who used drugs or alcohol during pregnancy, but as with AIDS, if a woman was pregnant and sought treatment for her substance abuse, the doors often slammed shut. A 1990 General Accounting Office report found that of the approximately 280,000 pregnant women who needed drug-abuse treatment in 1989, only 11 percent received it. It was the same old party line: With a lack of prenatal and obstetrical care and fears of legal liability should a treatment medication harm a developing fetus, programs couldn't possibly treat these women.

Substance-abuse researchers were appalled. When Wendy Chavkin, M.D., was head of the New York City Bureau of Maternity Services, her staffers complained that they were having difficulty finding slots for pregnant women in local drug treatment programs. So Chavkin decided to conduct a study. She had her staff call seventy-eight drug treatment centers and say they were pregnant and on drugs and wanted treatment. More than half of the programs turned the women down flat. Two-thirds refused women who said they were on Medicaid, and 87 percent refused women who were pregnant, on crack, and on Medicaid.

Says Chavkin, now an associate professor of public health and obstetrics and gynecology at the Columbia-Presbyterian Medical Center, "I was not only disturbed because here was yet another example of gender bias against women. I was also particularly struck by the cruelty of punishing women for their drug use while simultaneously precluding their options to do anything about it."

The clinical experiences of Wendy Chavkin, Margaret Jensvold, and others suggest that women—whether chemically dependent or suffering from depression—may need to be treated differently from their male counterparts. In terms of depression, for instance, programs need to be sensitive to the fact that in women the disorder tends to be associated with lowered self-esteem, unrealistic expectations for physical perfection, feelings of helplessness, conflict in interpersonal relationships, physical and sexual abuse, reproductive-related events, discrimination, and poverty.

"Historically, psychiatry has ignored, minimized, or misinterpreted the profound biological, social, economic, and power differences between women and men, all of which greatly affect individual psychological development," writes feminist psychiatrist Karen Johnson, M.D. "For now female patients cannot be assured of receiving the quality of psychiatric care that male patients can take for granted."

Karen Johnson and an array of feminist physicians and patients are sounding a call for woman-centered care. Their message is a simple one: the paternalistic treatment of women, the denigration of their emotional lives, must finally stop.

HEALING THE SYSTEM

12

DRUG MARKETING
Selling Women Out

In most businesses, products are tested on the segment of the population that will be using the product. Not so with the pharmaceutical industry. Although most of the prescription and over-the-counter drugs now on the market were tested primarily on men, women are the biggest customers. Women take more prescription drugs than men and buy more over-the-counter medications for themselves and their families.

The lack of knowledge about how drugs affect women's bodies and women's health has not stopped pharmaceutical manufacturers from encouraging physicians to prescribe their products to women. They also pitch advertising directly to women, who see doctors more than men and make up 70 percent of drugstore shoppers.

The magazine ads and television commercials that pharmaceutical firms produce, whether aimed at doctors or consumers, are just as manipulative in their imagery as ads for a new laundry detergent or brand of ketchup. The difference is the consequence: In the long run it matters little what brand of soap a woman buys. But how much and what kind of drugs she buys for herself and/or her family may matter a great deal and have a profound impact on health and well-being.

Studies show that physicians receive most of their information about new prescription medications from advertising and from the "detail men," representatives of the drug companies who visit medical offices to tout new products and offer incentives for physicians to prescribe their companies' drugs. Detail men give away free samples of the drugs, plus T-shirts, coffee mugs, pens, and notepads imprinted with the products' names. Pharmaceutical companies spend much of their budgets on lavish promotional schemes: gifts, dinners, and travel for doctors who prescribe the most drugs. For example, the maker of the estrogen skin patch flew gynecologists who had prescribed large numbers of patches to the Caribbean for a "conference" touting the benefits of supplemental estrogen. Pharmaceutical drug-promotion budgets can be as high as five thousand dollars per physician per year. One study found that three-quarters of physicians had received money from pharmaceutical companies within the preceding two years.

"Clearly because of the number of drugs on the market, no practitioner can keep up today," says Joellen W. Hawkins, RNC, Ph.D., a professor at Boston College's School of Nursing who has examined gender bias and sex stereotyping in pharmaceutical advertising. "So physicians rely very heavily on medication advertisements. And if the detail person has been in with something that week, they're very likely to use it, or if they have a pen or pad on their desk with the product's name." Studies show that even when doctors *think* they get their information on drugs from the medical literature, much of their information actually comes from advertisements. "Drug advertisements are simply more visually arresting and conceptually accessible than are papers in the medical literature, and physicians appear to respond to this difference," concluded one study. Three-quarters of physicians read the drug advertisements in medical journals, and about 80 percent of those physicians find the ads helpful.

Unfortunately the ads may be horribly inaccurate. An article in the professional journal *Annals of Internal Medicine* found that 92 percent of the ads examined did not meet the standards for fairness, accuracy, and balance set by the Food and Drug Administration. The study also found that nearly half—44 percent—of the ads could lead doctors to prescribe the drugs inappropriately if they relied solely on the advertisements for information.

The pharmaceutical industry's hard-sell advertising tactics, coupled with the lack of good data on how drugs affect women, make it highly unlikely that every prescription a physician writes for a woman is absolutely necessary and is the best drug for that individual's specific condition. Targeting drugs toward women is not altruism but capitalism, with serious consequences for women's health.

■ ADVERTISING IMAGES:
CRANKY OLD WOMEN AND SEXY YOUNG GIRLS

The medical information in pharmaceutical ads isn't all that is inaccurate. The images used to sell the product may also mislead. Pharmaceutical advertising tends to reinforce the beliefs that physicians have about female patients, for instance that women's symptoms are "all in their head" and that women patients are more demanding, more complaining, and more anxious about their health than men. Drug company advertising exploits these myths to encourage doctors to prescribe their product as a way of placating supposedly demanding women with supposedly psychosomatic symptoms. The drug ads in the professional journals read by physicians also tend to show older, depressed, anxious women, or very sexy and voluptuous young women.

Joellen Hawkins and colleague Cynthia Aber did several studies looking at gender images in medical ads. What they found were ads filled with white male doctors and white female nurses (generally wearing short white uniforms), and women patients looking up at godlike father-image physicians. "Interestingly, we did not find one ad with a woman physician and a male consumer," says Hawkins. In fact, there were hardly any women physicians in the ads at all, and when there were, "they were usually only in ads having something to do with women, such as contraceptive drugs or yeast medications. Heaven forbid they show a woman surgeon or pathologist."

Ronda Macchello, M.D., an internist at the Palo Alto Medical Clinic, has also examined medical advertising. She does a presentation at medical conferences, complete with dozens of slides of offensive drug ads, hoping to show other physicians the bias inherent in the messages that bombard them. She found that the advertisers "seem to feel that the only doctor who is going to have any credibility for other doctors is someone who looks like Marcus Welby. When there are women physicians in the ad, they are quite strikingly young and pretty—they look like models with white coats and stethoscopes on."

Women in drug ads are more likely than men to be naked, with full body exposed. When men are naked, it is generally from the waist up only. "Not one ad portrays a man as a sex object, nor do many portray men with negative characteristics," says Hawkins. When men in these ads are stressed, it's from work, but women are stressed from family, housework, and menial tasks. Men are active, women passive. The women are often posed provocatively. Write Hawkins and Aber, "Some of the women have obviously dyed or bleached hair. Many have exaggerated makeup, long painted nails, long flowing hair, low-cut, sheer, or nude-tone outfits."

Hawkins is particularly appalled by ads in orthopedic journals for equipment such as hip-pinning machines. Pandering to the libidos of predominantly male orthopedic surgeons, these ads use sex to sell expensive medical equipment. "These ads show very young models in skintight outfits, even though young women are not the patients getting their hips replaced. In one ad there's a young woman on a hip-pinning machine with the post jammed into her crotch. If there are men in the ads, they're always in loose-fitting running shorts, but the women in the same ads are wearing skintight exercise clothes."

Macchello found an ad for a bowel prep (a liquid patients drink before having diagnostic images of the gastrointestinal tract) that used a subliminal sex image to sell the product. "Bowel preps are about the least sexy thing you can imagine," she says. "They really taste foul. The ad shows a woman with her mouth open, ready to drink the stuff. And in the glass, in a bubble, is an image of a penis. She's drinking a penis."

Sex may sell, whether the product is medicine or blue jeans, but the predominant image of the woman patient in pharmaceutical ads is the cranky old woman.

One popular ad for an antianxiety drug shows three different photographs of the same late-middle-aged woman. She is wearing a different outfit in each picture, but with similar pained, unpleasant expressions. The headline reads: "Varied complaints . . . Repeat visits . . . Negative workups . . . Suspect persistent anxiety." The implication is that this woman has visited her doctor at least three different times, complaining of a medical problem. The doctor has not been able to figure out what is wrong. Therefore the problem must be all in her head. The copy reads, "You probably see patients like this every day." Says Dr. Macchello, "The implication is that the patient is a horrible, whiny woman who keeps coming back to you with no problem, and if you give her this medicine, she'll be out of your face."

Women make up 80 percent of the "patients" in ads for psychotropic drugs, and the advertisers' message is obviously getting through to physicians, who write women more prescriptions than men for antidepressant drugs and tranquilizers (see chapter 11). "There's a real abuse of women patients. The idea is, 'Give her something to shut her up,' " says Ann R. Turkel, M.D., assistant clinical professor of psychiatry, Columbia University College of Physicians and Surgeons.

The ads for these drugs seem to confirm something physicians already believe, or plant a mental seed that perhaps women really do complain for no reason. The result for women may be too many prescriptions for psychoactive drugs, but men's health care may also be affected.

"If a woman comes in and you can't find anything wrong, they think it must be something in her mind. But if a man comes in, it must be something physical," says Hawkins. "So men get disserviced too. They get overtested, and nobody ever thinks it may be something psychological. Their psychological needs sometimes get ignored, although they certainly don't get mistreated in the way that women do."

Macchello found that women were overrepresented in ads for psychotropic drugs but underrrepresented in ads for drugs to treat physical conditions such as high blood pressure, heart disease, arthritis, ulcers, and diabetes. Eva Lynn Thompson, who published another study of sex bias in drug ads warns, "By showing patients of a particular age or sex group, a drug advertisement is implying that the age or sex group is likely to have the condition which the advertised drug ameliorates." Biased ads can mislead by omission, too. For instance, because of the male bias in advertisements for cardiovascular drugs, "some physicians might be less likely to note early signs of these conditions in women," says Thompson. As chapter 4 showed, underdiagnosis of women's heart problems is rampant. Drug ads may be partly to blame.

Hawkins describes another ad, for Tenormin, a hypertension medication. The photograph shows a group of six people. The sex ratio is equal—three men and three women—but that's about all that's equal. Two of the men look like businessmen; one is a construction worker. The women include an old lady in hair curlers and a bathrobe with a sour expression, an overweight woman sitting down to a large meal, and a masculine-looking woman clutching a cat.

And these ads are not isolated examples. "There was a series of ads that told physicians the drug would allow patients to 'get on with their lives,'" says Hawkins. "The man would be portrayed as being able to get back to his job, but the woman would be sitting on a bench knitting. In another ad one side showed a man as a truck driver. The caption said the drug allowed him to 'follow normal daily routines.' But the caption near the woman in the ad, who doesn't seem to have a job, reads, 'enhance patient compliance.'"

The theme of compliance—how well patients follow doctors' orders—runs through many ads for prescription drugs. Convenience is stressed for the man, compliance for the woman. That's because drug ads suggest that most women are too stupid to follow directions. "It's very typical to portray women as dumb," says Hawkins. "There are drug ads that call women pill-skippers, suggesting that they're not bright enough to remember to take their medicine."

Hawkins and Macchello's findings are particularly discouraging when compared with similar studies done in the 1970s, all of which came to conclusions nearly identical to those of the more recent work.

In one of the earliest studies of how pharmaceutical advertising affects physicians' perceptions of their patients, in 1971, Robert Seidenberg, M.D., found that advertisements for mood-altering drugs seemed to exploit the boredom that many women felt as housewives. He wrote, "The burden of giving a child a bath at night, or a distaste for washing dishes might be converted into medically treatable syndromes . . . one often sees women portrayed in their humdrum environment with the recommendation that they be drugged to become adjusted to their lot. The drug industry openly acknowledges the enslavement of women, as shown in an ad with a woman behind bars made up of brooms and mops. The caption reads, 'You can't set her free but you can help make her feel less anxious.' "

By making everyday boredom into a psychological illness, drug manufacturers have created an enormous market for tranquilizers and antidepressants. Many of these ads still show women as unable to handle daily life without their bottle of pills. If washing dishes were really causing major depression, it might make more sense for women to avoid the expensive medication and spend their money on a dishwasher instead.

Jane Prather and Linda S. Fidell found in 1975 that ads for mood-altering drugs tended to show women while those for other drugs showed men, and that women tended to be shown as suffering from primarily emotional illness while men are shown as having primarily organic illness. "That is, women may display (or be interpreted as displaying) emotional symptoms when the problem is organic, while men show (or are thought to show) organic symptoms when the 'cause' is emotional. The possibility for misdiagnosis of both sexes would appear therefore to be increased."

In another study from the 1970s, psychiatrists were asked about the images in psychotropic drug ads. They admitted that physicians' thinking might be affected by seeing women portrayed as the majority of patients. Some of the comments were: "Tends to perpetrate general trend of thinking of women as weaker, more sick," "subliminally might indicate women are crazier," "might imprint male M.D.'s with the impression that mental illness and femaleness go together."

Some of the same characters that inhabited drug advertisements in the 1970s still grace the pages of medical journals. One early study listed such female stereotypes as the irritable old lady, the overwrought mother, the depressed housewife, the complaining matron, and the attractive seductress—a cast familiar to any casual reader flipping through the medical literature. More than other types of advertising, the pharmaceutical ads that appear in professional journals still seem to rely on these outdated depictions of women.

■ THE DRUG ADS THAT PATIENTS SEE

Both prescription and over-the-counter drugs are advertised directly to patients. But the drug ads shown in women's magazines are very different from those in the medical journals. All of a sudden the young sexpots and old sourpusses have metamorphosed into efficient, capable working women and mothers who intelligently weigh all the information before purchasing medicine for themselves and their families. Ironically, while professional ads exploit negative images of women patients to encourage physicians to prescribe more drugs, consumer ads exploit the idea of women's greater health knowledge and concerns to get women to buy more drugs for themselves and their families.

Since 1986 the FDA has allowed makers of prescription drugs to advertise their products directly to consumers, mainly women. "It takes a certain amount of confidence to have a dialogue with the doctor rather than accept everything he says, to talk to him rather than go for the over-the-counter drug," says Joan Lemler, an account supervisor at Medicus Consumer-DMB&B, who has worked on advertising campaigns for Seldane (an antihistamine), Nicorette (a nicotine chewing gum to help smokers quit), Cardizem (a drug to treat angina), and Peridex (an oral rinse to treat gum disease). "I think there's been a lot of respect for that audience because it's been a progressive audience."

Market research indicates that even when a drug is for a medical condition that affects men and women equally, the ads will be most effective when aimed at women. "Women are an easier group to target if the drug is appropriate," says Lemler. "They tend to accept treatment more than men, and they're more proactive, more into preventive medicine." So even though the incidence of allergies is pretty much equal, most of the advertising for Seldane was aimed at women and advertised in women's magazines. These ads were "nonbranded," meaning that the manufacturer, Merrell Dow, did not mention the drug by name but advised women to ask their doctors about prescription medicine for hayfever.

So great is women's appeal for advertisers that even drugs taken exclusively by men are often advertised to women. A woman who has worked in the art department of a pharmaceutical agency says, "When we were deciding what to do with Proscar [a drug used to treat enlarged prostate glands], there was a campaign geared toward women, even though it's a drug for men. Women tend to be the ones who make lots of decisions in the household and who get their husbands to go to the doctor."

This woman, who asked not to be named, says that advertising, whether for medical products or any other kind of product, is still a male-dominated business. While male copywriters and art directors work on campaigns for female products such as tampons and birth control pills, "I was only allowed to work on the Proscar campaign aimed at women. I was told I wouldn't understand the campaign for men."

Ads for over-the-counter (OTC) medications also play on women's greater health knowledge. These ads—for cold and cough medicines, analgesics, and so on—often feature capable homemakers happily medicating their families. "Advertisers of over-the-counter drugs have no problem exploiting the homemaker mythology, the idea of the woman as being the person in the home who is responsible for medical care, and who is knowledgeable about it," says R. Stephen Craig, Ph.D., a communications professor at the University of Maine.

Craig's study of over-the-counter drug commercials found that women were significantly more likely than men to appear in drug ads than in ads for other products. He writes, "This supports the hypothesis that drug advertisers take advantage of stereotypical images of women as home medical caregivers. It also raises the question of whether female consumers are being encouraged by these ads to overuse OTC medications as a way of gaining the family's love and respect."

Some of the commercials, says Craig, are quite explicit in their imagery. "There is one commercial for a cough syrup [Robitussin] that has a woman's family lined up outside a door, waiting for her to give them medicine, just like in a doctor's office. In this glorification [of women's knowledge of health care] women are being encouraged to use more over-the-counter medications. What I'm suggesting is that women who feel alienated in the home and relish being experts in the few things they're allowed to be experts in, use medications as a way of confirming their value and their personal worth."

Unlike the men in prescription drug ads, the men in OTC drug commercials "were either absent altogether or appeared to be unrealistic exaggerations, relying on the wife/mother to make even the simplest decisions on home medical care."

Another TV commercial Craig describes starts with an announcer asking, "Home alone?" while the screen shows a father and son. The father is in a quandary because his child is sick and he doesn't know how to medicate the problem . . . until the mother comes home. "She's explicitly portrayed as the expert in the family," says Craig.

In yet another, a man and woman are in bed. She's sleeping, but he's coughing, and nudges her awake for some medicine.

Milk of Magnesia even uses the initials M.O.M.

In these ads, women give medication to others—husbands, children— more often than to themselves. "There's an analogy with food commercials. Instead of being shown eating their own food, women are shown preparing food which is then eaten by a husband or child," says Craig. "It's reaffirming the mother's value both to herself and to her family. [The commercials imply that] it's more important to the woman that her family enjoys her cooking than that she does. And more important that she care for her family than care for herself."

Again there's a medical danger to such lopsided messages. While most physicians would agree that less medicine is better, these ads encourage women to medicate their partners and children as a way of showing love. There may even be a more subtle message. According to Craig's study, "Such commercials may encourage women to use OTC medications as a way of establishing a limited power over husband/children, and therefore as a path of self-actualization. Should this be the case, such advertising may . . . reinforce the model of drug-taking as a solution to problems."

There's even been a suggestion in drug abuse circles that the promotion of OTC medications in commercials tends to glorify the use of all drugs and may increase the use of all drugs—legal and illegal, safe and dangerous. Some over-the-counter drug ads practically turn women into drug pushers for their families, creating a future generation of potential drug abusers.

As with prescription drugs, the advertising for over-the-counter health products is aimed at women even when the product is used by men. When condoms' main purpose was to prevent pregnancy and sexually transmitted diseases, there was little advertising. But in this age of AIDS, condoms are suddenly the best protection men and women have against HIV transmission. Most condoms (with the exception of the new, so-called female condom) are worn by men, but much of the advertising is designed to get women to purchase them and to bear the responsibility for having their partners wear them.

"I never understood the concept of targeting condoms at women," says Janet L. Mitchell, M.D., MPH, chief of perinatology at Harlem Hospital in New York. "It's a male device. It also puts women in a precarious position in the bedroom. It blames women, telling them it's their fault if they can't get their man to wear a condom. Historically in this country, in bedrooms, men are in control. But condom messages are directed at women. Why not target *men*? It's their responsibility."

Women's greater concern about health care means they are more susceptible to appeals that tout the *preventive* benefits of some medications. This may be the case with ads for female hormones—both estrogen replacement therapy and oral contraceptives. One way that companies have tried to widen the market for these products is to advertise that they prevent disease as well as treat menopausal symptoms and prevent pregnancy.

Women are currently getting a hard sell on both postmenopausal replacement therapy and oral contraceptives. Manufacturers are trying to convince women and their physicians that all, or most, women should be taking hormones for the health benefits. For instance, oral contraceptives have been shown to help prevent ovarian and endometrial cancer. Postmenopausal hormone replacement therapy can help prevent osteoporosis. Advertisements for these drugs stress their preventive effects, while putting the side effects and health risks—stroke and breast cancer for the birth control pill, endometrial cancer for hormone replacement therapy—in small print. The idea is that you don't need to have any menopausal symptoms to take estrogen, and you don't even have to be sexually active to benefit from oral contraceptives.

One brochure for a birth control pill claims "Added Noncontraceptive Benefits," including cycle regularity, reduced blood loss and anemia, and more comfortable periods. And, boasts the ad, there's no generic equivalent (meaning that women do not have a lower-cost alternative).

Another ad has a woman saying, "I always knew the Pill was effective birth control. . . . Now I know it can give me more." The copy promises "extra noncontraceptive health benefits for the days ahead" (including reduction of irregular menses, dysmenorrhea, pelvic inflammatory disease, ectopic pregnancy, benign breast disease, ovarian cysts, endometrial and ovarian cancer).

In an ad for estrogen replacement therapy, which runs in many women's magazines, the copy reads, "Menopause is the reason most women start on Premarin. Ask your doctor if osteoporosis is a reason to stay on it." It continues, "Symptoms of menopause will pass. The risk of osteoporosis won't." But the ad doesn't mention that neither will the risk of cancer from taking the drug.

In an attempt to create a bigger market for their products, the manufacturers may be going too far. It is now possible for teenage girls to start taking birth control pills, continue on them without a break until menopause (since the FDA recently ruled that oral contraceptives are safe after age thirty-five), and then switch to hormone replacement therapy at menopause. Encouraged by physicians and pharmaceutical manufacturers, women may wind up taking hormones for nearly their entire lives, although there are no studies to show that this kind of long-term use is safe. At some point health has to win out over hype.

■ THE WOMAN CONSUMER

Advertisements aren't the only way pharmaceutical firms are biased against women. Just as dry cleaners often take advantage of women by charging more to clean a woman's shirt than a man's, drug companies may also overcharge women. A casual look around the neighborhood drugstore shows some obvious instances. Many "women's" deodorant formulas cost more than men's. Cortisone creams (for treating minor skin itches and irritations) cost more when they have the prefix *gyne*, meaning they can be used on the female genitals. Yet the less expensive, regular cortisone cream is perfectly safe for use in the vaginal area.

In general, drugs are more expensive in America than in most other countries. A General Accounting Office study found that drugs cost an average of 60 percent less in the United Kingdom. Since women receive more prescriptions, live longer, and are sicker and poorer, the price-gouging affects them most. In addition, women buy medicines for their families as well as for themselves. So the burdens of drug and contraceptive costs fall squarely on women.

While many drugs are overpriced, medicines taken by women seem to be especially costly. Premarin (estrogen), for example, costs twenty-eight cents a pill in the United States, but only nine cents in Great Britain.

Norplant, the recently approved contraceptive implant, was selling in Sweden and some developing countries for as little as $23. When the drug became available in the United States in 1991, Wyeth-Ayerst started charging $365. The cost to make and market the drug is estimated to be just $16 per implant. Additionally, $17 million of taxpayers' money was used to help develop the device, along with another $25 million from foundations. Under pressure from family-planning groups, the pharmaceutical company agreed to cut the price to public clinics as of December 1995—but did not specify by how much.

When Upjohn began marketing Depo-Provera—a drug that has been

sold for two decades to treat cancer—as a contraceptive in 1992, the price
went from $12 to $29 per dose. Upjohn claimed it was recouping development costs, but critics argued that research had ended years ago and that
the drug was already available as a contraceptive in many countries.

There is a sense among health care reformers and physicians that drug
company prices are out of control. At one recent conference of the American College of Obstetricians and Gynecologists, a doctor who had just attended an elegant breakfast and received a leather briefcase and tape
recorder from a company that manufactured birth control pills muttered,
"I wish they'd keep the briefcases and lower the cost of the pills." (Of
course the price of drugs doesn't just affect women. For instance, when
Levamisole, a veterinary medication used to cure worm infestations in
sheep, was approved to treat colon cancer in humans, the price of a dose
went from six cents to six dollars.)

Drugs with cosmetic rather than medical uses are especially lucrative
for manufacturers. Just as with cosmetic surgery, these drugs may be heavily advertised and steeply priced. One example is Rogaine Topical Solution
for growing hair. Although few studies have been done on the effectiveness
of Rogaine in women, when sales to men were disappointing, the manufacturer went after the women's market.

The Food and Drug Administration approved Rogaine in August 1988
as a treatment for androgenic alopecia, also called male-pattern baldness.
Analysts predicted first-year sales of $500 million, but they overestimated
men's desperation. First-year sales were only $70 million, and men seemed
to find the drug expensive, messy, inconvenient, and ultimately ineffective.
But Upjohn figured out a way to double the potential market for the drug.
They got it approved for women in August 1991.

"That nod of approval increased the product's target market from 30
million men to 50 million people and made Rogaine available to an entire
universe of customers who are already comfortable with hair treatment
products and who feel enormous social pressure to do something, anything,
to stop hair loss," said an article in *American Druggist*. An advertising campaign appeared in women's magazines. The pictures show just the back of
a woman's head. Her medium-length blond hair is tied in a ponytail, and
a floppy hat with flowers covers her head. The copy says she is twenty-five
years old—hardly the product's typical user.

Upjohn admits the drug doesn't work for everyone, that it must be
used for six months to a year before the results are known. If the product
does work, it must be applied twice daily for life, or the effects reverse. But
when Rogaine *does* work and *is* used for life, the profits to the company are

enormous. The average cost of treatment is seven hundred dollars a year. U.S. sales of the drug are now $84 million per year, with 25–30 percent of sales—about $21–25 million—to women.

The *American Druggist* article cites pharmacists as saying Rogaine doesn't work at growing hair for many people, although it does seem to halt hair loss or thinning. Instead of purchasing thousands of dollars' worth of Rogaine, perhaps the young woman in the ad should just keep her hat.

■ TARGETING AGING BABY BOOMERS

Another way drug companies increase profits is by focusing on small market niches to sell products. The idea is that wherever a problem can be identified, a drug solution can be manufactured.

The best example of this trend is the growing market for vaginal "moisturizers" for postmenopausal women. There used to be vaginal lubricants designed primarily for sexual purposes, and prescription estrogen creams for postmenopausal women. Now there's a new category of "personal" moisturizers that can be purchased over-the-counter. While K-Y jelly, the old standard, still commands over 50 percent of the market, new products are aimed directly at postmenopausal women: Parke Davis's Replens, and Schering Plough's Gyne-Moistrin are two examples. As the first wave of baby boomers, who came of age in the sexual revolution reach menopause, pharmaceutical manufacturers see an ever-expanding population of customers with uncomfortably dry vaginas, willing to buy expensive products to remedy the problem. An estimated forty million women baby boomers will reach menopause in the next twenty years.

Another article in *American Druggist*, titled "The New VD," equates vaginal dryness with sexually transmitted diseases. Of course, sexually transmitted diseases are caused by pathogenic organisms and require medical treatment; vaginal dryness is a normal part of aging. But the manufacturers of the new moisturizers stress that vaginal dryness is a medical problem with an easily purchased solution—much as the manufacturers of expensive facial moisturizers try to convince women that the normal aging of human skin is a pathological condition, too.

According to the article, "The $40 million personal lubricant market has grown 30% in the last year and is one of the 10 fastest-growing health and beauty aid categories." Says Georgia Witkin, Ph.D., clinical instructor of obstetrics and gynecology at Mount Sinai School of Medicine in New York, "Vaginal dryness is the new VD. The symptoms make women feel like their bodies have betrayed them."

Manufacturers stress that the new moisturizers are superior to the old lubricants, which simply eased friction during intercourse. New products supposedly suffuse vaginal tissues with moisture. Women will have to decide for themselves whether a simple, inexpensive product like K-Y jelly is as effective as the high-tech, much-hyped newcomers.

Because the FDA classifies these products as cosmetics, not drugs, the manufacturers can't make specific medical claims on the label. But they can expand their market by emphasizing that not only postmenopausal women need extra vaginal moisture. Those who may suffer from vaginal dryness include: women who are postpartum, breast-feeding, undergoing certain cancer treatments, exercising, under stress, or taking antibiotics, fertility drugs, endometriosis drugs, or oral contraceptives. The market is estimated at between twenty-five and fifty million women. In one study 90 percent of women with vaginal dryness who wanted to have more comfortable sex said the moisturizers helped. The researchers even got grateful phone calls from the women's husbands.

Because the products have the potential for big sales, manufacturers are urging *pharmacists* to counsel women. "Traditionally, vaginal dryness has not been covered well in pharmacy schools, and pharmacists are poorly prepared to counsel about it," said an expert quoted in the article. "But it just takes a little initiative." By selling moisturizers as medical rather than recreational relief, "lubricants will never be a neglected category again."

■ OVER-THE-COUNTER DRUGS: BETTER FOR WOMEN OR NOT?

Pharmaceutical profits can be greatly increased by getting rid of the middle man, that is, the physician. When a drug switches from prescription to over-the-counter sales, profits rise dramatically. For instance, in early 1991 when Monistat 7 and Gyne-Lotrimin, two treatments for vaginal yeast infections, went over the counter, yearly sales soared. One pharmacy industry newspaper referred to the feminine hygiene category as one of the OTC department's "shining stars. Strong sales in recent years, largely attributable to the Rx-to-OTC switch of the antifungal preparations, are expected to continue."

To pharmaceutical companies and many consumers, prescriptions are like censorship, blocking people's access to the medications they desire. Shouldn't people have the right to take an antibiotic when they feel like it, the same way they can buy aspirin and antihistamines? When vaginal yeast medications were sold by prescription only, was it denying women control over their own health, or protecting them from potential harm? The answer depends on whom you ask.

"There are advantages to women in having access, but the problem I am concerned about is misdiagnosis or mistreatment of what they think is vaginitis," says Joellen Hawkins. "We get a lot of women who have tried a fungicide, but they didn't have a fungus infection. Or they had some concomitant infection that the medicine didn't touch. We're also seeing overtreatment. At the first little glimmer of something, if they think they're a little itchy, they'll use the medication. And then you kill off a lot of organisms in the vagina, change the pH, and something else can move in or overgrow." Physicians are also concerned that women will treat recurrent vaginal yeast infections by simply buying more tubes of medicine, not finding out until later that the recurrent infections are due to underlying diabetes or HIV infection.

In fact, when yeast medications went over-the-counter, the decision was prompted less by concerns about women's health and more by worry that the patent on the medication was running out. The pharmaceutical companies had a limited amount of time to make as much money as possible before lower-priced generic versions reached the market. Commercials for the drugs—Monistat, Gyne-Lotrimin, and others—stress what a breakthrough the over-the-counter availability is for women. But the companies are still charging high prices for the medications, and insurance companies will no longer reimburse women, since they pay only for prescription drugs. The sole party to benefit may be the manufacturers.

One pharmacy journal ran an article by the man responsible for the marketing campaign for Gyne-Lotrimin, who wrote, "We knew that approximately 22 million women are diagnosed with vaginal yeast infections every year; that 14 percent of the female population suffer from the ailment; but we couldn't target any particular group. We decided, therefore, to address *all* adult women [emphasis added]." Although, as mentioned earlier, female physicians rarely appear in the ads that run in medical journals, the company decided to use female gynecologists as spokespeople for Gyne-Lotrimin, because of their greater credibility with women.

Now the biggest controversy in the prescription versus over-the-counter debate is birth control pills, which some women's health advocates believe should be sold in drugstores nationwide as a remedy for the epidemic of teen pregnancies. But encouraging millions of teenage girls to skip seeing the doctor and begin taking hormones daily may not be the best way to promote women's health.

In 1993 the FDA's Fertility and Maternal Health Drugs Advisory

Committee voted to change the labeling on oral contraceptive pills. The old labels read that a physician should take a medical history and perform a physical exam, including pelvic exam and Pap smear, before prescribing birth control pills, and then at least yearly while the pills are being taken. The new label would be revised to reflect the lower doses of hormones now in oral contraceptives. It would say that the physical exam could be deferred if the patient requested it and the physician agreed. In other words, anyone who wanted birth control pills could just request a prescription. This labeling change would open the door for OTC status.

Advocates for making the Pill available without a prescription say that unintended pregnancies will decline, while health risks will be negligible. The new low-dose pills, they say, are safe enough to sell without a doctor's permission. Some of these health advocates argue that from a public health standpoint it would make more sense to sell birth control pills in vending machines and cigarettes by prescription only.

Those who oppose selling oral contraceptives over-the-counter believe that unintended pregnancies may actually *rise* if women don't receive a health professional's instructions on pill taking, and that women's general health may suffer if they no longer have to check in with the doctor to get their prescription refilled. Women might have gone to their gynecologist for a Pill prescription, but while they were there they also received a Pap smear, breast exam, and so on.

"European countries have had birth control pills over-the-counter for a long time," says Hawkins. "The problem is, how are we going to monitor women who are at risk for taking birth control pills because they have a bad family history or bad personal history or are heavy smokers? How are we going to make sure they don't have high blood pressure or a high risk for thrombophlebitis? And how are we going to get them in for Pap smears? We're seeing so many abnormal Pap smears now in young women."

How do women feel about it? The National Women's Health Network, a feminist advocacy group, opposes the sale of birth control pills without a prescription. And the American College of Obstetricians and Gynecologists commissioned a Gallup survey in 1993 to discover the public's views on this controversial issue. The poll, of 997 women ages eighteen and over, found that 86 percent do *not* believe that oral contraceptives are safe enough to buy without first seeing a doctor.

In January 1993 the FDA canceled a meeting to discuss the proposal to allow over-the-counter sales of birth control pills, citing the need to consult with a wider range of interest groups. Right now the issue is on hold, but selling the Pill over-the-counter would mean enormous profits for pharmaceutical manufacturers, so it's a safe bet that the discussion is far from over.

■ MAKING DRUG MARKETING WOMEN-FRIENDLY

While the Pill's status is still being debated, there are signs that other aspects of the pharmaceutical industry may become more women-friendly. For one thing, health care reformers have already put pharmaceutical firms on notice that they must curb their exorbitant prices.

Pharmaceutical manufacturers are also showing interest in developing and testing drugs specifically for women. In 1993, jumping on the new women's health bandwagon, the Pharmaceutical Manufacturers Association placed stories in several medical and pharmaceutical journals boasting that 301 new drugs were in development for use by women. They defined women's drugs as those for treating diseases that affect only women, that disproportionately affect women, or that are among the top ten causes of death in women.

While the association's announcement is welcome, it is not as altruistic as it seems. The top ten causes of death are nearly identical for men and women, with heart disease, cancer, and stroke at the top of the list. And the majority of these drugs heralded for women were simply new drugs for women *and* men that were finally being tested on women.

One drug that would make a real difference in women's lives, RU-486, is not on this list. So far no pharmaceutical manufacturer has shown any interest in manufacturing and marketing the drug for sale in the United States. The drug is not only an abortifacient, but may also be a treatment for breast and brain cancer, uterine fibroids, endometriosis and Epstein-Barr virus. In addition, RU-486 may be useful for inducing labor, or as an oral contraceptive. But fear of the vocal anti-abortion minority prevents pharmaceutical manufacturers from testing and marketing the drug.

Now that pharmaceutical manufacturers are generally embracing the women's market, their advertising campaigns are finally showing some signs of change. Rather than show photographs of "patients," ads now use fewer people and more abstract images: diagrams, drawings of molecules, photographs of the product, and so on. "This may be the way the companies are skirting the whole issue of gender bias," says Dr. Macchello.

Ads that do use models are starting to use fewer stereotyped images and less degrading copy. For instance, a new ad for Tums antacid, which can be used as a calcium supplement to prevent bone loss in postmenopausal women, shows a healthy-looking older woman under the slogan "This woman is going through a major loss." The old slogan read, "This woman is a loser." "I have a feeling there must have been a lot of complaints," says Dr. Macchello.

An ad for Procardia, a heart medication, also underwent a transformation. The old ad showed three men and a woman. The men were a construction worker in a hardhat, a man in overalls who obviously engaged in some kind of outdoor labor, and a business executive. The only woman in the picture was a waitress with bleached hair and carmine lips.

The first page of the new ad is a composite photograph of eight faces—five men and three women. The two-page spread that follows shows a group portrait of all eight, shown only from the shoulders up. Their occupations are impossible to discern, but all are smiling.

Even ads for psychotropic drugs are improving. An ad for Zoloft, a popular antidepressant, shows a woman patient, but instead of looking depressed she's pictured dancing, playing with her grandchildren, giving a business presentation, having a dinner date, and jogging.

The men in drug ads aren't all hardhats and business executives anymore. Campaigns for Proscar (to treat enlarged prostate glands) and Cognex (an anti-Alzheimer's drug) show men hugging their grandchildren. Lodine, an arthritis drug, features a man returning to his gardening. There seems to have been a conscious decision to change outdated stereotypes and make new ads reflect today's reality rather than the 1950s' rigid gender roles. After one of Dr. Macchello's presentations a woman representative from one of the pharmaceutical companies came up to her and said, "I wish we could videotape this and send it to my marketing people. I've been telling this to them for years."

Gender bias has been a part of pharmaceutical advertising for so long that it's impossible to sort out which came first, physicians' biased attitudes toward women patients or the pharmaceutical ads that reflect them. But the recent change in advertising may finally portend a shift away from biased treatment and prescribing.

At least when drugs are advertised directly to the public, women can disregard them or regard them with healthy skepticism. But in the case of ads directed toward physicians, the images and text may alter a doctor's prescribing habits without patients having any knowledge of their influence.

Although the pharmaceutical industry is becoming more sensitive to women's health needs, it still has a long way to go. In spite of some recent changes, much of the medical information in drug ads is inaccurate, and many of the images are still biased. And, of course, most of the drugs being advertised were never adequately tested in women. Continued change is essential to ensure that the medications women receive from their doctors or buy for themselves are safe, effective, and appropriate.

13

WOMEN AND THE LAW
Unhealthy Judgments

T he battle over women's bodies continues in doctors' offices and hospitals. But it has also moved to a new arena: the courtroom. While health care has traditionally been a private affair between a woman and her doctor, increasingly governmental and judicial forces are inserting themselves into medical decision making.

"Sometimes the unfairness women face in the health care system is also illegal," says Marcia Greenberger, copresident of the National Women's Law Center. "Sometimes it can be a form of illegal sex discrimination. Or it may be denial of a woman's right to privacy. Sometimes it's violation of a statutory right—access to health care. Or it could be violation of contract rights or a tort, such as malpractice." The legal influence may be direct—as in the case of court-ordered cesarean sections—or indirect, as when physicians perform more tests or do more procedures because of fear of malpractice. Fewer gynecologists now deliver babies, for instance, because the risk of lawsuit and financial loss is too high.

■ MEDICAL MAL(E)-PRACTICE

When most people think of the intersection of law and medicine, they think of malpractice suits. Obstetrical suits are the most common, and failure to diagnose cancer—often breast or cervical cancer—is next. Along with articles on how to *cure* breast cancer, medical journals now contain articles on how to avoid malpractice suits for failing to diagnose it early. Miscommunication between doctor and patient is a major factor in many malpractice cases, and as the next chapter will show, miscommunication is most common when the patient is a woman. Thus, women probably bring more malpractice suits against physicians than men do.

In an attempt to characterize the plaintiffs in malpractice suits, one study compiled data on the patients who called six different law offices in five states, claiming to have suffered an injury caused by medical negligence. The study found that over half the callers had had a poor relationship with their health care provider *before* their injury. Of 502 potential plaintiffs, 58 percent were female. While not all of these initial phone calls resulted in the patient bringing a malpractice suit (the lawyers often felt the damages were not sufficiently serious to justify proceeding), it is significant that more women than men felt themselves wronged by the medical profession.

Indeed, there is a perception among the lawyers who handle these cases that women are treated more cavalierly by the medical profession. Harvey F. Wachsman, a practicing attorney and president of the American Board of Professional Liability as well as a practicing neurosurgeon and medical adjunct at the State University of New York, is currently representing forty-one women in their malpractice cases against James Burt, M.D., the so-called "love surgery" doctor who rearranged the genitals and reproductive organs of thousands of women, believing he would improve their sex lives. Dr. Burt surrendered his license in 1989 after performing his surgery for twenty-two years.

According to Dr. Wachsman, other physicians knew about Burt's questionable surgical techniques for years, yet none took steps to stop him. "Women were being destroyed wholesale for years, and nobody did anything. Other doctors would put women in stirrups, take a look and say, 'Ha, ha, looks like Jim Burt got ahold of you.' If somebody was doing something to men's genitals, something would have been done about it in an hour. Or if Burt had cut someone's arm on the street, he would be in jail. But because the victims were women, he was able to mutilate them and still be free." Burt's butchery is an extreme case, but still indicative of women's second-class status as patients.

The financial awards in malpractice cases are also related to gender. "If a woman who has been medically injured doesn't work outside the home, she will have a lot smaller damage award than a man," says attorney Karen H. Rothenberg, professor and director of the law and health care program at the University of Maryland School of Law. "Damages are often tied to lost earnings and value." And in a society where women earn only about three-quarters of what men do, their bodily injuries are worth less, too.

But malpractice suits are just one example of how the law may be called in to mediate disputes between women and those responsible for providing their health care. Women may also sue pharmaceutical and other health manufacturers for product liability or personal damages. It's difficult to believe that coincidence alone accounts for why all recent health scandals involving medications and pharmaceutical or medical products primarily affect women. Consider the Dalkon Shield IUD, which caused pelvic inflammatory disease and infertility in women who used it; the superabsorbent Rely tampon, which led to life-threatening toxic shock syndrome; silicone breast implants, which are believed to cause a spectrum of immune disorders; or the drugs thalidomide and diethylstilbestrol, given to unsuspecting women who harmed their children by taking them.

For women, another of the disturbing ways in which the legal system may be called in to decide their care falls under the misleading rubric "maternal-fetal conflict"—times when doctors and/or the courts take it upon themselves to determine that a woman's rights and those of her fetus do not coincide. In these cases, laws may be used to impose health care decisions on women—for instance, forcing a competent pregnant woman to have an IV inserted or undergo a cesarean section against her wishes. "The real conflict isn't between mother and fetus, but between pregnant women and physicians or hospitals. That's a better way of putting it," says Lawrence J. Nelson, a bioethics consultant and attorney in San Francisco. Others suggest that the dispute be relabeled maternal-fetal *relations*, or maternal-fetal *issues*.

Ironically, medical advances are at least partly responsible for this artificial conflict. High-tech diagnostic equipment, such as ultrasound machines, and new surgical techniques that enable doctors to directly treat and even operate on the fetus, have changed the way obstetricians think about pregnant women.

Not long ago, obstetricians considered the pregnant woman and her fetus one unit, one patient. But since there are interventions now to treat the fetus, obstetricians increasingly talk about their *two* patients. And the supposed conflict occurs when the obstetrician feels that the mother is somehow standing in the way of the fetus's well-being.

Pitting the interests of these "two" patients against each other, obstetricians have usurped responsibility for the fetus's welfare. Not only doesn't Mother know best anymore, but she may even be her fetus's biggest enemy. Enter the heroic doctor—aided by a sympathetic judge if necessary—to save the unborn child, even if it means ignoring a woman's wishes for her own care.

The problem with this reasoning is that the *mother* is a legal individual with a right to privacy and autonomy. The fetus, in spite of what antiabortionists would have people believe, is *not* a legal person until birth. There's a distinction between having a moral obligation to the fetus and having a legal responsibility. "If you start talking about fetal rights, it's easy to act as if the fetus exists independently of the woman. And to have any fetal rights that are enforceable, you have to take action against the pregnant woman. That's where I think the argument breaks down," says Nelson.

There are only a few circumstances where a fetus can have any legal rights. "What would fetal rights be?" asks Lynn Paltrow, director of special litigation for the Center for Reproductive Law and Policy. "You can leave money to an unborn child. And you can sometimes prosecute for murder when a pregnant woman and her fetus are killed. But under federal law there are no legal rights for the fetus. It's an argument of the antiabortionists."

The antiabortion groups have taken the concept of fetal rights to an extreme, believing in some cases that the unborn child has more rights than the woman who carries it. But their effort to treat fetuses as legal people may backfire and harm more babies than it saves. Pregnant women fearing loss of autonomy or even prosecution (for harming a fetus through substance abuse, for example) might avoid prenatal care or even opt for abortion to preserve their own freedoms.

Roe v. *Wade*—the landmark court decision that ensures women's right to abortion—is also the basis for ensuring their right to privacy while pregnant. "*Roe* v. *Wade* is an opinion that established more than any other that pregnant women have a right to bodily integrity," says Paltrow, "that the fetus is not a person, even after viability."

According to Lori B. Andrews, professor of law at Chicago-Kent College of Law, "*Roe* v. *Wade* is that thin thread holding women's autonomy, that says that the fetus is *not* independently alive, is not a person." Overturning *Roe* v. *Wade* would have implications far beyond a woman's right to abortion. *Roe* v. *Wade* also ensures that women don't lose their autonomy for the nine months they are pregnant.

The cases that challenge women's autonomy can take many forms, but three of the most common are court-ordered cesarean sections, prosecution of pregnant substance abusers for endangering the fetus, and gender inequities in living wills and right-to-die cases.

■ TIE HER DOWN AND CUT HER OPEN: COURT-ORDERED CESAREAN SECTIONS

In 1987 Angela Carder, twenty-seven, was pregnant with her first child. After years of battling leukemia, she had been in remission for three years, but when she was twenty-five weeks into her pregnancy, she began having back pain and shortness of breath. Tests showed a lung tumor, and the prognosis was terminal. Because of Angela's frail condition and the unlikelihood of the child surviving, Angela, her husband, her parents, *and* her doctors decided against a cesarean section. But the hospital went to court for a decision, and the judge ultimately determined that a cesarean section should be performed. "The wording of the decision was frightening," says Paltrow. "It begins with condolences to the family, an admission that the judges know they may have shortened her life. The people arguing this case were arguing that Angela's rights didn't matter."

Angela had the operation. Her baby died almost immediately, and Angela died barely two days later, with the cesarean listed as a contributing cause of death. Later—too late for Angela or her child—a federal district court overturned the decision and reiterated the principle of a woman's autonomy.

The infamous "AC" case, as it was referred to in the press and the legal journals, may be the most dramatic, but it is hardly the only instance of pregnant women being taken to court by overzealous physicians or hospitals wanting to impose their recommendations for a cesarean section. In 1987 the *New England Journal of Medicine* reported on a review of cases where physicians went to court in order to force pregnant women to undergo cesarean sections, hospitalization, and intrauterine transfusions against their will. The study found that 86 percent of physicians' requests were granted by the courts. In most of these cases the patients were poor, black, Asian, or Hispanic. The disenfranchisement factor is disturbing, but the legal principles used to defend the court decisions could be used against any woman, no matter what her race or socioeconomic status.

Only a few of these cases have come to trial, but no one knows how many more are unreported, either because they are never fully litigated (they never go to court before a jury), or because a woman simply caved in and gave permission for the operation. Sometimes just the threat of legal action is enough to make a woman follow a physician's recommendations. Or an insurance company may refuse to pay unless the doctors' orders are obeyed.

The rarity of these cases can be better put in context by understanding that the vast majority of women are incredibly altruistic when it comes to the well-being of their unborn children. "In 99.9 percent of cases, the woman is going to do whatever is necessary for the best outcome of the pregnancy," says Ann Allen, legal counsel for the American College of Obstetricians and Gynecologists. "A lot of times she will do more than what the obstetrician says."

Far from ignoring physicians' recommendations, most women embrace them wholeheartedly. Hundreds of thousands of women willingly submit to cesareans sections each year, in spite of evidence that half or more of these operations may be unnecessary. Considering that cesarean sections are major surgery with very real risks to the mother and questionable benefits to the fetus, it's amazing that more women aren't flatly refusing the operation. That they aren't is evidence of their altruism when it comes to their babies' health.

When women do refuse cesareans, it may be because of the danger to their own health (as in the Angela Carder case), or because of cultural or religious beliefs. "In some cultures having a cesarean section means that a woman becomes basically dead in the eyes of her family and community," says Rothenberg. "There needs to be an inclusion of cultural and religious accommodation in these decisions."

Other women, because of language difficulties or lack of education, refuse permission without a real understanding of the risks and benefits of the surgery. Some of these cases might be avoided with better communication. But the bottom line is that whatever decision a woman makes, it must be hers and hers alone, no matter what the final outcome. "If we take freedom seriously, then people have to have the freedom to make bad choices," says Nelson. "I heard a woman tell about refusing her obstetrician's recommendation for a cesarean. She wanted to deliver vaginally, and her baby died. She has to live with that decision. Physicians and nurses may have strong feelings about this, but it's not their choice."

Adds Paltrow, "Other people shouldn't do things to you that interfere with your intentions. That includes killing the fetus if you want the baby, or locking you in a room if you want an abortion." Or operating on you if you have refused permission for the surgery.

Major medical organizations, including the American Academy of Obstetricians and Gynecologists, have affirmed this right. "We say that a woman's autonomy has to be respected, that she is the decision maker," says Allen. "We argue strongly against physicians or hospitals going to court for a court order. A lot of times physicians call us up with difficult situations and say, 'What do we do?' We say, 'Explain everything to the woman and help her make the decision.' We always come down on the side of not going to court."

But not all obstetricians concur. And when they decide to seek legal authority for their medical recommendations, they have a distinct advantage over the patient. "It's difficult for a pregnant woman to get due process," explains Andrews. "She's not represented. The call to the judge may be in the middle of the night. The medical witness is usually very credible, telling the judge that this baby, and maybe this woman, will die if an immediate cesarean is not performed." Andrews says she knows of a California obstetrician who says he's gone to court *fifty* times to force pregnant women to follow his medical recommendations—and won in all but one case. When the court-ordered surgery is done, the women have little recourse. The physicians and hospitals are protected (granted judicial immunity) by the court order, and unless the woman can prove negligence or malpractice, she cannot sue them.

Still, this California obstetrician is clearly the exception. Most physicians recoil at the idea of taking legal action against their patients. "Going to court is not the answer," says Richard H. Schwarz, M.D., a past president of the American College of Obstetricians and Gynecologists and interim president, provost and vice president for clinical affairs at the State University of New York Health Science Center at Brooklyn. "What are you going to do? Tie a woman down and do surgery? That's repugnant to most physicians. It's a complete dissolution of the doctor-patient relationship. What I would do is do the best I could without going against the autonomy of the patient."

There's also the fact that medicine is not an exact science. "Physicians have to understand that there may be more flexibility in a situation than they feel," says Allen. No matter how good the intentions of the obstetrician or how credible the medical witness, there's no way to determine how many of the babies would be born healthy without the cesarean. In several of these cases a woman facing a court-ordered cesarean simply walked out of the hospital, and her baby was later born healthy. "It's very hard for physicians when their training is to get the best possible outcome, and they really believe that the fetus would be compromised if they don't do a cesarean. For physicians, cesarean sections are not a big deal, but women may feel differently," says Allen.

In 1981, Jessie Mae Jefferson, a Georgia woman, refused a doctor's recommendation of a cesarean for religious reasons. She was taken to court, where her physician was given permission to perform the operation (after telling the judge there was a 99 percent certainty that the child would not survive a vaginal delivery and a 50 percent chance that the mother would die, too). Because Jessie Mae and her husband believed that whatever happened to the child was God's will, she went into hiding and did not report to the hospital as ordered. Instead she vaginally delivered a healthy baby several days later.

While many court-ordered cesareans are still decided by emergency judicial order, when the cases do go to court there is a growing legal consensus supporting a woman's right to privacy and autonomy. "There's a small body of law, a handful of cases, and the assumption is that *all* people have the right to determine what happens to their own bodies," says Paltrow. The highest level of court law is confirming women's autonomy.

One case that is often cited as legal precedent concerns a man who was asked to donate bone marrow to save a relative's life. The man refused, even though the risk to him was small. The dying relative went to court, which, although deploring the man's decision not to give his marrow, affirmed his right to make it. The court clearly stated that an individual could not be forced to undergo any kind of surgical or medical procedure to save another individual's life. The decision stated:

> For our law to *compel* defendant to submit to an intrusion of his body would change every concept and principle upon which our society is founded. To do so would defeat the sanctity of the individual.... For a society which respects the rights of *one* individual, to sink its teeth into the jugular vein or neck of one of its members and suck from it sustenance for *another* member, is revolting to our hard-wrought concepts of jurisprudence. Forceable extraction of living body tissue causes revulsion to the judicial mind. Such would raise the spectre of the swastika and the Inquisition, reminiscent of the horrors this portends.

Translated to maternal-fetal cases, it is legally unsupportable to order a woman to undergo a cesarean section to save her unborn child's life.

Yet in spite of the legal consensus, new cases continue to emerge. In mid-1993, an Illinois hospital contacted a state attorney who went to court to force a twenty-two-year-old Pentecostal Christian woman to have a cesarean two weeks before her due date. The woman had refused the operation on religious and personal grounds. The fetus, according to the woman's physician, was being deprived of oxygen and would be born either severely brain damaged or dead. But the lower court refused to issue the order, and the Supreme Court refused to hear the case, allowing the lower court's decision *not* to force the cesarean to stand. The baby, a boy, was born at full term, low-weight but apparently healthy.

■ CAN A CHILD BE ABUSED BEFORE BIRTH?: PREGNANCY AND SUBSTANCE ABUSE

A woman's autonomy during pregnancy may also be challenged if her lifestyle is thought to jeopardize the health of her fetus. Consider the case of a pregnant woman in Wyoming who was badly beaten by her boyfriend. When she arrived in the emergency room for treatment, the staff checked her blood-alcohol level. Based on the results, the woman was prosecuted for endangering her fetus. The man who abused her was never charged with a crime.

Some people believe that a woman who finds herself pregnant, whether by choice or by chance, has two options: either abort the fetus or do everything possible to ensure a perfect pregnancy outcome. Morally these two choices may make sense, but as legal sanctions they lead to a horrifying slippery slope that threatens women's independence—and does little to ensure healthy babies.

If a woman can be prosecuted for taking drugs or drinking alcohol while pregnant, can she be prosecuted for smoking cigarettes? What about drinking coffee? What if she decides to go downhill skiing? Paint a room and be exposed to toxic fumes? Forget to wear her seatbelt? Not take her vitamins? Refuse to drink milk? All these activities can potentially threaten a pregnancy, but few would argue that the "pregnancy police" should attempt to prosecute pregnant women for every gestational transgression. Yet in 1986, after her child was born brain-damaged, a California woman was prosecuted for not following her doctor's advice to stay off her feet while pregnant.

The same medical and judicial paternalism responsible for court-ordered cesarean sections dominates the legal efforts to make pregnant women virtual prisoners, unable to make their own decisions about what to eat or how much exercise to get. The zealots argue that the well-being of a pregnancy is a public health concern, and that society has a stake in a woman's delivering a healthy child. The expense of caring for children who have been harmed in utero, these advocates say, is too large to ignore.

Fortunately, the majority of health experts—including the American College of Obstetricians and Gynecologists—believe that prosecuting pregnant women causes more harm than good, and that treatment is a better option than prison. "ACOG is against the prosecution of pregnant women. We feel that it's right for physicians to help pregnant substance abusers get treatment, but not to prosecute them," says Allen. "We're also concerned about the deterrent effect. Women may not get prenatal care if they're concerned about being prosecuted." Many drug abusers who find themselves pregnant do seek treatment and are turned away by programs that exclude them (see chapter 11 for more on this). "Treatment programs say they're afraid of liability if the fetus is harmed," says Rothenberg. "But there's no case law to support that. It's a perception of liability, but not reality. It would be nice if the public—and the treatment programs—supported pregnant women."

Lawmakers finally seem to be conceding the point. In 1993 there were fifty-one bills introduced in state legislatures pertaining to the abuse of potentially harmful substances during pregnancy. The majority sought to offer testing, counseling, referral, and treatment services, or to require the posting of warning signs or the establishment of task forces. The remainder dealt with whether criminal charges could be brought against pregnant or postpartum women involved with substance abuse. Of the nine bills finally enacted, none imposed criminal sanctions.

State laws still vary widely. For example, a new law in Virginia gives pregnant substance abusers priority status for treatment in rehabilitation facilities. Minnesota, however, still defines child abuse or neglect as including substance abuse during pregnancy.

The legal distinctions also lead to legal games. Since the fetus is not a legal person, prosecuting a pregnant woman for child abuse or neglect, or for delivering drugs to a minor, can usually be successfully challenged by the defense. So in some instances the prosecution charges a woman with a crime immediately *after* birth. The charge is "trafficking in drugs to a minor," defined as delivering drugs to the newborn child through the still-attached umbilical cord. Hundreds of these criminal cases have been brought nationwide, after doctors or hospitals notified law enforcement authorities, although most legal decisions have found the prosecutions illegal and/or unconstitutional.

There's a frightening Big Brother aspect to state-enforced pregnancy-behavior codes. In 1991 two Washington State waiters were fired for refusing to serve a pregnant woman the raspberry daiquiri she had ordered. The restaurant's management fired the waiters because they did not treat the customer with respect. But the public's sympathy seemed to be with the waiters, and the case set off a statewide campaign to allow restaurants to refuse serving alcohol to pregnant women. Not only would such a law be an insult to women—akin to establishments refusing to serve people on the basis of skin color—but as a fetal-protection policy it would fall far short of its goal. Alcohol can do the most damage to unborn children in the first trimester of pregnancy, well before an outside observer could possibly see that a woman is pregnant.

Cases of prosecuting pregnant women are rare—although not as rare as they should be. In mid–1994 a group of women instituted a class action suit against the Medical University of South Carolina for their unwilling participation in a prenatal care program that seemed to have run amok. Physicians at the university had taken it upon themselves to test pregnant women for drug abuse. If the results were positive, the women were given an ultimatum: Either enter the university's treatment program or be reported to the authorities. The women, virtually all African-Americans, had never given their consent for the testing or waived their right to confidentiality. Since the program began in 1989, more than forty women have been arrested, sometimes within a day of giving birth. Some of the women were put in leg shackles or handcuffed to hospital beds during their arrests. It's hard to see how this type of rough handling could possibly help the women's children, which was ostensibly the intention of the arrests.

■ DYING AS A GENDERED ACTIVITY

Pregnant women may have to legally defend not only their lifestyle, but their deathstyle, too. All fifty states now have laws allowing individuals to establish advance directives such as living wills, specifying their care should they become terminally ill or comatose and unable to make their decisions known. But in thirty-four states, a woman's living will is automatically invalidated if she is pregnant. In two of these states, the living will is invalidated if the fetus is viable. In twelve states, life support cannot be removed if it is probable that the fetus could develop to the point of live birth. And in twenty states, the living will is invalidated no matter what the stage of pregnancy. The laws making exceptions for pregnant women were pushed by antiabortion advocates, even though live births from comatose women are exceptionally rare.

According to David A. Smith, former director of legal services for Choice in Dying, most of these laws that deprive pregnant women of their treatment-refusal rights and compel them to be maintained on life support are unconstitutional. The only laws that may hold up constitutionally are those that specify restrictions on living wills only when the fetus is considered viable. Seeking a way to preserve women's rights when they are pregnant, several states (including Arizona, New Jersey, and Maryland) now ask women to specify in their living wills what treatment they want should they become irreversibly comatose or brain-dead while pregnant. "It makes women think about the question but doesn't take any rights away," says Rothenberg.

Not just pregnancy but gender itself may influence end-of-life treatment. One disturbing survey reported in a legal journal found a strong gender bias in right-to-die cases. In twenty-two right-to-die cases from appeals courts in fourteen states (the bulk of the appellate decisions involving patients who had been mentally competent but left no written directives for their care), the courts showed a strong tendency to accept evidence of men's preferences with regard to life-sustaining treatment, but to reject or fail to consider evidence of women's preferences. Men who were now mentally incompetent and being kept alive by hospital equipment were granted the right to die if family and friends testified in court that this is what they would have wished. But the evidence of family and friends was not accepted for women. The study found that in cases involving women, the courts denied petitions for removing life support in twelve of fourteen cases; but for men, petitions were denied in only two of eight cases.

Even more disturbing than the court decisions was the biased reasoning used to arrive at them. The study found that women were consistently portrayed as less capable of making rational decisions. A thirty-one-year-old woman's comments on life support were characterized as "offhand remarks made by a person when young," while a thirty-three-year-old man's comments were seen to express a "deeply held," "solemn, intelligent determination." Says study author Steven Miles, M.D., faculty associate at the University of Minnesota, Center for Biomedical Ethics, "Women were referred to by their first names, and constructed as emotional, immature, unreflective and vulnerable to medical neglect, while men were called by their last names, and constructed as rational, mature, decisive and assaulted by medical technology. Only women were described as curled in a fetal position, while men were described as having contractures, the medical term."

Dr. Miles is not the only one to notice that dying is often treated as a gendered activity. "Women live longer, and women live with more and more morbidity," says Rothenberg. "Most people in nursing homes are women. So clearly these end-of-life decisions are having more of an impact on women than men."

■ WHOSE LIFE IS IT, ANYWAY?

There seems to be a disturbing double standard in both law and medicine with regard to women's health care decisions. Much of the distinction occurs when a woman is pregnant, when her physical condition is wrongly seen to compromise her independence. In spite of the growing legal consensus of the courts and professional agreement among medical organizations, challenges to women's autonomy keep popping up.

In 1993 a study reported that pregnant women infected with HIV who took the drug AZT were able to greatly reduce the risk of passing the AIDS virus to their offspring. Reacting to this finding, some public health authorities believe that pregnant women should undergo mandatory AIDS testing and should be legally required to take AZT if they test positive for the virus. Some of the issues of autonomy involved in this scenario are the same as in the cesarean-section and substance-abuse cases. Can you force a competent adult woman to have a medical test? Can you force her to relinquish confidentiality and make the results of the tests known? And, based on the results of the test, can you legally force her to take a drug?

"No money will be saved by forcing HIV-infected pregnant women to take AZT if the effect is to scare them away from prenatal care," says Lynn Paltrow. "Then you wind up with sick babies. If you do test pregnant women and they won't take AZT, do you hospitalize them? AZT has serious, serious side effects. It's balancing one person's life against the other."

It's disturbing to see medical advances, which should be used to improve quality of life, mobilized to take away a woman's autonomy the instant she conceives. It's equally disturbing to think that men and women are equal under the law *except* when a woman is pregnant.

Now that medical advances are beginning to show the effects that a *man's* actions have on his unborn children, there may be even more legal challenges to lifestyle restrictions. What if it were shown that men with HIV could avoid passing the virus to their partners and unborn children if they took AZT? Would anyone attempt to force men to be tested for HIV and take AZT before engaging in any act of heterosexual intercourse?

Certainly studies have shown that a man's lifestyle, including substance abuse, can affect his sperm, and consequently the health of any children conceived with it. In 1991 the *Journal of the American Medical Association* published an article showing evidence that men who took cocaine may actually deliver the drug via sperm cells to their offspring. Commenting on the study, a bioethics journal noted, "This could produce an embryo damaged even before implantation, without the woman's ever having touched the substance." The author then began to speculate whether a man could ever be arrested for delivering drugs to a minor via his sperm cells and concluded sarcastically, "Oh, never mind." Clearly the idea of holding a man responsible for his unborn child's well-being is too absurd for our society even to consider.

"Often fetal protection comes up in connection with women, but it's frequently just as important for men," says Marcia Greenberger of the National Women's Law Center. Not only men's lifestyles, but also their employment can affect their fertility or pose reproductive hazards. Yet only women have been barred from specific jobs because of reproductive hazards.

In 1982 the Johnson Controls company, a lead battery manufacturing plant, adopted a "fetal protection" policy that barred all potentially fertile women from jobs that exposed them to lead. The women sued—successfully—for their jobs and their right to make their own decisions about whether they wanted to risk lead exposure. One man was also part of the lawsuit. He, too, claimed that the company's policy was discriminatory. He had been fired after requesting a transfer so that he would *not* be exposed to lead. According to the ACLU's Joan Bertin, "When the corporate medical director at the company was asked why men with high levels of lead in their blood weren't warned that they shouldn't conceive a child, his answer was, 'Because I can't control the situation.'" The implication was that he *could* control the women.

These fetal-protection policies have now been ruled illegal, instances of gender discrimination. In most cases they don't protect fetuses, but do exclude women from certain jobs. Yet the men who do these jobs may be just as much at risk. Employers and courts have ignored a growing body of medical evidence showing that most of these same hazards—cigarettes, alcohol, drugs, industrial solvents, lead, pesticides, petroleum products, paint—can affect men's sperm and can also cause birth defects in offspring. Though men are more likely to work at jobs that expose them to dangerous chemicals, there has so far been no effort to prevent men who may father children from taking these jobs. Rather than force men to have vasectomies, employers should provide both men and women with information about possible reproductive hazards, and should develop clothing and equipment to help them reduce exposure to toxins.

Protecting babies isn't the only motivation behind these so-called fetal-protection policies. The cases seem to come up only when women infiltrate relatively high-paying, formerly all-male jobs. There have been no attempts to "protect" women from exposure to hazardous dry-cleaning fumes, beauty-salon chemicals, computer radiation, and so forth. Not long after the U.S. Supreme Court ruled that employers could not discriminate against potentially fertile women, there were reports that women in the former East Germany were having themselves sterilized in hopes of finding better work.

Obviously fertility and pregnancy protectionism is just one of the legal issues in women's health care. Chapter 3 showed how government paternalism kept not just pregnant women but *all* women of reproductive age out of many clinical research trials, with devastating effects on women's health care. Under the old system, even women of reproductive age who weren't pregnant and had no intention of becoming pregnant couldn't volunteer for medical research because of possible hazards should they become pregnant. Scientists were afraid of lawsuits if a fetus was harmed.

Recently there has been an attempt to legally correct this paternalism and restore decision making to the woman. The National Institutes of Health and the Food and Drug Administration are taking steps to allow women of any age or reproductive status to make their own decisions about whether to volunteer for medical research. One powerful argument: Manufacturers of drugs and medical devices might be more legally liable for excluding women than for including them. For instance, women who are injured by a drug or treatment could sue for having been exposed to something that had not been adequately tested on women.

Ideally and ultimately, the law shouldn't have to get involved in a woman's personal medical decisions. Deciding whether to participate in medical research, for example, involves weighing the potential risk of an experimental treatment versus the potential benefit to one's own health, as well as the benefits that may accrue to other women as a result of the study. While research rules are finally changing, other medical decisions may still involve the court system in what should be a private relationship between a woman and her doctor.

Women have a right to absolute autonomy during pregnancy, safe treatments from physicians, safe products from medical manufacturers, and respect at the end of life. Unfortunately, as in the cases of court-ordered cesareans, prosecutions of pregnant women for substance abuse, and biased decisions regarding euthanasia, women are not only second-class patients, they are often second-class under the law, as well.

14

WOMEN AND DOCTORS
A Troubled Relationship

Most women who visit physicians aren't aware of the lack of research into women's health, the difficulties in diagnosing women with cardiac disease, or the discrimination against women in medical school. What they *are* aware of is dissatisfaction with their physicians and with their health care in general. They base these opinions on what goes on in the doctor's office and the respect—or lack of it—they receive there. "The usual experience for a woman going to a gynecologist includes humiliation, depersonalization, even pain, and too seldom does she come away with her needs having been met," asserts gynecologist John M. Smith, M.D., author of *Women and Doctors*. And gynecologists are certainly not the only physicians guilty of this mistreatment.

Marianne J. Legato, M.D., associate director of the Center for Women's Health at Columbia–Presbyterian Medical Center, has toured the country talking with women about their experiences as patients. "The general mood is anger," she says. Women complained to her that their physicians were insensitive, uninterested, rushed, arrogant, and uncommunicative. Because women's health care is fragmented, with women seeing a gynecologist for reproductive health, an internist for a general physical, and other specialists for more specific problems, one woman told her she felt "like a salami, with a slice in every doctor's office in town."

None of this surprises Dr. Legato, who says that medicine is a mirror of the rest of society and its values. "Women, the old, the poor, children, and minority groups as a whole who haven't achieved economic power are taken less seriously and held in less regard . . . which kind of leaves the emphasis on white males."

Many physicians interact with their women patients based on a view of the female sex that was already archaic decades ago. "If she's premeno-pausal, she is dismissed as suffering from PMS; if she's postmenopausal, then she obviously needs hormone replacement therapy; if she's a home-maker, she has too much time on her hands; if she's a business executive, then the pressure of her job is too much for her. She just can't win," writes Isadore Rosenfeld, M.D.

Medical school textbooks from only two decades ago portray women not much differently from the "walking wombs" that physicians treated in the 1800s. In this century gynecologists embraced the idea that hormones were the long-suspected link between the uterus and the brain. This theory led them to believe that a pelvic exam could help diagnose mental prob-lems. Conditions such as painful or irregular periods, excessive morning sickness or labor pain, and infertility became indications that a woman was battling her femininity. One 1947 obstetrics textbook, still on a practicing physician's shelf, introduces a chapter on such pregnancy problems as heartburn, nausea and vomiting, constipation, backache, varicose veins, and hemorrhoids with the sentence "Women with satisfactory self-control and more than average intelligence have fewer complaints than do other women."

Things still hadn't improved by the 1970s. A 1973 study of how women were portrayed in gynecology textbooks found that most textbooks were more concerned with the well-being of a woman's husband than with the woman herself. Wrote the authors, "Women are consistently described as anatomically destined to reproduce, nurture, and keep their husbands happy." A popular 1971 ob-gyn textbook portrayed women as helpless, childlike creatures who couldn't survive sex, pregnancy, delivery, or child raising without their doctors and added, "The traits that compose the core of the female personality are feminine narcissism, masochism, and passiv-ity."

While current textbooks seem generally more sensitive and realistic, the physicians who trained on the older books are still in practice. When *JAMA*, a leading medical journal, ran an article in 1991 about gender dis-parities in medical care, they received a letter from a physician in Ohio who wrote that perhaps women's "overanxiousness" about their health and their greater use of health services "may be due to temperamental differ-ences in gender-mediated clinical features of depression, which are mani-fested by women's less active, more ruminative responses that are linked to dysfunction of the right frontal cortex in which the metabolic rate is higher in females." In other words women are more anxious about their health because they are somehow brain-damaged. With doctors like this, no wonder women are unhappy.

■ WOMEN AS PATIENTS

Surveys show that women are more dissatisfied with their physicians than men are. And the dissatisfaction is not necessarily due to the quality of the medical care women receive, but to the lack of communication and respect they perceive in the encounter. In a 1993 Commonwealth Fund survey of twenty-five hundred women and a thousand men on the subject of women's health, women reported greater communication problems with their physicians, and were more likely to change doctors because of their dissatisfaction. One out of four women said she had been "talked down to" or treated like a child by a physician. Nearly one out of five women had been told that a reported medical condition was "all in your head."

The perception nationwide is that doctors and patients just don't understand each other. A study of one thousand complaints from dissatisfied patients at a large Michigan health maintenance organization found that more than 90 percent of the problems involved communication. "The most common complaints had to do with a lack of compassion on the physician's part," says Richard M. Frankel, Ph.D., associate professor of medicine at the University of Rochester School of Medicine and Dentistry. "Patients would complain their physician never looked at them during the entire encounter, made them feel humiliated or used medical jargon that left them confused."

As an example, Frankel describes the case of a nineteen-year-old woman who was told during a routine office visit that she had a mild vaginal infection. Although the infection is only sometimes spread sexually, the physician told the patient the infection was *usually* spread through intercourse. When she began to ask questions, he cut her off and went on to another subject. "I don't think he knew how much it upset me," she said later. "Because of that I broke up with my boyfriend, and because of the way he told me I quit the H.M.O. [health maintenance organization]." Frankel has found that patients of both sexes have an average of only eighteen seconds before being interrupted by their doctors.

Besides communication, a sexual dynamic may also make women's visits to the doctor uncomfortable or unpleasant. Real sexual abuse, which can occur in any profession, will not be discussed in this chapter; when male physicians abuse female patients, it has little to do with institutionalized gender bias and everything to do with criminal activity. But there are more common and subtle forms of gender bias that take place in the doctor's office and may have just as dire consequences on women's health and psyches. "Physicians often experience role conflict and sometimes confusion," says Frankel. He describes the case of a physician who finds himself attracted to a female patient. "Because he feels some conflict, he doesn't do a breast exam or a pelvic exam. The woman's health is sacrificed because of a sexual tension." The physician may have avoided sexual abuse, but at a high cost to his patient.

Although most women patients will never be sexually abused by their physicians, many times there is a sexual dynamic at work between the doctor and his patient. The majority of physicians in this country are males, and the majority of patients are females. Women visit physicians more often than men do and make more use of health care services. They report more acute symptoms and illnesses and suffer from more chronic conditions.

Any other kind of business would go out of its way to satisfy its biggest customers, catering to their needs and providing quality service. But the attitude of many physicians toward the majority of their patients/clients is arrogant and scornful.

"Women are patronized and treated like little girls," says Ann R. Turkel, M.D., assistant clinical professor of psychiatry, Columbia University College of Physicians and Surgeons. "They're even referred to as girls. Male physicians will call female patients by their first names, but they are always called 'Doctor.' They don't do that with men. Women are patted on the head, called 'dear' or 'honey.' And doctors tell them things like, 'Don't you worry your pretty little head about it. That's not for you to worry about; that's for me to worry about.' Then they're surprised when women see these statements and reactions as degrading and insulting."

That's what happened to Eleanor, who went to see a new gynecologist on the recommendation of her husband, an internist. The new physician seemed pleasant and thorough, taking her history and performing the usual tests. But when it came time to speak with him afterward he was dismissive. "I'll call your husband and discuss your results with him when the tests come back," he said.

"I was furious," she recalls. "I told him that *I* was his patient, not my husband, and that he should discuss my results with *me*."

There is also a perception among women that physicians don't take women's time seriously. How else to explain what happened to Roberta, a busy magazine editor who was on a tight deadline schedule the day of her doctor's appointment. "My office was just one city block from the doctor's office, so I called them five minutes before my appointment time to see if the doctor was running on schedule," she recalls. The receptionist assured her he was, so Roberta left her office and arrived at her appointment on time—only to be kept waiting for nearly an hour. "When I finally saw the doctor, I was practically shaking with rage, and my blood pressure was sky high," she says. Even though the doctor apologized and spent a lot of time talking with her after the checkup, Roberta decided to find another doctor.

"I think women are kept waiting longer for an appointment than men are," says Dr. Turkel. "I wouldn't go to a gynecologist who kept me waiting in the waiting room for an hour and a half, but I hear these stories all the time from women patients about their gynecologist's office."

Advice columnist Ann Landers even gave a rare interview to *JAMA* to let physicians know how dissatisfied women are with their doctors. "I can't say too often how angry women are about having to wait in the doctor's office," she said. "And, who do they complain to? The office manager, who is also a woman. Then, when the male doctor finally sees them—an hour later—the woman is so glad to see him that she soft-pedals the inconvenience. She wants to see the doctor as a 'knight in shining armor.' This should change. The doctor's time is no more important than the patient's and, while I can understand special circumstances, I can't understand why a doctor is *always* running late."

Doctors may treat women as if they are inferior patients, but studies show that they are anything but. Women tend to ask more questions—and receive more information because of their inquisitiveness. Women also show more emotion during office visits and are more likely to confide a personal problem that may have a bearing on their health to their physicians. Men, on the other hand, ask fewer questions of their physicians, give less information to the doctor, and display less emotion. During a typical fifteen-minute office visit, women ask an average of six questions. Men don't ask any.

"Practice makes perfect, and my hunch is that women have many more chances to practice being patients," says Sherrie Kaplan, Ph.D., codirector of the New England Medical Center's Primary Care Outcomes Research Institute. "They go for reproductive care, take their children for pediatric care. By the time they themselves develop chronic diseases, they're more familiar with how the process works."

She continues, "Men often don't have an opportunity to practice patienthood until it's time to make a decision—prostate in or prostate out? Should they take high blood pressure medication, which can cause impotence, or risk a stroke instead? And men don't get a lot of support for being concerned about their health care."

Although physicians should be thrilled to have patients who are interested in their health, ask questions, and volunteer personal information, women's concerns are often dismissed as symptoms of anxiety, their questions brushed aside. In business, successful executives are often seen as having forceful, take-charge personalities, while women with similar attributes are described as aggressive or bitchy. In medicine, male patients seem to describe symptoms, while women complain. Instead of valuing women as active, informed patients, doctors are more likely to prefer patients who don't ask questions, don't interrupt, don't question their judgment, and—perhaps most important—get in and out of the office as quickly as possible. Researchers have actually found that physicians *like* male patients better than female ones, even when factors such as age, education, income, and occupation are controlled for.

Perhaps because of these attitudes, women often feel frustrated when they try to ask questions and receive explanations. One study reported that women received significantly more explanations than men—but not significantly more explaining *time*. Wrote the authors, "It is possible that many of the explanations they received were brief and perfunctory. Or, put differently, the men may have received fewer but fuller explanations than the women." The study also found that women were less likely than men to receive explanations that matched the level of technicality of the questions they asked. Doctors tended to talk down to women when answering their questions.

In an attempt to get the answers to their questions within the time constraints of a typical office visit, many women have followed the advice doled out in women's magazines, that to maximize the efficiency of a medical visit, they should write down their questions and concerns. But not only do many physicians dislike what they see as a "laundry list" approach, they may actually consider it pathological. "Medical textbooks from around the turn of the century to the 1950s described a syndrome called 'patient with a small list,'" says Frankel. "There was a supposition that patients who made lists of concerns were psychiatrically impaired." Tell that to the busy professional woman who efficiently scribbles some questions for her doctor into her Filofax so as not to waste her time or his during the appointment.

So ingrained are the problems of communication between physicians and their women patients that even women whose business is health care may not overcome them. Kaplan runs a program to help train patients to get the most out of their doctors' visits. She reviews their medical histories and records with them, explains their options, and helps them put their questions and concerns in order of importance before seeing the physician. Yet, she admits, "Even though I teach this stuff, when I'm a patient, I wimp out the same way anybody else does."

■ MISCOMMUNICATION OR MISTREATMENT?

Far more serious than patronizing attitudes and lack of consideration for women's time are the myths about women patients' complaints that jeopardize women's health care.

"Physician folklore says that women are more demanding patients," says Karen Carlson, M.D., an internist at Massachusetts General Hospital in Boston. "From my experience women are interested in health and prevention, desire to be listened to and treated with respect, want the opportunity to present and explain their agenda, and want their symptoms and concerns taken seriously."

But all too often women's symptoms are not taken seriously because physicians erroneously believe that these symptoms have no physical basis and that women's complaints are simply a sign of their demanding natures.

A 1979 study compared the medical records of fifty-two married couples to see how they had been treated for five common problems: back pain, headache, dizziness, chest pain, and fatigue. "The physicians' workups were significantly more extensive for the men than they were for women," reported the authors. "These data tend to support the argument that male physicians take medical illness more seriously in men than in women."

Another study found that women were shortchanged even in general checkups. Men's visits are more likely to include vision and hearing tests, chest X rays, ECGs, blood tests, rectal examinations, and urinalyses.

Dr. Carlson, speaking to a roomful of women physicians at an annual meeting of the American Medical Women's Association, cited evidence to show that women may actually complain *less* than men. "The myth is that women complain more, but studies show another truth," she says. Carlson cited studies showing that, compared with men, women with colon cancer are more likely to delay care and experience diagnostic delay. That women with chronic joint symptoms and arthritis are less likely to report pain. That women have more severe and frequent colds, but men are more likely to overrate their symptoms. That women delay seeking help for chest pain or symptoms of a heart attack. These studies point to women as being more stoic, yet when they finally do show up in the doctor's office, they are apt to be met with skepticism.

Betsy Murphy (not her real name) had been seeing the same doctor for years. "We had a perfectly fine relationship as long as I just went for my yearly checkups and didn't ask a lot of questions," she recalls. "But then I got my first yeast infection and had to go see him for a prescription—the medicine wasn't available over-the-counter then." Betsy told her doctor what she thought she had—she had talked to enough friends and read enough magazine articles to recognize the distinctive cottage-cheeselike discharge, yeasty odor, and intense itching. "But he ignored me when I told him what I thought was wrong. After he took a culture and examined it under the microscope, he sneeringly said, 'Well, Ms. Murphy, it seems as if your diagnosis is correct.' " Although he diagnosed the problem and prescribed the medication, Betsy left his office feeling insulted and patronized.

At a recent workshop on the patient-physician partnership, an auditorium full of physicians was asked how they would handle a "problem" patient. One of these "problems" was the patient who comes in and announces his or her own diagnosis. The physicians, almost unanimously, ridiculed the patient for daring to speculate what was wrong. They preferred that someone just present a description of symptoms, as specifically and articulately as possible. "It's no help for someone to come to me and say, 'I have a cold and I just need some medicine,' " said a participating doctor to a journalist in the audience. "Instead the patient should describe how they feel as specifically as possible. And obviously some people are more articulate and some less; that's where the doctor's skill comes in." In other words, a patient should show up for an appointment and tell the doctor, "I have a stuffy nose and I keep sneezing," and then wait for the doctor, in his infinite wisdom, to pronounce, "You have a cold." For a patient, male or female, who is reasonably certain what is wrong, the suggestion seems ludicrous.

Women's dissatisfaction with their medical care can lead to serious health consequences. They may switch doctors so frequently that they receive no continuity of care. Or they may simply avoid seeing doctors altogether because they find the experience humiliating. When men without a regular source of health care are asked why they don't have one, they tend to reply that they don't need a doctor. But women are more apt to say that they cannot find the right doctor, or that they have recently moved, or that their previous doctor is no longer available. In the Commonwealth Fund poll, 41 percent of woman (compared with 27 percent of men) said they had switched doctors in the past because they were dissatisfied. "If you brought your car in to be fixed and the person who fixed it did an okay but not great job, but was nasty, wouldn't you go to another mechanic? The same is true of physicians," says Frankel.

Physicians seem to realize there's a problem, but many of their efforts to remedy it are laughable. One 1993 article in the medical newspaper *American Medical News* advised doctors that if they wanted to make their practice "women-friendly," they should "create an atmosphere similar to that of a living room. This includes the seating, lighting and wall decorations." Yet it's difficult to imagine any woman listing "ugly wallpaper" as a reason for being dissatisfied with her health care. It's not the decor women are complaining about when they complain about doctors' offices.

Ob-gyn John Smith lists padded stirrups and speculum warmers as among the improvements women have gotten their doctors to make since the 1960s. But even these superficial improvements are not enough. What women really want are doctors who will listen to them, talk to them, and treat their medical questions and problems with respect and empathy.

■ ARE WOMEN DOCTORS THE ANSWER?

It would be ludicrous to state that all male doctors are cold and unemotional and all women physicians are empathetic and nurturing. Such gender stereotypes may apply to groups, but certainly not to individuals. There are plenty of concerned, communicative male physicians and plenty of callous, uncaring women.

That said, it is also true that studies show a significant difference in the way that male and female physicians practice their profession. A study of nearly 100,000 women in a Minneapolis health plan found that women received better preventive care from women physicians, who are more likely to recommend mammograms and take a Pap smear than male physicians. The differences were more pronounced among family practitioners and internists than among gynecologists.

Those results wouldn't surprise Nellie, who switched from a male to a female gynecologist when she was sixty-one years old. At her first appointment, the new physician began to take a complete health history. When she asked about mammograms, she was stunned to find out that not only had Nellie never had the screening test but "my old doctor had never even mentioned it to me."

Other studies show further differences between male and female physicians:

- Male physicians are more likely to label their patients "demanding, bitchy, noncompliant."
- Male doctors tend to interrupt their patients, but female doctors are more likely to *be* interrupted by their patients.
- Women physicians are more inclined to care for the indigent.
- Women doctors show more emotion, and their patients perceive that as caring, whether the emotion is positive or negative.
- Most dramatic, but perhaps least surprising, are the differences in communication skills between male and female physicians. Women doctors seem to communicate better with their patients, just as women in general communicate better with other people. After all, before there are male physicians and female physicians, there are men and women. "Gender isn't something you can take off and put on like a doctor's white coat," says Candace West, Ph.D., professor of sociology at the University of California, Santa Cruz.

When a woman visits a male physician, it's not just a doctor-patient relationship, but a male-female relationship as well. Many women find talking to another woman easier than talking to a male doctor, especially about personal or intimate problems such as abuse or battering, rape, and eating disorders that may affect physical and emotional health. "From the patient's point of view it comes down to, 'What are you willing to tell Mom as opposed to Dad?'" says Deborah Allen, M.D., professor and chairman of the Department of Family Practice at Indiana University School of Medicine. "I think that generally women are more comfortable revealing their sexual problems and histories, and their concerns about childbearing and birth control, to another woman, because they don't feel they're going to be judged. Just as most men aren't going to talk about their sexual dysfunction with a woman."

Elizabeth had been seeing the same gynecologist for years. One night she was raped when a man broke into her apartment in the middle of the night. At the emergency room, after the staff examined her for injuries and tested for pregnancy and sexually transmitted diseases, they advised her that she should have a follow-up visit in six weeks. Thinking she'd be more comfortable with her own doctor, Elizabeth made an appointment and told the receptionist the reason for the visit. "But when I got there, my doctor was clearly uncomfortable and embarrassed," she recalls. "He didn't even ask me how I was, and he didn't seem to know what to check for. He made me feel dirty and ashamed—something the police and the emergency room staff definitely *didn't*. Those people were complete strangers to me, but the physician I'd been visiting since I was right out of college treated me as if *I'd* done something wrong."

Julie was twenty-three years old when she learned that she would have to have her vagina surgically removed because of cancer. Her mother had taken the drug diethylstilbestrol (DES) during pregnancy, before the dangers were known. Her doctor, in an awkward attempt to help his patient cope with the devastating loss of her sexuality, said to her, "Look at me—I'm in my 50's and I've lived my whole life without one." If nothing else, a woman physician could never make such a tactless and insensitive remark.

When women patients are paired with women physicians, the visits last longer, there is greater rapport, and there is more talk. Women seem more willing to report symptoms and divulge personal information to female doctors. And because female physicians show more emotion and interrupt patients less, they are seen as more caring and empathetic, and less authoritarian.

Male and female physicians also issue their "doctor's orders" quite differently. Male physicians tend to issue imperatives or commands. But women physicians couch their recommendations in the form of proposals: "Let's try this." "Why don't we check this and then you can come back and tell me how it's going two weeks from now." "Let's talk about this." The relationship between a woman physician and her patient is less hierarchical and more of a partnership, regardless of whether the patient is male or female. Candace West, whose work is being used in medical schools to train the next generation of doctors, also found that patients were much more likely to comply with these mitigated proposals than with outright commands.

For all these reasons, many women show a strong preference for seeing a female physician. John Smith believes that nearly all women would prefer a woman gynecologist; other health care providers believe the preference carries over into primary care as well. The caseload of female doctors is 72 percent female, compared with an average 60 percent for male physicians.

Interestingly, women physicians' better communicating skills may not just make them more attuned to the health care needs of other women; they may also do better at treating men. "Women doctors spend more time with their patients. Men doctors spend more time with women patients. And the least time is with men doctors and men patients," says Steven A. Cohen-Cole, M.D., a psychiatrist at Emory University Medical School.

Sherrie Kaplan and Sheldon Greenfield, M.D., of Tufts University

Medical School, found that the more actively patients were involved in communicating with their doctors, the better their health outcomes. And men who have female physicians take a more active role in their care. "When you listen to tapes of doctors and patients, you hear men say things like 'How's the old ticker, Doc?' They tend to blow off their concerns and say they're fine," says Kaplan. "But when men see women health providers, they do much better. It may be that the women are better at responding to the 'old ticker' question. They may be able to say, 'Are you worried that you're having a heart attack?' "

Men who might not expect or even want to be questioned by a male doctor about psychological concerns might welcome such a discussion when initiated by a female physician. Kaplan goes so far as to say she thinks that men who join HMOs should be required to see women providers for the first six months "to practice patienthood. They may have issues about genital exams, but women have been dealing with that for years."

■ CAN'T WE ALL JUST GET ALONG?

It's *not* true that only women can care for women. And it's *not* true that only women have the communication skills necessary to be a good doctor. "The studies on how male and female physicians communicate with their patients report the mean, the general case," says Debra Roter, Dr.P.H., Johns Hopkins University School of Hygiene and Public Health. "Obviously some male doctors are better at communicating than some females. There's no guarantee that if you go to a female doctor she's going to be better in all of these things." Roter takes her children to a male pediatrician who she says is "a good example of a male physician who has superb skills. I think I'd be hard pressed to find a better doctor, male or female, who is a better communicator."

Most of the researchers studying doctor-patient relationships believe that communication skills are something that can be taught to both sexes. Recognizing that these skills are essential for practicing clinical medicine, nearly all of the nation's accredited medical schools now offer some kind of training in doctor-patient communication.

Professional medical organizations are urging their members to make better communication with patients a priority, too. In 1993 the American College of Obstetricians and Gynecologists urged their member physicians to go "back to basics" and "re-affirm the doctor-patient relationship and the very values and traditions on which it is based." Said Richard S. Hollis, M.D., then the organization's president, "I believe we need to rethink what it means to care, to take a hard look at ourselves and how we deliver health care." Dr. Hollis's program to "put the patient first" included stressing better communication skills for physicians.

The aim of all these efforts is to help the majority of doctors, who truly care about their patients, show their interest more effectively. Too often doctors mean well but fail to communicate their concern to patients. They may seem brusque or businesslike rather than compassionate. Kaplan tells the story of one physician-patient encounter that illustrates the problem of good intentions but bad communication:

A woman with breast cancer was waiting to be examined by her physician. When he walked into the examining room, he was practically bent over double from back pain. Concerned, the woman asked if he was okay. "I'm fine," he replied abruptly, then began the examination. Afterward the woman told Kaplan she was very upset by how her doctor had dismissed her concerns about him. Confronted with his patient's feelings, the doctor got very choked up and said, "But you have breast cancer. How can I possibly complain to you about my back problems?" She replied, "You made me feel like I was a breast rather than a person. I may have breast cancer, but I'm still a woman. And I don't want to be deprived of my opportunity to care about other people." Training programs for medical students hope to ensure that exchanges like this no longer take place.

It's ironic that this new emphasis on teaching medical students such traits as bedside manners comes at a time when (admittedly much needed) health reforms threaten to destroy what little remains of an "old-fashioned" doctor-patient relationship. "We're doing funny things to the doctor-patient relationship," says Kaplan. "We're constraining the time doctors can spend with patients. We tell them, 'We want you to see six patients an hour . . . but we also want you to be the most wonderful and compassionate person you can be.' "

Women physicians, who tend to be more attentive to their patients and spend more time with them, may find these time constraints particularly onerous. Conversely, health maintenance organizations may be leery of hiring women doctors because they see fewer patients an hour. "From one perspective women physicians are less efficient," says Frankel. "Because they take a little more time to complete their visits, they may be providing higher quality care, but at a lower cost return for the health maintenance organization." Others counter these charges by saying that women physicians' greater rapport with patients means that patients can get their concerns out in one visit and then may need fewer visits in the future.

Physicians are also concerned that health care reforms will mean less of a chance for a long-term doctor-patient relationship, because patients may not be able to choose their physicians, and health maintenance organizations may have patients see different doctors with each visit. "Continuity of care is an invaluable part of the doctor-patient relationship," says Dr. Allen. "The more I know about my patients, the easier it is to take care of them."

One woman patient with vague pelvic complaints recently consulted a colleague of Dr. Allen's. "As soon as I heard the name, I knew that she was having a stress reaction," says Dr. Allen. "This patient had called me the week before to tell me that her boyfriend had killed himself because they had broken up. She wasn't sick or anything; she just wanted me to know what was happening in her life."

Allen had cared for this woman since she was a teenager, "and you couldn't pay for the knowledge I have about her. Nor could another physician gain it in ten office visits. It's good to be a good communicator, but if you're starting cold with someone each time, it's hard. Knowledge about a patient, and the establishment of a good doctor-patient relationship, is accumulated over time."

Health care reforms may jeopardize medical communication, but the solution is not just more female physicians, but more *good* physicians, skilled in all aspects of healing, including relating to patients respectfully and humanely. Dr. Lillian Gonzalez-Pardo, past president of the American Medical Women's Association, hopes that as more women enter medicine, male and female physicians will adopt each other's best qualities: "From my viewpoint, the ideal doctor combines traits considered as masculine—such as assertiveness and decisiveness—with feminine traits, such as empathy and a spirit of cooperation." Regardless of their sex, physicians with these attributes may be able not only to heal patients' ills but also to ease the troubled relationship between women and their doctors.

15

THE FUTURE OF
WOMEN'S HEALTH

This book began with the assertion that women can only be informed medical consumers up to a point. That ultimately they are limited by the lack of research on women's health. Since we started work on this book, the National Institutes of Health, the nation's premier research institution, responded to the criticism that it had been neglecting women in clinical trials by funding a number of important studies, including the Women's Health Initiative (WHI), the Heart and Estrogen/Progestin Replacement Study, and the first AIDS trial to look at the course of the disease in women. These and myriad other smaller efforts should finally provide answers about how to prevent and treat some of the biggest killers of women.

But it's not time to rest on our laurels, to declare the job done. For one thing, results from the largest of these studies, the WHI, will not be available until the turn of the century. And even if all the results could somehow magically appear tomorrow, they would not be sufficient to eliminate all the gaps.

"It isn't enough to gather more research information on women," says San Francisco psychiatrist Karen Johnson. "We need to ensure the clinical profession's medical translation of science to direct patient service. Otherwise cardiologists will integrate the new data into their practice, bone specialists will integrate it into theirs." But this will serve only to take women out of the context of their lives and to look at their health as it applies to a specific organ. It doesn't address the next part of the equation, what many consider the culmination of the decades-long women's health movement. That is, the integration of all of this new knowledge into every speciality so that it affects the clinical care of all women, young and old.

This is a crucial next step. For woman's health care, as it currently exists, is characterized by fragmented, uncoordinated care. Because women's health needs have traditionally been categorized as either "reproductive" or "all other," women have been forced into seeing at least two providers, frequently a gynecologist and a generalist, such as a family practitioner or internist. Typically one doctor doesn't know what the other is doing. One study found that, after excluding obstetric services, physicians in family practice, internal medicine, and gynecology provided overlapping services to women. Carolyn Clancy, M.D., director of the division of primary care at the Agency for Health Care Policy and Research, describes the care of women as "a patchwork quilt with gaps."

Uncoordinated services are not only a waste of time and money, they result in inadequate care, as evidenced by the low cancer screening rates for women. In one telling study, researchers at Dartmouth sent actresses in their mid-fifties posing as patients to hundreds of family physicians and internists for checkups. More than one-third of the doctors did not perform clinical breast exams unless prompted by the women. In another study more than one-third of the women had not had a Pap smear, pelvic exam, or breast exam in the previous year. There's even evidence, as discussed in the previous chapter, that the sex of the physician makes a crucial difference in the type of preventive care a woman gets, something women have always intuitively felt but couldn't quite prove.

In light of this fragmentation, women's health advocates charge that no single specialty is qualified to provide comprehensive primary care to women. From our perspective this analysis is on the mark, although you wouldn't know it by talking to internists, family practitioners, or ob-gyns, who claim they're already serving as the gatekeepers of women's health.

Let's take a closer look at ob-gyns. At the turn of the last century, when the field of obstetrics and gynecology was created, it made sense to entrust women's health to a reproductive specialty. After all, women were dying in childbirth, delivery injuries were leaving them incontinent, and women were suffering from chronic pelvic pain due to undiagnosed pelvic inflammatory disease. "Medicine responded to the need to provide health care for women by creating a specialty," says Karen Johnson. "At the time it was a perfectly reasonable approach to take. But in the ensuing century medical science has changed dramatically. We now understand it's erroneous to assign women's health to a reproductive surgical specialty. Women's health is much more broad-based than that." Still, more than half of all women use their ob-gyn as their primary care provider.

But these women may not be getting true primary care. In terms of services performed, a Gallup poll commissioned by the American College of Obstetricians and Gynecologists found that ob-gyns did far fewer cholesterol tests compared with other doctors and were less likely to discuss emotional or mental health problems, diet and exercise, and the use of medication—hardly what anyone would call comprehensive care. Ob-gyns are also responsible for subjecting women to far too many cesarean sections and hysterectomies. They've had to be dragged kicking and screaming into the AIDS epidemic, and many still resist providing routine obstetrical care to HIV-infected women. Not only have ob-gyns abdicated their responsibility for providing abortions, we can also thank the specialty for medicalizing almost every aspect of women's health, from menstruation to childbirth to menopause.

Now gynecologists are discussing creating a new discipline in climacteric medicine. The demographics belie a market too rich to ignore: In the next two decades some forty million American women will pass through menopause; by the year 2012, women over fifty will make up about half of the patients visiting ob-gyns. Many women gynecologists, who are about to enter menopause themselves, are undoubtedly attempting to be more responsive to their female patients. But we can guarantee, based on the field's past legacy, that many gynecologists will make it their mission to fix all these poor estrogen-deficient women. "By focusing on the menopause," says internist Eileen Hoffman, M.D., of New York University, "gynecologists are trying to mark it as theirs."

This may be so, but it's not all they are doing. On the cusp of health care reform, which promises to place a premium on primary care, ACOG is helping its members position themselves as—what else?—primary care providers. In 1993 the college published a set of guidelines encouraging members to offer patients a wide range of screening tests and immunizations and to counsel them about such things as high-risk sexual behaviors, sexual functioning, breast self-examination, domestic violence, injury prevention, depression, and substance abuse. These guidelines were followed in early 1994 with a new ACOG-sponsored medical journal, *Primary Care Update for Ob/Gyns*. In the introduction to the first issue, then-president Richard S. Hollis, M.D., wrote, "The need to fill the demand for primary care in obstetrics/gynecology cannot be overestimated. For the majority of women of reproductive age, we are not only their primary physicians, but often the only physicians they see."

The move toward primary care is a step in the right direction. But if gynecology truly plans to meet the needs of women, it must do more than offer its members optional guidelines for care. It must go all the way and restructure its training program to include general medicine training for all residents. For instance, gynecology residents will have to be trained in infectious and chronic diseases, cardiology, and endocrinology, the same disciplines in which internists and family practitioners receive training.

This isn't to imply that these other specialties are pulling their weight. While family physicians receive interdisciplinary training, they are limited in that they divide their attention among women, men, and children. Nor are internists prepared to address all of women's health needs. Although two-thirds of internists' patients are women—and 80 percent when the doctor is a woman—they receive almost no training in the female reproductive tract. Yet there's no anatomical separation between the abdomen and the pelvis. "The intestines come all the way down into the pelvis, and they can stick onto an ovary," says Hoffman. "Endometriosis can migrate up to the lung and cause pain when you take a deep breath. It can actually migrate out of the abdominal cavity to your nose and give you nosebleeds during your period."

An internist who sees mostly women, Hoffman was moved by the lives of her female patients but felt frustrated at how inadequately trained she was to care for them. "Medicine had divvied up the professional turf," she says. "Breasts and other reproductive organs went to gynecologists, and the rest of us didn't have to worry about it. I sensed there was a woman's way toward health and illness that I wasn't privy to because I wasn't taught it."

Like Hoffman, Vivian Terkel, M.D., was struck by how disadvantaged she was when it came to providing comprehensive care to women. "I knew next to no gynecology when I finished my training," says Terkel, an internist and codirector of the University of California, San Diego, Center for Women's Health. Like Hoffman she did on-the-job training in Pap smears and pelvic exams, in part because her female patients demanded the service. Interestingly male internists rarely perform Paps and pelvics, even though they routinely examine the genitalia of their male patients.

Arbitrarily parceling out women's body parts has had dire consequences. All medicine that didn't get assigned to obstetrics and gynecology became men's health—hence the advent of the 70-kilogram male as the medical model, rendering the health needs of women invisible. As Carolyn Clancy says, "Women's health needs have come to be defined by providers rather than by women, which means that a lot of issues important to women aren't addressed well by any provider group."

Domestic violence is a case in point. The emergency room physician deals with a woman's black eye or broken bone. The gynecologist handles her pelvic pain. The internist her stomachache. The psychologist or psychiatrist her depression or substance abuse. Social workers or lawyers may get involved. "Nowhere does the team come together around the phenomenon of violence against the woman in the context of her life," says Hoffman.

"If medicine was woman-centered, we would see that violence is epidemic in our culture. The medical research establishment would be devoting millions of dollars to look for a cure. They'd be looking for the cure not in women but in men, and there would be all sorts of diagnostic labels in the DSM for problems of male aggression. It wouldn't be a disease of women, it would be a disease of men. But if you were to research the literature on domestic violence, battering, sexual abuse, incest, and rape, you would only find descriptions of the victims and very, very little literature on how to effectively deal with this problem in men."

If health care was woman-centered, all the conditions that have been neglected in research or written off as psychiatric would be integrated into primary care. Rather than simply treating the aftereffects, doctors would get at the cause of a woman's problem, a principle Hoffman has built into her practice.

"My antenna goes up every time I see someone come back into my office with multiple complaints that don't add up to a diagnosis," she says. "For instance, a headache or a backache that may be a metaphor for something else. It could be trouble at home, stress on the job, or a history of incest being incorporated into the woman's persona, so she takes on these symptoms. Alcohol and substance abuse, eating disorders, irritable bowel syndrome, chronic pelvic pain syndrome, and multiple personality disorder describe women's behaviors as they interact with the health care system, but the etiology is never got at."

For all its shortcomings, the practice of medicine is changing to fill the gaps in knowledge about women's bodies. Granted, the modifications are not simply a result of a sudden case of altruism. The growing threats of health care reform, congressional pressure on the research community to be accountable to women, and market forces are all conspiring to shape medicine for perhaps the next millennium.

Health care reform, one of the priorities of President Clinton's administration, will have far-reaching implications for women's health. "There's nothing more important for women's health in this country than the way the medical care is delivered," says Marcia Greenberger, copresident of the

National Women's Law Center. "Health care reform will go to the heart of what's considered basic health care. As such, it will affect the kind of care women and their families get."

For instance, women may have more at stake in the debate over *how* people are covered by health insurance. Right now some 12 million women have no health insurance, and millions more have inadequate coverage. "When women are employed, they're disproportionately employed by companies that don't provide health care coverage," says Greenberger. "Or they may be employed part-time. If they're covered as dependents and there's a change in their marital status, they may lose their health care coverage. And many employers are looking to cut costs by dropping dependent coverage entirely. If health care reform is really going to provide universal coverage without regard to employment, women will be major beneficiaries of that coverage."

To be women-friendly, any new system must ensure universal access, affordability, and coverage for care by nurse-practitioners and nurse-midwives, and for preventive services, reproductive health—including screening tests, contraception, and abortion as well as pregnancy—and long-term care, since women live longer than men. In addition, women must be included on all planning boards and committees that make determinations about access and coverage. Only if these requirements are met will women truly have government-insured, equal access to decent health care.

As Leslie Wolfe, executive director of the nonprofit Center for Women Policy Studies, says, "Women make up more than half the U.S. population, but our health needs have been relegated to second place. If I were in the White House, I would be building a health care reform package that starts with women's health as its bedrock." So far the Clinton administration appears responsive.

There is another sea change that will directly affect the kind of care women receive: the burgeoning movement toward comprehensive women's health centers, one-stop shopping where practitioners with training in such areas as ob-gyn, general medicine, menopause, cardiology, oncology, infectious diseases, endocrinology, and bone metabolism gather under one roof. Instead of a woman having to make the rounds to two or three different doctors, the doctors make themselves available to her during a single appointment. While such centers may regrettably take the onus off individual specialities to expand, they nonetheless offer women an integrated health care experience.

There are no good statistics on the number of women's centers or clinics in this country. But it's clear the range and number of these services are growing. At the new clinical center at the Yale–New Haven hospital, women come in for an initial one-day program that includes risk-factor assessment, nutrition and lifestyle counseling, and, if necessary, treatment recommendations. The program has a strong emphasis on disease prevention and health promotion.

In late 1993 the University of California, San Diego, opened its Center for Women's Health, with a multidisciplinary team that gathers in an outpatient building near the UCSD hospital in downtown San Diego. Codirectors Terkel and Elaine Hansen, M.D., an ob-gyn, dreamed up the idea for the center while watching their kids play soccer one afternoon. So far patients are beside themselves with gratitude. "Women are starving for comprehensive care in one place," says Terkel. "They're tired of their complaints not being addressed and they're worried about having too much done to them that they don't need."

In fact both Yale and UCSD are adamant about individualizing care. Even though they have mammography, ultrasound, and bone density machines on site, they won't give new patients every high-tech test in the book. In California this approach can be explained by two words—*managed care*, which pays doctors for doing less, not more. In states without this mandate there may be too great an incentive for women's health centers to turn the big technological guns on every woman who walks in the door.

One can't help but worry that some of these centers exist solely to market services to women, to apply technology to their bodies. As Hoffman says, "A mammogram, a bone density test, a medical consultation, an endometrial biopsy, a pelvic ultrasound. Again, it's maintaining that model of women as illness that needs to come under constant scrutiny and be monitored and screened and studied. We have to be very careful that we don't turn ourselves into profit centers."

In other cases the point isn't to turn a profit but to get women, who hospital administrators know make all the health care decisions for their families, to identify with the medical institution. When family members need care, the idea is that women will be more likely to direct them to the woman-friendly hospital in her neighborhood.

Just as researchers who have had no interest in women's health have begun to clamor to study women now that the funding is there, so a cadre of conservative hospital administrators has suddenly discovered a lucrative market in women's health as well. So far no one knows what a model women's health center should look like or whether this type of practice is doing a better job at meeting the health care needs of women. One thing seems certain: It's going to be easy to attract educated, high-income women who are tired of orchestrating their health care. But these centers also have an obligation to make their services available to the economically disadvantaged women in their communities who are normally locked out of the health care system. Yale is planning to do this. A study is currently under way at Johns Hopkins to find out whether these centers are more than mere marketing vehicles.

As more and more hospitals contemplate repackaging their women's health services, the nursing profession is undergoing its own quiet revolution. At a time when primary care physicians are in short supply, women are discovering they can get many of their health care needs met by registered nurses, who can offer preventive services (such as nutrition and smoking-cessation counseling), routine screening tests, gynecological exams, and basic primary care. Studies show that nurses spend more time with patients, offer more health-promotion counseling, charge less per visit, and achieve results comparable to doctors. What's more, nurses in more than thirty-five states can write prescriptions.

To meet women's increasing demands for nursing services, the University of California, San Francisco, School of Nursing now offers a woman's primary care program, one- and two-year courses of study for nurse-practitioners interested in graduate training in women's primary health care.

"The public has been led to believe that the only person who can provide health care is the physician," says Muriel Shore, R.N., a member of the American Nurses Association's board of directors. "There's been reluctance on the part of doctors to share the arena, but that's beginning to change."

Not, of course, if the American Medical Association has anything to say about it, and it has plenty. Many physicians believe nurses should not be allowed to write prescriptions and are against independent practice. Doctors have about twelve years of training, they argue, while nurse-practitioners are registered nurses with up to two years' additional training in a specialty, such as gynecology, family practice, or now women's health. Women who are cared for by nurses in independent practice also have difficulty getting their medical bills reimbursed by insurance. The AMA strongly opposes efforts by the nursing profession to eliminate this barrier, although health care reform, with its emphasis on alternative providers, may change this.

Nursing practices and women's health centers may have plenty to offer women, but, again, if they exist in a vacuum, they're not enough. By themselves they are only stopgap measures. For what is still lacking in America is a standardized model for the comprehensive care of women. If medicine was woman-centered, it would "reflect women as whole human beings with minds, bodies, and spirits," write Hoffman and Johnson.

Consider, for example, the perimenopausal woman with borderline hypertension who's suffering from increasingly severe migraines, a common scenario. Asks Janet Henrich, an associate professor of medicine at the Yale University School of Medicine, "How do you take into account what effect her hormonal status is going to have not only on her increasing problem with migraines but on how that might interfere with the metabolism of some of the antimigraine drugs? And this just addresses the questions she walks into the office with.

"One of the considerations in starting her on estrogen replacement therapy before she actually has her last menstrual period involves another whole set of questions about the risks and benefits of estrogen to the bones, heart, breasts, to the protection of the uterus.

"Not only are most physicians not comfortable in addressing the multitude of health issues in women, especially as they age, but they don't have the background in clinical epidemiology to be able to look at all the conflicting information that's in the literature and be able to interpret that and discuss it with the patient."

Eileen Hoffman and Karen Johnson argue that the way to integrate all this knowledge into practice is by creating a new medical specialty devoted solely to women's health. "As medical curricula are structured, no single physician, unless they've taken it upon themselves to obtain additional training, is qualified to offer anything approaching comprehensive woman-centered care," says Johnson. "Most physicians are practicing men's health and providing it to women as if they're the same."

Physicians do not take a field of medicine seriously unless it's an integral part of their training, Johnson convincingly argues. A specialty would also translate into an academic department devoted to women's health, which would give the field even more credibility and provide a central arena from which to study women's health issues.

Sue Rosser, Ph.D., director of Women's Studies at the University of South Carolina, Columbia, says that the debate about a woman's health specialty mirrors the one a decade ago over whether there should be separate departments of women's studies. The solution at most institutions has been to create departments and at the same time integrate the content into the traditional disciplines. Likewise in medicine, Rosser argues, a specialty would ensure the inclusion of women's health in all aspects of medicine.

So far the medical profession has not warmed up to the idea. When Carolyn Clancy wrote about the gaps in women's health care for the *Journal of the American Medical Association* and broached the subject of a specialty, four of the six people reviewing the article said, "You've got to be kidding. The last thing people need is another specialty."

Even Clancy is on the fence about the best approach to take. In fact the issue is as divided as any, with feminists on both sides forcefully stating their cases. Psychiatrist Michelle Harrison is convinced that women and men are more alike than different. As we know from experience, defining women by their differences is dangerous, since women's differences have traditionally been used against them. A specialty poses the danger of further ghettoizing women's health and creating another poorly paid primary care specialty.

A better approach may be to have all physicians train in women's health. Currently fewer than 20 percent of medical schools teach women's health, and much of what they offer is elective. Yet women are asking for residencies and fellowships in this area—and finding little available. Typically they must customize programs themselves.

"I shared my students' and residents' frustration and disappointment at how few opportunities there were for them to do special clinical work, let alone research, in this area," says Janet Henrich. So Henrich, an internist, helped develop the Program in Women's Health at Yale University, a collaboration between the departments of medicine and ob-gyn, which has established a core curriculum in women's health for residents.

Albert Einstein College of Medicine in New York is also starting a residency program in internal medicine that includes training in Pap smears, pelvic exams, routine gynecological programs, the management of menopause, and such psychiatric issues as depression, anxiety disorders, and domestic violence. Women's health programs have also popped up at the University of Louisville, the State University of New York at Stony Brook, Stanford, and the Mount Sinai School of Medicine in New York.

"I refer to this as trickle-down curriculum," says Henrich. "It's an important effort, but if we're truly going to change the way women are cared for and have their issues addressed appropriately by research as well as clinical care, we have to influence minds when they're fertile, and that's when they're in medical school." To that end, in 1993 the Medical College of Pennsylvania became the first medical school in the nation to integrate women's health into all its medical school curricula. At the same time NIH is conducting a review of medical school curricula to identify gaps in women's health care and recommend ways to fill them.

On a larger scale, the American Medical Women's Association is offering to practice physicians a continuing medical education course on women's health. The first three-day session focused on the medical care of midlife and older women. A follow-up course will deal with the health care of women of reproductive age.

Most professional organizations, however, have been slow to pick up the gauntlet. "When I called the American College of Physicians [which represents internists] and asked them, 'What are your efforts in this area, what are your plans?' there was absolute silence at the other end," says one health care provider. All of which is testament to the fact that most specialties believe they're already doing a good job taking care of women. If only that were true.

Despite helter-skelter improvements in the care of women, the move toward special centers, nurse-run practices, and medical school curricula in women's health suggests a larger trend: the feminization of medicine. More women than ever are entering medical school. By the year 2010 the AMA estimates that one-third of all doctors will be women. As we've previously discussed, there's evidence that women physicians communicate better and spend more time with their patients than male physicians. Not surprisingly these women are bringing a feminine, and sometimes feminist, sensibility to the practice of medicine.

"Feminism is about empowering all our patients—men, women, and children—and treating them with respect," says Laura Helfman, M.D., an emergency room doctor in North Carolina. "We're doctors, we're not gods up on high." To Helfman this means taking the opportunity to do "a gentle and warm pelvic exam so I can reeducate the person receiving it that it doesn't have to be awful." To a gynecologist friend of hers it means making sure that patients never have to wait and that they always get to speak with the doctor. To a surgeon friend it means holding the patient's hand in the recovery room.

Unlike the traditional medical encounter, in which patients are given a paucity of information about their condition, feminist doctors are committed to sharing the knowledge. At the Breast Service at the Columbia-Presbyterian Medical Center, surgeons Alison Estabrook and Freya Schnabel give all patients copies of their medical records, including pathology reports. "Doctors used to say these were confidential," says Estabrook. "But women are interested in knowing all they can about their condition. In our office we let patients set the tone. It's more 'Our Bodies, Ourselves.'"

These practitioners are putting the rest of the health care system on notice. Women, both as physicians and as patients, are primed to transform the way medicine is practiced in this country. And so we celebrate the new female norm: the 60-kilogram woman. She has breasts and a uterus and a heart and lungs and kidneys. But she's much more than that. No longer a metaphor for disease, she's the model for health. To modify the statement we made three-hundred-plus pages ago: The time is right for a new woman-centered health care movement. It's the least women should demand.

NOTES

INTRODUCTION

p. 3   "Says Elaine Borins, M.D. . . ." Personal interview, 29 June 1990.

p. 3   "In the early . . ." Mary Lou Ballweg, *Overcoming Endometriosis* (New York: Congdon & Weed, 1987), p. 18.

p. 3   "Although endometriosis . . ." David L. Olive and Lisa Barrie Schwartz, Review Article, "Endometriosis," *New England Journal of Medicine* 328.24 (1993): 1761. In the article Olive and Schwartz note a prevalence of 10 percent. In a personal interview, 8 July 1993, Olive said that amounts to "about five million women walking around with endometriosis."

p. 3   "In 1984, in a required . . ." Adriane Fugh-Berman, "Tales Out of Medical School," *The Nation*, 20 Jan. 1992, pp. 55–56.

p. 4   "In 1988 a study . . ." The Steering Committee of the Physicians' Health Study Research Group, "Preliminary Report: Findings from the Aspirin Component of the Ongoing Physicians' Health Study," *New England Journal of Medicine* 318 (1988): 262–64.

p. 5   "Says Florence Haseltine, M.D. . . ." Personal interview, 29 June 1990.

p. 5   "For instance, when the Food . . ." Linda Meredith, "Community Perspectives," National Conference on Women and HIV Infection, Washington, D.C., 14 Dec. 1990. Also M. A. Fischl, et al., "The Efficacy of Azidothymidine (AZT) in the Treatment of Patients with AIDS and AIDS-Related Complex: A Double-Blind Placebo-Controlled Trial," *New England Journal of Medicine* 317 (1987): 185–91.

p. 5   " 'The elegant studies . . .' " Howard Minkoff, "Clinical Manifestations of HIV-Infected Women," National Conference on Women and HIV Infection, Washington, D.C., 14 Dec. 1990.

p. 5   "As of this writing . . ." Joan Kuriansky, press conference, Campaign for Women's Health, a project of the Older Women's League, Washington, D.C., 24 Sept. 1993.

p. 5   "Over a twelve-month period . . ." *The Commonwealth Fund Women's Health Survey* (New York: Louis Harris and Associates, 1993), p. 6.

p. 5   "Women are twice . . ." *The Commonwealth Fund Women's Health Survey*, p. 7. The report found that 17 percent of women, versus 7 percent of men, had been told that a medical condition was "all in their head."

p. 5   "A stunning capper . . ." Nicole Lurie, et al., "Preventive Care for Women: Does the Sex of the Physician Matter?" *New England Journal of Medicine* 329.7 (1993): 478–82.

p. 6   "In the Commonwealth . . ." *The Commonwealth Fund Women's Health Survey*, p. 7.

p. 6   "Rhoda Kupferberg . . ." Rhoda Kupferberg, personal interview, 15 May 1993.

p. 7   "Although women have hearts . . ." "Poll Shows Women Rely on Ob-Gyns for Primary Care," press release, American College of Obstetricians and Gynecologists, 29 Oct. 1993. According to a Gallup poll commissioned by ACOG, of over a thousand women ages eighteen to sixty-five, 54 percent of the women questioned said they considered their ob-gyn to be their primary physician. In addition, over one-third of the women polled said they visit their ob-gyns specifically for preventive health care or other nongynecological health problems.

p. 8   "Most gynecologists . . ." Carolyn Westhoff, et al., "Residency Training in Contra-ception, Sterilization, and Abortion," *Obstetrics & Gynecology* 81 (1993): 311–14. In this survey of obstetrics and gynecology chief residents, 47 percent had never performed a first-trimester-induced abortion, and 45 percent had performed fewer than ten procedures. Also, "Abortion Attitudes: Little Change in 14 Years," press re-lease, American College of Obstetricians and Gynecologists, 21 Aug. 1986. In a survey of 1,300 ob-gyns, 84 percent supported a woman's right to abortion at least in some circumstances, but only 34 percent said they ever performed abortions themselves.

p. 8   " 'What benign condition . . .' " Karen Johnson, personal interview, 13 Sept. 1993.

p. 8   "Referring to some . . ." Felicia Stewart, speaking at "Contraceptive Technology," a conference cosponsored by the Association of Reproductive Health Professionals and the National Association of Nurse-Practitioners in Reproductive Health, Vir-ginia, 1989.

p. 9   " 'The medical system . . .' " Barbara Ehrenreich and Deirdre English, *Complaints and Disorders—The Sexual Politics of Sickness* (Old Westbury, N.Y.: The Feminist Press, 1973), p. 5.

1: A BRIEF HISTORY OF MEDICINE
A Legacy of Ignorance

Note: The historical picture put together in this chapter was culled from a wide va-riety of sources. In addition to the books, journal articles, and interviews listed be-low as citations for quotes and facts, other background sources for the chapter and good sources of information on women's health history are:

Biological Woman—The Convenient Myth, eds. Ruth Hubbard, Mary Sue Henifin, and Barbara Fried (Cambridge, Mass.: Schenkman Publishing Company, 1982).
First of All: Significant "Firsts" by American Women, Joan McCullough (New York: Holt, Rinehart and Winston, 1980).
The Mind Has No Sex? Women in the Origins of Modern Science, Londa Schiebinger (Cambridge, Mass.: Harvard University Press, 1989).
The Politics of Women's Biology, Ruth Hubbard (New Brunswick, N.J.: Rutgers Uni-versity Press, 1990).
Seizing Our Bodies: The Politics of Women's Health, ed. Claudia Dreifus (New York: Vintage Books, 1977).
Sympathy and Science: Women Physicians in American Medicine, Regina Markell Morantz-Sanchez (New York: Oxford University Press, 1985).
Women and Health Psychology: Biomedical Issues, Cheryl Brown Travis (Hillsdale, N.J.: Lawrence Erlbaum Associates, 1988).
Women and Health: The Politics of Sex in Medicine, ed. Elizabeth Fee (Farmingdale, N.Y.: Baywood Publishing Company, 1983).
Women, Health and Medicine in America: A Historical Handbook, ed. Rima D. Ap-ple (New York: Garland Publishing, 1990).
Women's Bodies: A Social History of Women's Encounter with Health, Ill-Health, and Medicine, Edward Shorter (New Brunswick, N.J.: Transaction Publishers, 1991).

p. 14   " 'She [Woman] has a head . . .' " Charles Meigs, *Females and Their Diseases* (Phila-delphia, 1848). Meigs was professor of obstetrics and diseases of women and children at Jefferson Medical College in Philadelphia, and his quote has become the archetypal example (cited in most histories of women's health care) of early doctors' opinion of women.

p. 14   " '[It was] as if the Almighty . . .' " M. L. Holbrook, addressing a medical society in 1870, cited in Barbara Ehrenreich and Deirdre English, *For Her Own Good: 150 Years of the Experts' Advice to Women* (Garden City, N.Y.: Anchor Press/Doubleday,

1978), p. 108. Ehrenreich and English's book is an excellent history of women's health care in America, filtered through a 1970s feminist sensibility. See also Ehrenreich and English's *Complaints and Disorders—The Sexual Politics of Sickness* (Old Westbury, N.Y.: The Feminist Press, 1973) and *Witches, Midwives and Nurses: A History of Women Healers* (New York: The Feminist Press, 1973).

p. 14   " 'The Uterus, it must be remembered . . .' " Frederick Hollick, *The Diseases of Women, Their Cause and Cure Familiarly Explained* (New York: T. W. Strong, 1849).

p. 14   " 'Thus, women are treated . . .' " M. E. Dirix, *Women's Complete Guide to Health* (New York: W. A. Townsend and Adams, 1869), pp. 23–24.

p. 14   " 'We cannot too emphatically urge . . .' " W. C. Taylor, *A Physician's Counsels to Women in Health and Disease* (Springfield, Ill.: W. J. Holland & Co., 1871).

p. 14   " [We must recognize] the gigantic power . . .' " W. W. Bliss, *Woman and Her Thirty-Years' Pilgrimage* (Boston: B. B. Russell, 1870), p. 96.

p. 14   "Physicians who attended the forty-fourth annual meeting . . ." Charles P. Noble, "The Causation of the Diseases of Women," *Journal of the American Medical Association* 21 (1893): 410–15, reprinted in "*JAMA* 100 Years Ago" 270.11 (1993): 1288.

p. 15   "Doctors at that same conference . . ." George H. Rohe, "Lactational Insanity," *Journal of the American Medical Association* 21(1893): 325, reprinted in "*JAMA* 100 Years Ago" 270.10 (1993): 1180.

p. 15   "Even singing while menstruating . . ." "Impairment of the Voice, In Female Singers, Due to Diseased Sexual Organs, *Journal of the American Medical Association* 19 (1892): 36–37, reprinted in "*JAMA* 100 Years Ago," 268.2 (1992): 163.

p. 16   "The president of the British Medical Association . . ." Mrs. H. M. Plunkett, *Women, Plumbers and Doctors, or Household Sanitation* (New York: D. Appleton, 1897), p. 11, cited in Ehrenreich and English, *For Her Own Good*, p. 142.

p. 16   "Tight lacing of corsets . . ." Ehrenreich and English, *For Her Own Good*. pp. 100–101.

p. 17   " 'Among the indications . . .' " G. J. Barker-Benfield, "The Spermatic Economy: A Nineteenth Century View of Sexuality," *Feminist Studies* 1 (Summer 1972): 45–74.

p. 17   "Mary Livermore, a women's suffrage worker . . ." *Complaints and Disorders*, p. 25.

p. 18   "The regular physicians were scathing . . ." Mary Roth Walsh, *"Doctors Wanted: No Women Need Apply"* (New Haven: Yale University Press, 1977), p. xiii.

p. 18   "With the slogan . . ." Caroline Bird, *Enterprising Women* (New York: W. W. Norton & Company, Inc., 1976), pp. 124, 126.

p. 18   "According to the manufacturer . . ." Personal interview, 17 Sept. 1993, with Bob Stites, vice president of Numark Laboratories, which currently owns the rights to Lydia Pinkham's tonic.

p. 19   "By the turn of the century . . ." *For Her Own Good*, p. 84.

p. 20   "By 1930 midwives had practically disappeared . . ." *For Her Own Good*, p. 88.

p. 20   "Today just 4 percent . . ." National Center for Health Statistics, "Advance Report of Final Natality Statistics, 1990," *Monthly Vital Statistics Report* 41.9 (Hyattsville, MD: Public Health Service, 1993): 7.

p. 20   " 'With the elimination of midwifery . . .' " *For Her Own Good*, p. 88.

p. 21   "Concerned with the . . ." Harold Speert, *Obstetrics and Gynecology in America: A History* (Baltimore: Waverly Press, 1980), p. 142.

p. 21   "By 1912 these nurses . . ." *Obstetrics and Gynecology in America*, p. 142.

p. 21   "Largely as the result of . . ." *Obstetrics and Gynecology in America*, p. 142.

p. 21   "Dr. Augustus Gardner . . ." Gena Corea, *The Hidden Malpractice*, updated ed. (New York: Harper Colophon Books/Harper & Row, 1985), p. 99.

p. 21   "The American Medical Association . . ." *The Hidden Malpractice*, p. 137.

p. 21   "Sanger's call for motherhood . . ." Ellen Chesler, *Woman of Valor: Margaret Sanger and the Birth Control Movement in America* (New York: Simon & Schuster, 1992), p. 204.

p. 22   "One of the most egregious . . ." The questionable practices of Dr. J. Marion Sims are culled from a variety of sources, including Durrenda Ojanuga, "The Medical Ethics of the 'Father of Gynaecology,' Dr. J. Marion Sims," *Journal of the Institute* of Medical Ethics 19 (1993): 28–31. And G. J. Barker-Benfield, *The Horrors of the Half-Known Life* (New York: Harper Colophon Books/Harper & Row, 1976).

p. 23   "Less well known . . ." *The Hidden Malpractice*, p. 13.

p. 23   "Even more recently . . ." Saundra Sturdevant, "The Bar Girls of Subic Bay," *The Nation*, 3 April 1989, p. 444.

p. 24   "Today most people take women doctors . . ." Judith Mandelbaum-Schmid, "Women & Medicine: An Unequal Past, A Common Future," *MD*, May 1992, p. 87.

p. 24   "In 1896, 33 percent . . ." *"Doctors Wanted,"* p. 205.

p. 24   ". . . (although across the country . . ." Regina Morantz-Sanchez, "So Honored, So Loved? The Women's Medical Movement in Decline," *"Send Us a Lady Physician" Women Doctors in America, 1835–1920*, ed. Ruth J. Abram (New York: W. W. Norton & Company, 1985), p. 231.

p. 24   " 'There have been instances . . .' " Edward H. Clark, *Sex in Education, or, A Fair Chance for Girls* (Boston and New York: Houghton Mifflin and Company, 1873), p. 39.

p. 25   "He describes one studious young female . . ." *Sex in Education*, p. 82.

p. 25   "Becoming a doctor was her mission . . ." Elizabeth Blackwell, *Pioneer Work in Opening the Medical Profession to Women: Autobiographical Sketches by Dr. Elizabeth Blackwell* (New York: Schocken, 1977, reprint of 1895 ed.), pp. 27–29.

p. 26   "Johns Hopkins Medical School . . ." *"Send Us a Lady Physician,"* p. 231.

p. 26   " 'We should give to man . . .' " Proceedings of the Women's Rights Convention, cited in *"Send Us a Lady Physician,"* p. 17.

p. 26   " 'How many men do we find . . .' " "The Necessity for Women Physicians," Medical College of Pennsylvania Archives, 1871, cited in *"Send Us a Lady Physician,"* p. 17.

p. 26   "Mary Walsh quotes a woman physician . . ." *"Doctors Wanted,"* p. 144.

p. 26   "And in 1894 a disgusted doctor . . ." Mary A. Spink, ed., *Women's Medical Journal* 2 (1894): 18.

p. 27   "In 1881 three female physicians . . ." Emily F. Pope, Emma L. Call, and C. Augusta Pope, *The Practice of Medicine by Women in the United States* (Boston, 1881).

p. 27   "Those medical schools that remained . . ." *"Doctors Wanted,"* p. 205.

p. 28   "In 1930 M. Esther Harding, a psychiatrist . . ." Harding to Van Hoosen, May 6, 1930, Van Hoosen Papers, Medical College of Pennsylvania, cited in *In Her Own Words: Oral Histories of Women Physicians*, eds. Regina Markell Morantz, Cynthia Stoloda Pomerleau, and Carol Hansen Fenichel (Westport, Conn.: Greenwood Press, 1982), pp. 29, 38n.

p. 28   "Dr. Emily Barringer . . ." *"Doctors Wanted,"* p. 229.

p. 29   "The immediate result of this victory . . ." *"Doctors Wanted,"* p. 230.

p. 29   "In 1970 Congress' Special Subcommittee . . ." *"Doctors Wanted,"* p. 244.

p. 29   "Between 1970 and 1975 . . ." Mandelbaum-Schmid, *MD*, May 1992, p. 89.

p. 29   ". . . and today 40 percent . . ." Leigh Page, "Class Portrait: A Decade of Change at Med Schools," *American Medical News*, 22 Feb. 1993, p. 12.

p. 29   "In 1974 the *New England Journal of Medicine* . . ." Sonia Bauer, "Correspondence," *New England Journal of Medicine* 291.21 (1974): 1141–42.

p. 30   "For twenty-two years . . ." Ellen Hopkins, "Doctor of Love," *In Health*, Nov.–Dec. 1990, pp. 79–84. Also, personal interview with Harvey Wachsman, an attorney who is representing forty-one women in malpractice cases against Dr. Burt, 2 March 1994.

p. 30   "Nearly 550,000 hysterectomies . . ." E. J. Graves, "1991 Summary: National Hospital Discharge Survey," *Advance Data from Vital and Health Statistics* 227 (Hyattsville, MD: National Center for Health Statistics (1993): 7.

p. 30   " 'If they want to do that . . .' " Michelle Harrison, M.D., speaking as part of a panel discussion on "Women's Health: A Medical Specialty?" at The First Annual Congress on Women's Health, Washington, D.C., 3 June 1993.

2: SCIENCE AND MEDICINE
Where Are the Women Now?

p. 32   "After a distinguished ..." Susan Leeman, personal interviews, 28 Jan. 1993 and 21 April 1994.

p. 33   "A generation later ..." Kym Chandler, personal interview, 23 Jan. 1993.

p. 34   " 'Any woman patient ...' " Frances Conley, personal interview, 12 Jan. 1993.

p. 35   "In 1992 the federal ..." "Women in Biomedical Careers: Dynamics of Change," National Institutes of Health, Office of Research on Women's Health, Bethesda, MD, 11–12 June 1992. Also based on personal interviews.

p. 35   "Later that same ..." Roundtables, "Women in Academic Medicine and Health Science," Society for the Advancement of Women's Health Research, New York, 5 Oct. 1992, and Palo Alto, 1 Jan. 1993.

p. 35   " 'We've all had mentors ...' " An obstetrician-gynecologist who asked to remain anonymous, personal interview, 4 Feb. 1993.

p. 36   "Willa Drummond ..." Willa Drummond, personal interview, 27 Jan. 1993.

p. 36   "... a field of only ..." Drummond.

p. 36   " 'As a woman ...' " Nadine Bruce, personal interview, 16 Feb. 1993.

p. 37   "When an instructor ..." Adriane Fugh-Berman, "Tales Out of Medical School," *The Nation*, 20 Jan. 1992, p. 54.

p. 37   "... only 8 percent of women ..." Janet Bickel, Luncheon Keynote, "Women in Academic Medicine—A Literature Review," Roundtable, New York.

p. 37   " 'No one had told her ...' " Sharyn Lenhart, "Sexual Harassment and Gender Discrimination in Medicine," 78th annual meeting, American Medical Women's Association, New York, 6 Nov. 1993. Also personal interview, 29 Jan. 1993.

p. 37   "Women who attempt ..." Lynn Gerber, comment made at conference on Women in Biomedical Careers.

p. 38   "Women receive only 21.5 percent ..." "Women in NIH Extramural Grant Programs," Fiscal Years 1981 to 1992, Division of Research Grants, National Institutes of Health.

p. 38   " 'Women are less apt ...' " Bernadine Healy, presentation, Women in Biomedical Careers, 11 June 1992.

p. 38   "When she was ..." An associate professor of medicine who asked to remain anonymous, personal interview, 23 April 1993.

p. 38   "When Phyllis Gardner ..." Phyllis Gardner, personal interview, 12 Jan. 1993.

p. 38   "Gardner says. ..." Gardner.

p. 39   "... the seven-year tenure track ..." David Brown, Panel II, "Advancement and Workplace Climate," Women in Biomedical Careers, 11 June 1992.

p. 39   " '... seventy-kilogram career ...' " Lenhart, 6 Nov. 1993.

p. 39   "The Yale ..." Merle Waxman, director, Office for Women in Medicine, Yale University School of Medicine, phone conversation, 5 April 1994.

p. 39   "Some schools have ..." Janet Bickel, "The Changing Faces of Promotion and Tenure at U.S. Medical Schools," *Academic Medicine* 66.5 (1991): 251–52.

p. 39   " 'Tenure is an anachronism ...' " Brown.

p. 39   "... 81 percent of ..." Nancy M. Bennett and Katherine G. Nickerson, "Women in Academic Medicine: Perceived Obstacles to Advancement," *Journal of the American Medical Women's Association*, July–Aug. 1992, p. 116.

p. 40   " 'The lack of adequate ...' " Bennett and Nickerson, p. 117.

p. 40   "78 percent of women ..." Laurie Jones, "Is Medicine Doing More to Accommodate Families?" *American Medical News*, 4 Jan. 1993, p. 13.

p. 40   " 'For women the presumption ...' " Bernice Sandler, *The Campus Climate Revisited: Chilly for Women Faculty, Administrators, and Graduate Students*, Project on the Status and Education of Women, Association of American Colleges, Oct. 1986, p. 5.

p. 40   " 'Medicine is very conducive ...' " Drummond.

p. 40   "In 1988, female physicians ..." "Empowering Women in Medicine," the Feminist Majority Foundation, 1991, p. 2.

p. 40   "In family practice ..." American Medical Association, 1994.

p. 40   "... the average net income ..." *Women in Medicine in America* (Chicago: American Medical Association, 1991), p. 23.

p. 40   "An associate professor ..." Lenhart.

p. 41   "In 1992, black women ..." Association of American Medical Colleges, Section for Student Services, "Fall Enrollment Questionnaire and Reported Graduates Report," 1992. Cited in *Women in Academic Medicine and Health Sciences*, Roundtable Findings, 1993, Society for the Advancement of Women's Health Research, p. 9.

p. 41   " 'For many minority women ...' " Public hearing on Recruitment, Retention, Re-Entry, and Advancement of Women in Biomedical Careers, National Institutes of Health, Office of Research on Women's Health, Bethesda, MD, 2–3 March 1992. Cited in the Report of the National Institutes of Health: Opportunities for Research on Women's Health, Sept. 1992, p. 26.

p. 41   " 'The criteria seem to change ...' " Susan Blumenthal, Roundtable, Women in Academic Medicine and Health Science, Society for the Advancement of Women's Health Research, Palo Alto, 1 Jan. 1993.

p. 41   " 'It must be biological ...' " Michelle Harrison, personal interview, 14 March 1993.

p. 41   "A search committee's top ..." Carol Nadelson, personal interview, 2 March 1993.

p. 41   "Although women comprise half ..." Janet Bickel and Renee Quinnie, "Women in Medicine Statistics," Table 1, Association of American Medical Colleges, June 1992.

p. 41   "In some of the highest-paying ..." Bickel and Quinnie, Table 4.

pp. 41–42   "Of the more than almost two thousand ..." Association of American Medical Colleges, 1994.

p. 42   "... the majority of women are clustered ..." Bickel and Quinnie, Figure 1, "Full-Time Medical School Faculty by Rank & Gender." Fifty percent of women versus 34.5 percent of men are at the assistant professor level. At the senior levels 19.7 percent of women but 25.4 percent of men are associate professors. Full professors consist of only 9.5 percent of the women, but 31.5 percent of the men.

p. 42   " '... academic ghettos.' " Bernadine Healy, presentation, "Women in Biomedical Careers," 11 June 1992.

p. 42   "In pediatrics ..." Jane Schaller, presentation, Panel II: Advancement and Workplace Climate, "Women in Biomedical Careers," 11 June 1992.

p. 42   "Of 126 academic ..." Bickel and Quinnie.

p. 42   "The American College ..." Alice Kirkman, American College of Obstetricians and Gynecologists, 1994.

p. 42   "The American Medical Association ..." Mark Stewart, AMA, 1994.

p. 42   "Of the 2,028 members ..." National Academy of Sciences, 1994.

p. 42   "Although the National Institutes ..." Office of the Director, NIH, 1994.

p. 42   "Women make up 17 percent ..." Report of the Task Force on the Status of NIH Intramural Women Scientists, 1993.

p. 43   " 'When women demonstrate ...' " Lenhart.

p. 43   "In a 1992 report ..." Bennett and Nickerson: 115–118.

p. 43   "Another survey, of 133 ..." Miriam Komaromy, et al., "Sexual Harassment in Medical Training," *New England Journal of Medicine* 328.5 (1993): 322–26. See also editorial by Frances Conley, "Toward a More Perfect World—Eliminating Sexual Discrimination in Academic Medicine," pp. 351–52.

p. 43   "One of the female residents ..." Komaromy.

p. 43   " 'I owe them ...' " Lenhart.

p. 44   "... the Stanford Faculty Senate meeting ..." Conley.

p. 44   "... that Gerald Silverberg was ..." Gerald Silverberg declined to be interviewed for this book.

p. 45   " 'Fran realizes she is ...' " Margaret Billingham, personal interview, 13 Jan. 1993.

p. 45   "... 'you can practically smell ...' " Chandler.

p. 46   "... these microinequities ..." Mary Rowe, phone conversation, 5 April, 1994.

p. 46   " 'They're tough ...' " Lenhart.

p. 46   "At one extreme ..." Rowe.

p. 47   " '... a defensive persona ...' " Drummond.

p. 47   " 'Most women grieve . . .' " Sharyn Lenhart and Clyde Evans, "Sexual Harassment and Gender Discrimination: A Primer for Women Physicians," *Journal of the American Medical Women's Association,* May–June 1991, pp. 79–80.

p. 47   "From early childhood . . ." Heidi Weissmann, personal interview, 10 Dec. 1992.

p. 48   "Weissmann 'has repeatedly . . .' " Personal correspondence from Donald Blaufox to Ernst Jaffe, 26 Sept. 1983.

p. 48   "Her trouble started . . ." Weissmann.

p. 48   " 'At that point . . .' " Weissmann.

p. 48   "Weissmann says that . . ." *Heidi S. Weissmann v. Albert Einstein College of Medicine of Yeshiva University; Montefiore Medical Center; M. Donald Blaufox; and Leonard Freeman,* Second Amended Complaint, United States District Court, Southern District of New York, 18 May 1989.

p. 49   "In 1988, she filed . . ." Weissmann, Second Amended Complaint.

p. 49   ". . . Weissmann, who previously won . . ." Decision handed down by United States Court of Appeals, Second Circuit, Feb. 1989.

p. 49   "While Freeman's legal fees . . ." "Are Scientific Misconduct and Conflicts of Interest Hazardous to Our Health?" Nineteenth Report by the Committee on Government Operations, 10 Sept. 1990, p. 40.

p. 49   "Not only has Freeman . . ." News Briefs, Montefiore Staff & Alumni Association, 7.1 (1991): 9.

pp. 49–50   " 'It's incredibly depressing . . .' " Walter Stewart, personal interview, 17 Dec. 1992.

p. 50   ". . . women are kept from top . . ." Judith Lorber, presentation at Roundtable, Women in Academic Medicine and Health Science, Society for the Advancement of Women's Health Research, New York, 5 Oct. 1992.

p. 50   " 'The reason men are so . . .' " Lorber, Roundtable. See also Judith Lorber, *Paradoxes of Gender* (New Haven: Yale University Press, 1994), p. 242.

p. 50   ". . . the 'Salieri phenomenon . . .' " Lorber.

p. 50   ". . . 'skewed groups' . . ." Lenhart.

p. 50   "In a 'tilted' group . . ." Lenhart.

pp. 50–51   " 'Individuals are still . . .' " Lenhart.

p. 51   ". . . 'balanced' group . . ." Lenhart.

p. 51   ". . . the American Medical Association . . ." AMA, *Women in Medicine in America,* p. 33.

p. 51   "Other researchers say . . ." Lenhart.

p. 51   "Little did she know . . ." Margaret Jensvold, personal interviews, 22 Sept. 1991 and 4 April 1994.

p. 51   " 'I knew my mother's . . .' " Jensvold.

p. 52   "In a suit filed . . ." Jensvold.

p. 52   "Jensvold says her boss . . ." David Rubinow declined to be interviewed for this book.

p. 52   ". . . Rubinow told Jensvold she would . . ." During the course of the trial Rubinow denied all of Jensvold's charges.

p. 52   " 'I'd gone to NIMH . . .' " Jensvold.

p. 53   "Her plan was to study . . ." Jean Hamilton, personal interview, 27 March 1993. Also sworn statement by Jean Hamilton, 27 July 1983.

p. 53   "A superior, Fred Goodwin . . ." Hamilton, sworn statement.

p. 53   ". . . Hamilton says, she had higher . . ." Hamilton, sworn statement.

p. 53   ". . . she had the first approved protocol . . ." Hamilton, personal interview and sworn statement.

p. 53   " 'I was invisible . . .' " Hamilton, personal interview.

p. 54   ". . . it has an annual budget . . ." Robert Taylor, "WHEW! A Healthy Budget Boost for NIH," *The Journal of NIH Research,* Nov. 1993, p. 36.

p. 54   ". . . three-fourths of academic chairs . . ." Jensvold.

p. 54   " 'What goes on internally . . .' " Personal interview with a female administrator at NIH who asked to remain anonymous, 3 March 1993.

p. 54   ". . . including one in . . ." Margaret F. Jensvold, et al., "Menstrual Cycle-related Depressive Symptoms Treated with Variable Antidepressant Dosage," *Journal of Women's Health* 1.2 (1992): 109–15.

p. 54   " 'People think researchers . . .' " Billie Mackey, personal interviews, 19 Feb. 1993 and 8 March 1994.

p. 55   " 'It's total greed . . .' " Female administrator.

p. 55   ". . . women make up only . . ." Report of the Task Force on the Status of NIH Intramural Women Scientists, 1993.

p. 55   "Women make up 18 percent . . ." Report of the Task Force.

p. 55   "At NIMH, as of . . ." Jensvold.

p. 55   "Maureen Polsby . . ." Maureen Polsby, personal interviews, 20, 21, and 23 Dec. 1992. Also see "Harassment Linked to Fraud, Lawsuit Alleges," *Journal of the American Medical Association* 267.6 (1992): 783–84.

p. 55   " 'I got assigned . . .' " Polsby.

p. 55   "Female whistleblowers . . ." Mackey.

p. 55   "After filing her complaint . . ." Jensvold.

p. 56   "Rubinow, for instance . . ." The NIH Record, XLIV.12 (1992): 16. The article noted that the "award is given each spring to the institute or clinical physician who, by votes of the clinical associates, has been an outstanding bedside teacher in the best traditions of clinical medicine."

p. 56   "Before his departure . . ." Margaret Jensvold, Deborah Brower and Billie Mackey, Report: "Women Harmed by the National Institute of Mental Health," Submitted to Vice President Al Gore, July 1993, p. 16.

p. 56   "In 1994 Thomas . . ." Press Advisory, "Neurologist Under Investigation for Scientific Fraud and Sued for Sexual Harassment to be Given Prestigious $10,000 Award," Released jointly by Self Help for Equal Rights, Federation of Organizations for Professional Women, and People Against Fraud and the Abuse of Power in Public Institutions, May 1994.

p. 56   "And NIMH lab . . ." Jensvold, Brower, and Mackey, p. 16.

p. 56   " 'These men should not . . .' " Mackey.

p. 56   ". . . the Byzantine EEOC process . . ." Margaret Jensvold, Correspondence, *New England Journal of Medicine* 329.9 (1993): 661–62. Jensvold writes, "Currently, the Equal Employment Opportunity Commission (EEOC) has no sanctions for harassers. The EEOC and legal process are adversarial."

p. 56   "A complainant has . . ." Equal Employment Opportunity Commission, 1994.

p. 56   ". . . 'the process is set up . . .' " Female administrator.

p. 56   "If no resolution is reached . . ." EEOC, 1994.

p. 56   ". . . in 1992 only thirty-seven . . ." Mackey.

p. 57   "As of early 1994 . . ." Mackey.

p. 57   ". . . it took her until the spring . . ." Mackey. Bernadine Healy first talked publicly about issues of sexual harassment at NIH after the release of the Task Force report cited above.

p. 57   "At the time of . . ." Mackey.

p. 58   " 'We're witnessing . . .' " Jimmie Holland, Roundtable, Women in Academic Medicine and Health Science, Society for the Advancement of Women's Health Research, New York, 5 Oct. 1992.

p. 58   "Bernadine Healy . . ." Mackey.

p. 58   "The Office of . . ." Rosemary Torres, Office of Research on Women's Health, 1993.

p. 58   ". . . the lead of Harvard . . ." Brenda Hoffman, Roundtable, Women in Academic Medicine and Health Science, Society for the Advancement of Women's Health Research, New York, 5 Oct. 1992.

p. 58   " 'We're victims . . .' " Frances Conley, personal interview.

p. 58   " 'Nothing will change . . .' " Jacqueline Parthemore, Roundtable, Women in Academic Medicine and Health Science, Society for the Advancement of Women's Health Research, Palo Alto, 1 Jan. 1993.

pp. 58–59 "On March 11, 1994 . . ." Heidi Weissmann, personal interview, 4 April 1994.

p. 59   "Several weeks later . . ." Margaret Jensvold, 4 April 1994. For more on Jensvold's case, see Alisa Solomon, "Snake Pit," *Mirabella*, April 1993, pp. 140–144; Marcia Coyle, "A Scientist's Gender-Bias Case Centers on Mentoring," *The National Law Journal*, 21 March 1994: A14; and Scott S. Greenberger, "Science Friction: The Struggle of Female Researchers at NIH," *The Washington Post,* 11 July 1993: C3.

p. 59 "Maureen Polsby's . . ." Polsby.

3: THE RESEARCH GAP

p. 60 "The audit found . . ." Statement of Mark V. Nadel, "National Institutes of Health: Problems in Implementing Policy on Women in Study Populations," (Washington, D.C.: United States General Accounting Office), GAO/T-HRD-90-38.

p. 60 "In fact, most researchers . . ." "National Institutes of Health: Problems in Implementing Policy on Women in Study Populations," p. 8.

p. 60 " 'This was nothing but . . .' " Pat Schroeder, personal interview, 29 June 1990. This quote has previously appeared in: Beth Weinhouse, "The Significant Other," *Savvy Woman,* Oct. 1990, p. 13.

p. 61 " 'American women have been . . .' " Gina Kolata, "NIH Neglects Women, Study Says," *New York Times,* 19 June 1990, p. C6.

p. 61 "In the fifty applications reviewed . . ." "National Institutes of Health: Problems in Implementing Policy on Women . . . ," p. 8.

p. 61 " 'The [NIH] may win the Nobel prize . . .' " "The Latest Word: Women and Medicine," *Hastings Center Report,* Nov.–Dec. 1990, p. 47.

p. 61 "The Baltimore Longitudinal Study . . ." Nathan W. Shock, et al., "Normal Human Aging, The Baltimore Longitudinal Study" (Bethesda, MD.: U.S. Department of Public Health, 1984), NIH publication #84-2450. The information about the single toilet being used as a rationale for exclusivity comes from: Celia Hooper, "NIH Gets Serious About Inclusion of Women in Studies," *Journal of NIH Research,* Nov. 1990, p. 32.

p. 61 "Currently 40 percent . . ." "Vital Statistics," *Hippocrates,* Feb. 1993, p. 14.

p. 61 "The by-now-infamous . . ." The Steering Committee of the Physicians' Health Study Research Group, "Preliminary Report: Findings from the Aspirin Component of the Ongoing Physicians' Health Study," *New England Journal of Medicine* 318.4 (1988): 262–64.

p. 61 "The 1982 Multiple Risk Factor . . ." Edward B. Dietrich and Carol Cohan, *Women and Heart Disease* (New York: Times Books, 1992), p. 12.

p. 61 "A Harvard School of Public Health . . ." *Women and Heart Disease,* p. 12.

p. 62 "Perhaps most unbelievably . . ." Rebecca Dresser, "Wanted: Single, White Male for Medical Research," *Hastings Center Report,* Jan.–Feb. 1992, p. 24. Also, Patricia Aburdene and John Naisbitt, *Megatrends for Women* (New York: Villard Books, 1992), p. 134.

p. 62 "Said Congresswomen Olympia Snowe . . ." Judy Grande, "Cleveland Clinic Struggles to Find Women for Heart Study," *Cleveland Plain Dealer,* 5 Aug. 1990.

p. 62 "Only 13.5 percent . . ." "GAO Audit Reports NIH's Neglect of Women's Health Research," press release, The Society for the Advancement of Women's Health Research, 18 June 1990.

p. 62 "William F. Raub . . ." Celia Hooper, "NIH Gets Serious about Inclusion of Women in Studies," *Journal of NIH Research,* Nov. 1990, pp. 32, 34.

p. 62 "At the time of the GAO report . . ." Florence Haseltine, personal interview, 29 June 1990. Also: The Institute of Medicine, *Stengthening Research in Academic OB/GYN Departments,* Jessica Townsend, ed. (Washington, D.C.: National Academy Press, 1992), p. 111.

p. 62 "The National Institute of Child Health . . ." These statistics compiled from: "National Institutes of Health: Key Facts and History of Funding FY 1983-FY 1993," prepared by the Central Budget Office, Division of Financial Management, National Institutes of Health, p. 26. And: *Strengthening Research in Academic OB/GYN Departments,* p. 278.

p. 63 "Of over three thousand individuals . . ." *Strengthening Research . . . ,* p. 275.

p. 63 "A study of thirty years' . . ." Jerry H. Gurwitz, et al., "The Exclusion of the Elderly and Women from Clinical Trials in Acute Myocardial Infarction," *Journal of the American Medical Association* 268.11 (1992): 1421.

p. 63   "And at the National Cancer Institute . . ." Richard S. Ungerleider and Michael A.
             Friedman, "Special Report: Sex, Trials, and Datatapes," *Journal of the National Can-
             cer Institute* 83.1 (1991): 16–17.

p. 63   "The Institute of Medicine . . ." Institute of Medicine, *Strengthening Research in Ac-
             ademic OB/GYN Departments*, Jessica Townsend, ed. (Washington, D.C.: National
             Academy Press, 1992).

p. 63   " 'With no women's institute at NIH . . ." Wayne Burrows, M.D., assistant profes-
             sor of maternal-fetal medicine, University of South Carolina School of Medicine.
             Personal interview, 23 April 1993.

p. 63   "Ezra C. Davidson, Jr., M.D. . . ." "GAO Audit Reports NIH's Neglect of Women's
             Health Research," press release, Society for the Advancement of Women's Health
             Research, 18 June 1990.

pp. 63–64   " 'Our concern,' said the authors . . ." Council on Ethical and Judicial Affairs,
             American Medical Association, "Gender Disparities in Clinical Decision Making,"
             Journal of the American Medical Association 266.4 (1991): 559.

p. 64   " 'The overwhelming conclusion of . . .' " C. Roger Bone, et al., "NHLBI Work-
             shop Summary—Research Needs and Opportunities Related to Respiratory Health
             of Women," *American Review of Respiratory Diseases* 146 (1992): 534.

p. 65   " 'I gave Lesley . . .' " Florence Haseltine, personal interview, 24 Sept. 1993.

p. 65   "Congresswoman Snowe charged that . . ." Gina Kolata, "NIH Neglects Women,
             Study Says," *New York Times*, 19 June 1990, p. C6.

p. 65   "Said Congresswoman Schroeder . . ." Patricia Schroeder, personal interview, 29
             June 1990. This quote appeared previously in: Beth Weinhouse, "The Significant
             Other," *Savvy Women*, Oct. 1990, p. 14.

p. 65   " 'Who decides what ideas are . . .' " Elaine Borins, personal interview, 29 June
             1990.

p. 65   " 'Gender bias is not serious . . .' " Peter D. A. Warwick, "Sexism in Medical Test-
             ing," *Self*, Feb. 1990, p. 64.

p. 65   "Writing in a July 22 . . ." Marcia Angell, "Caring for Women's Health—What Is
             the Problem?," *New England Journal of Medicine* 329.4 (1993): 271.

pp. 65–66   " 'The typical study . . .' " Elaine Borins, personal interview, 29 June 1990.

p. 66   "They found that over 80 percent . . ." Karen Williams and Elaine F. Manace
             Borins, "Gender Bias in a Peer-Reviewed Medical Journal," *Journal of the American
             Medical Women's Association* 48.5 (1993): 160–62.

p. 66   " 'People think of *NEJM* . . .' " Elaine Borins, personal interview, 24 Aug. 1993.

pp. 66–67   " 'People thought that when researchers . . .' " Pam Charney, personal interview, 19
             July 1993.

p. 67   "Jean M. Mitchell, Ph.D., and . . ." Jean Mitchell, personal interview, 31 Dec.
             1992. Her unpublished paper, written with Christine M. Cushman, is titled, "Ev-
             idence of the Under-Representation of Women in Clinical Trials."

p. 67   " 'How we spend our research dollars . . .' " Irma Mebane-Sims, personal interview,
             20 May 1993.

p. 68   "Says current ORWH director . . ." Vivian W. Pinn, "Commentary: Women, Re-
             search, and the National Institutes of Health," *American Journal of Preventive Med-
             icine* 8.5 (1992): 325.

p. 68   "The NIH Revitalization Act ensures . . ." Public Law 103–43–June 10, 1993,
             "National Institutes of Health Revitalization Act of 1993."

p. 69   "The report stated that . . ." "Report of the NIH: Opportunities for Research on
             Women's Health," Hunt Valley, MD, 4–6 Sept. 1991, p. 7.

p. 69   "The report cited the . . ." "Opportunities for Research on Women's Health," p. 16.

p. 70   "For example, a recent study . . ." J. Claude Bennett for the Board on Health Sci-
             ences Policy of the Institute of Medicine, "Special Reports: Inclusion of Women in
             Clinical Trials—Policies for Population Subgroups," *New England Journal of Med-
             icine* 329.4 (1993): 290.

pp. 70–71   " 'I felt really special . . .' " Barbara S. Brown, "Testimony to the Office of Research
             on Women's Health, NIH," presented at the Scientific Meeting on Recruitment
             and Retention of Women in Clinical Trials, Bethesda, MD, 13 July 1993.

p. 71   "According to the Office of Research . . ." "Opportunities for Research on Women's Health," p. 15.

p. 71   "Evidence is now emerging . . ." "Opportunities for Research on Women's Health," p. 15.

p. 71   "For instance, recent studies suggest . . ." Ruby T. Senie, et al., "Timing of Breast Cancer Excision During the Menstrual Cycle Influences Duration of Disease-Free Survival," *Annals of Internal Medicine* 115 (1991): 337–42. Diana Swift, "Luteal Phase Best for Breast Surgery," *Medical Tribune*, 20 Jan. 1994.

p. 72   "When Proscar . . ." Diane Debrovner, "Of Mice and Men," *American Druggist*, Jan. 1993, p. 30.

p. 73   "But lawyers say that medical malpractice . . ." Institute of Medicine, *Women and Health Research*, Anna C. Mastoianni, Ruth Faden, and Daniel Federman, eds. (Washington, D.C.: National Academy Press, 1994), pp. 150–67.

pp. 73–74   "Only eleven drugs . . ." "Gender Differences in Pharmacokinetics," *The Female Patient*, April 1993, pp. 87–88.

p. 74   "One case often cited as precedent . . ." *Women and Health Research*, pp. 148–49.

p. 74   "The Food and Drug Administration's . . ." *Women and Health Research*, pp. 137–39.

p. 74   "The policy was supposed to be reevaluated . . ." Karen H. Rothenberg, University of Maryland School of Law. Ms. Rothenberg gave a presentation titled, "Legal and Ethical Issues," at the Office of Research on Women's Health Scientific Meeting, "Recruitment and Retention of Women in Clinical Studies," Bethesda, MD., 12 July 1993.

p. 74   "The GAO examined the clinical trials . . ." "Women's Health: FDA Needs to Ensure More Study of Gender Difference in Prescription Drug Testing," (Washington, D.C.: U.S. General Accounting Office, 1992), GAO/HRD-93-17.

pp. 74–75   " 'Practically all drugs . . .' " Diane Debrovner, "Of Mice and Men," *American Druggist*, Jan. 1993, p. 33.

p. 75   "As a result of the GAO audit . . ." Ruth Merkatz, et al., "Women in Clinical Trials of New Drugs: A Change in Food and Drug Administration Policy," *New England Journal of Medicine* 329 (1993): 292–96.

p. 75   "The GAO report found . . ." "Women's Health: FDA Needs to Ensure . . ." p. 11.

p. 75   "Women are the main consumers . . ." Jean A. Hamilton, "Biases in Women's Health Research," *Women & Therapy* 12.4 (1992): 98.

p. 75   " 'Researchers had the NIH telling them . . .' " Tracy Johnson, personal interview, 1 Sept. 1993.

pp. 75–76   "At a meeting in Bethesda . . ." "Scientific Meeting—Recruitment and Retention of Women in Clinical Studies," Office of Research on Women's Health, NIH, Bethesda, MD, 12–13 July 1993.

p. 76   " 'How many ways . . .' " Marcia Angell, "Caring for Women's Health—What Is the Problem?," *New England Journal of Medicine* 329.4 (1993): 272.

p. 76   "Recently NIH's requirements . . ." "NIH Guidelines on the Inclusion of Women and Minorities as Subjects in Clinical Research," *Federal Register*, 28 March 1994, pp. 14508–13.

p. 76   " 'But if you're going to examine . . .' " Judith LaRosa, personal interview, 27 Sept. 1993.

p. 77   " 'Scientists even use only male rat urine . . .' " Elaine Borins, personal interview, 24 Aug. 1993.

p. 77   "In the journal *Behavioral Neuroscience* . . ." Jeri Sechzer gave a presentation titled, "Gender Bias in Women's Health Research," at the Office of Research on Women's Health Scientific Meeting on the Recruitment and Retention of Women in Clinical Studies, Bethesda, MD, 12 July 1993.

p. 77   "The centerpiece of all these efforts . . ." "Protocol for Clinical Trial and Observational Study Components," WHI Clinical Coordinating Center, Fred Hutchinson Cancer Research Center, Seattle, 28 June 1993.

p. 77   "Some scientists argue . . ." Criticism of the Women's Health Initiative has come from many quarters, but a good, thorough discussion of the issues is contained in the Institute of Medicine's report, "An Assessment of the NIH Women's Health Initiative," Susan Thaul and Dana Hotra, eds. (Washington, D.C.: National Academy Press, 1993).

p. 78   " 'We've been using Premarin ...' " William Harlan, personal interview, 12 Oct. 1993.

p. 78   "Bernadine Healy, ex-director of NIH ..." Scott S. Greenberger, "Science Friction: The Struggle of Female Researchers at NIH," *Washington Post*, 11 July 1993, p. C3.

p. 78   "Yet only three of the first sixteen ..." "Science Friction," *Washington Post*, 11 July 1993.

pp. 78–79 " 'It will add some new information ...' " Florence Haseltine, personal interview, 24 Sept. 1993.

p. 79   " 'We can't make any assumption ...' " Beth Baker, "Medical Sleuths Study Older Women—At Last," *AARP Bulletin* (American Association of Retired Persons), June 1993, p. 5.

p. 79   " 'It's frightening a lot of researchers ...' " Nancy Reame, personal interview, 9 Sept. 1993.

p. 79   " 'Public pressure has to be maintained ...' " Florence Haseltine, personal interview, 24 Sept. 1993.

p. 80   "Oral contraceptives, for example ..." Gena Corea, *The Hidden Malpractice* (New York: Harper Colophon Books, updated ed. 1985), p. 151.

4: WOMEN'S HEARTS
The Deadly Difference

p. 85   "Though it has been ..." Jane E. Brody, "Personal Health: For Most of This Century, Heart Disease Has Been the Leading Killer of American Women," *New York Times*, 10 Nov. 1993, p. B9.

p. 85   "It wasn't until 1964 ..." Information on the 1964 "Hearts and Husbands" conference in Portland was provided by the American Heart Association press office, which sent a report of the conference from the the *Oregon Heart Herald* (Oct. 1964) entitled, " 'Hearts and Husbands' ... For Women Only." The AHA also sent a press release, "Hearts and Husbands," dated 6 Nov. 1964, from the Portland affiliate and the pamphlet "Eight Questions Wives Ask," which was printed by the Oregon Heart Association after the conference.

p. 86   " 'The conference was ...' " Mary Ann Malloy, personal interview, 23 May 1993. All subsequent quotes from Dr. Malloy are from this interview.

p. 86   "Yet many more women ..." "Heart and Stroke Facts: 1994 Statistical Supplement" (American Heart Association, 1993), p. 2.

p. 86   "Although women seem ..." "What Women Don't Know About Heart Disease and Cholesterol Could Hurt Them," press release, American Medical Association, 18 Dec. 1990. Numbers on lifetime risk of breast cancer and cardiovascular disease from the American Cancer Society and the American Heart Association, respectively.

p. 86   "And for those ..." "Heart and Stroke Facts," p. 2. According to the American Heart Association, in 1991 447,900 men died of cardiovascular diseases, versus 478,179 women.

p. 86   "Among women, 46 percent ..." Elaine D. Eaker, et al., "Cardiovascular Disease in Women," *Circulation* 84.4 (1993): 1999.

p. 86   "Because heart disease tends ..." Eaker, *Circulation*, p. 1999. Also Frank DeStefano, et al., "Trends in Nonfatal Coronary Heart Disease in the United States, 1980 Through 1989," *Archives of Internal Medicine* 153.21 (1993): 2489–94.

p. 86   " 'Women didn't die ...' " Nanette Wenger, personal interview, 7 June 1993. All subsequent quotes from Dr. Wenger are from this interview unless otherwise specified.

p. 86   "Yet despite these ominous ..." Dozens of articles began appearing in the early 1990s deploring the fact that research on coronary artery disease had ignored women. One example: Jerry H. Gurwitz, et al., "The Exclusion of the Elderly and Women from Clinical Trials in Acute Myocardial Infarction," *Journal of the Amer-*

ican Medical Association 268.11 (1992): 1417–22. The accompanying editorial also discussed the problem: Nanette K. Wenger, M.D., "Exclusion of the Elderly and Women from Coronary Trials: Is Their Quality of Care Compromised?" *JAMA* 268:11 (1992): 1460–61.

p. 86   " 'We're very much in an infancy . . .' " Irma Mebane-Sims, personal interview, 20 May 1993. All subsequent quotes from Dr. Mebane-Sims are from this interview.

p. 87   "It's true that . . ." Lawrence K. Altman, M.D., "Men, Women and Heart Disease: More than a Question of Sexism," the *New York Times*, 6 Aug. 1991, pp. B5, B8.

p. 87   "Many of the tests . . ." "Diagnosis of Heart Disease More Complicated in Women—Some Tests Less Reliable," *Internal Medicine News*, 1–14 Dec. 1991, pp. 1, 45.

p. 87   "The drugs used . . ." "Much Still Unknown About Heart Disease Drug Therapy in Women," *Internal Medicine News*, 15–31 Dec. 1991, p. 8. Also, the General Accounting Office's report "Women's Health: FDA Needs to Ensure More Study of Gender Differences in Prescription Drug Testing" (Oct. 1992) found an especially low representation of women in cardiovascular drug trials (pp. 9–10). One further example of how ignored women have been in cardiac drug trials came in early 1994, when the American Heart Association reported that a new study clearly demonstrated "for the first time" that the cholesterol-lowering drug lovastatin slows the progression of coronary disease and prevents development of new coronary lesions equally well in both women and men. ("Cholesterol-Lowering Drug Equally Effective in Women and Men, Canadian Study Shows," American Heart Association press release, 15 March 1994.)

p. 87   "When women do have heart attacks . . ." Philip Greenland, et al., "In-Hospital and One-Year Mortality in 1,524 Women after Myocardial Infarction," *Circulation* 83.2 (1991): 484–91. Also, Richard C. Becker, et al., "Comparison of Clinical Outcomes for Women and Men after Acute Myocardial Infarction," *Annals of Internal Medicine* 120.8 (1994): 638–45.

pp. 87–88   "Studies show . . ." Dozens of studies began looking at the differences in the diagnosis, treatment, and prognosis of men and women's heart disease. A few of the more notable ones:

- John Z. Ayanian and Arnold M. Epstein, "Differences in the Use of Procedures Between Women and Men Hospitalized for Coronary Artery Disease," *New England Journal of Medicine* 325.4 (1991): 221–25.
- Steven S. Khan, et al., "Increased Mortality of Women in Coronary Artery Bypass Surgery: Evidence for Referral Bias," *Annals of Internal Medicine* 112.8 (1990): 561–67.
- Charles Maynard, et al., "Gender Differences in the Treatment and Outcome of Acute Myocardial Infarction," *Archives of Internal Medicine* 152 (1992): 972–76.
- Leslie J. Shaw, et al., "Gender Differences in the Noninvasive Evaluation and Management of Patients with Suspected Coronary Artery Disease," *Annals of Internal Medicine* 120.7 (1994): 559–66.
- Richard M. Steingart, et al., "Sex Differences in the Management of Coronary Artery Disease," *New England Journal of Medicine* 325.4 (1991): 226–30.

p. 89   " 'That beats anybody . . .' " William Castelli, personal interview, 17 May 1993. Much of the information in the chapter about the Framingham findings comes directly from Dr. Castelli. All subsequent quotes from Dr. Castelli are from this interview. Information was also obtained from the "Framingham Study 30–Year Follow-Up" (Washington, D.C.: National Institutes of Health, April 1987).

p. 89   "A study in Scotland . . ." Christopher G. Isles, "Relation Between Coronary Risk and Coronary Mortality in Women of the Renfrew and Paisley Survey: Comparison with Men," *Lancet* 339 (1992): 702–6.

p. 89   "And a University of Pittsburgh . . ." "Older Women: Mortality Similar for High and Normal Cholesterol," *Geriatrics* 49.2 (1994): 54.

p. 90   "For instance, some scientists . . ." Carol Tavris, *The Mismeasure of Women* (New York: Simon & Schuster/Touchstone, 1992), p. 104. Also Elisabeth Rosenthal, "High Blood Pressure May Pose Less of a Danger for Women," *New York Times*, 4 Sept. 1991, p. C11.

p. 90   " 'We need information . . .' " JoAnn Manson, personal interview, 18 May 1993.
           All subsequent quotes from Dr. Manson are from this interview.

p. 90   "A study in New York hospitals . . ." Kathryn Anastos, et al., "Hypertension in
           Women: What Is Really Known?" *Annals of Internal Medicine* 115.4 (1991):
           287–93.

p. 90   "That's no surprise . . ." "Women's Health: FDA Needs to Ensure More Study of
           Gender Differences in Prescription Drug Testing," United States General Account-
           ing Office Report to Congressional Requesters, Oct. 1992.

p. 91   " 'You tend to hear . . .' " Audrey von Poelnitz, personal interview, 2 July 1993. All
           subsequent quotes from Dr. von Poelnitz are from this interview.

p. 91   "This last side effect . . ." Jane E. Brody, "Personal Health: The Fat to Fear, Experts
           Say, Is Around the Middle," *New York Times,* 20 Nov. 1991, p. C15.

p. 91   "And it's this 'yo-yo' . . ." I-Min Lee and Ralph S. Paffenbarger, "Change in Body
           Weight and Longevity," *Journal of the American Medical Association* 268.15 (1992):
           2045–49. Information on abdominal body fat and weight cycling was also obtained
           from Judith Rodin, Ph.D., dean, Graduate School of Arts and Sciences, Yale Uni-
           versity. Dr. Rodin spoke at a Weight Watchers press conference, "Women and Obe-
           sity . . . The Risks, The Reasons, Resolutions for Empowerment," New York, 4
           Feb. 1992.

p. 92   "Women with diabetes . . ." Information from Dr. Castelli and the Framingham
           study.

p. 92   "In one of the most ironic . . ." The Coronary Drug Project Research Group,
           "The Coronary Drug Project: Initial Findings Leading to Modifications of Its
           Research Protocol," *Journal of the American Medical Association* 214.7 (1970):
           1303–13.

pp. 93–94 "The old, high-dose . . ." R. Stan Williams, "Benefits and Risks of Oral Contracep-
           tive Use," *Postgraduate Medicine* 92.7 (1992): 155–71.

p. 94   "But because they are . . ." Trudy Bush, Ph.D., Johns Hopkins University, speaking
           at the session "Heart Disease," 1st Annual Congress on Women's Health, Washing-
           ton, D.C., 4 June 1993.

p. 94   " 'Similar to other research . . .' " Marianne J. Legato, personal interview, 23 May
           1993. All subsequent quotes from Dr. Legato are from this interview.

p. 94   "Other studies have shown . . ." Patrick Huyghe, "His and Her Solutions," *Health,*
           March 1991, p. 95.

p. 94   "In fact, studies have found . . ." "Despite Stress, Working Women May Have
           Lower Heart Disease Risk," *Medical World News,* Dec. 1993, p. 21. Also, Patricia
           Thomas, "Employment May Reduce Women's CAD Risk," *Medical World News,*
           April 1991, p. 15.

p. 95   "The Framingham study found . . ." Elaine D. Eaker, et al., "Myocardial Infarction
           and Coronary Death Among Women: Psychosocial Predictors from a 20-Year
           Follow-up of Women in the Framingham Study," *American Journal of Epidemiology,*
           135 (1992): 854–64.

p. 95   "The lowest risk . . ." "Women with Full Lives Have Less Risk of Heart Disease,"
           Medical Tribune, 2 May 1991.

p. 95   " 'Women in these kinds of jobs . . .' " Personal interview, Jane Sherwood, 17 June
           1993. All subsequent quotes from Ms. Sherwood are from this interview.

p. 95   "As Susan Faludi pointed out . . ." Susan Faludi, *Backlash* (New York: Crown,
           1991), pp. 38–9.

p. 96   "More than a third . . ." Nanette Wenger, M.D., speaking at the Annual Meeting
           of the American Medical Women's Association, New York, 31 Oct. 1993.

p. 97   "Bernadine Healy has coined . . ." Bernadine Healy, "The Yentl Syndrome," *New
           England Journal of Medicine* 325.4 (1991): 274.

p. 97   "One study found . . ." Pat Phillips, "Women's Angina Risk Probed," *Medical World
           News,* Oct. 1991, p. 10.

p. 97   "Yet women this age . . ." Pat Phillips, "Women's Angina Risk Probed," *Medical
           World News,* Oct. 1991, p. 10. Another study in older women also found that
           women with angina lived longer and had a lower risk of heart attacks than men: An-
           thony Orencia, et al., "Effect of Gender on Long-term Outcome of Angina Pectoris

and Myocardial Infarction/Sudden Unexpected Death," *Journal of the American Medical Association* 269.18 (1993): 2392–97.

p. 100   "Another problem is that . . ." "Poll Shows Women Rely on Ob-Gyns for Primary Care," news release, American College of Obstetricians and Gynecologists, 29 Oct. 1993.

p. 100   "The treadmill, or stress . . ." Nearly all of the cardiologists interviewed for this article bemoaned the lack of adequate testing for women. Also see: "Diagnosis of Heart Disease More Complicated in Women—Some Tests Less Reliable," *Internal Medicine News*, 1–14 Dec. 1991, pp. 1, 45.

p. 100   " 'Thirty-five percent . . .' " Linda Crouse, personal interview, 24 May 1993. All subsequent quotes from Dr. Crouse are from this interview.

p. 101   "Many women have a harmless . . ." Judith Hsia, M.D., George Washington University, speaking at the session, "Heart Disease," 1st Annual Congress on Women's Health, 4 June 1993, Washington, D.C.

p. 101   "One theory holds . . ." Judith Hsia, 4 June 1993.

p. 101   "Another hypothesis . . ." Judith Hsia, 4 June 1993.

p. 101   "The test is now . . ." Judith Hsia, 4 June 1993.

p. 101   "Studies have shown . . ." Steingart, *New England Journal of Medicine* 325.4 (1991): 226–30. And Shaw, *Annals of Internal Medicine* 120.7 (1994): 559–66.

p. 101   "They cited a 1987 study . . ." Council on Ethical and Judicial Affairs, American Medical Association, "Gender Disparities in Clinical Decision Making," *Journal of the American Medical Association* 266.4 (1991): 560.

p. 102   "Of the patients . . ." *JAMA* 266.4 (1991): 560.

p. 102   "Just because men and women . . ." Daniel B. Mark, et al., "Absence of Sex Bias in the Referral of Patients for Cardiac Catheterization," *New England Journal of Medicine* 330.16 (1994): 1101–06. And Nina A. Bickell, et al., "Referral Patterns for Coronary Artery Disease Treatment: Gender Bias or Good Clinical Judgment?" *Annals of Internal Medicine* 116.10 (1992): 791–97.

p. 102   " 'There's a lot of . . .' " Judith Hochman, personal interview, 17 June 1993.

p. 102   "Nearly forty percent of women's . . ." "Heart and Stroke Facts: 1994 Statistical Supplement," p. 10.

p. 102   "In the first year . . ." Rosalie F. Young and Eva Kahana, "Gender, Recovery from Late Life Heart Attack and Medical Care," *Women & Health* 20.1 (1993): 11–31.

p. 102   "Age alone . . ." Philip Greenland, et al., "In-Hospital and 1-Year Mortality in 1,524 Women after Myocardial Infarction," *Circulation* 83.2 (1991): 484–91.

p. 104   "One study reported . . ." Charles Maynard, et al., "Gender Differences in the Treatment and Outcome of Acute Myocardial Infarction," *Archives of Internal Medicine* 152 (1992): 972–76. A later study found that even when their conditions were identical, 69 percent of men and 57 percent of women received clot-busting drugs: "Asking Why Heart Treatments Fail in Women," *New York Times*, 18 March 1993, p. A18.

p. 104   "A Senate committee meeting . . ." "Heart Drug Response in Women," *New York Times*, 1 July 1992, p. C12.

p. 104   "Women's blood may also contain . . ." "TIMI-II: Women May Respond Differently to Thrombolytics," *Geriatrics* 47.9 (1992): 15–16.

p. 105   "According to the American Heart Association . . ." Sheryl F. Kelsey, et al., "Results of Percutaneous Transluminal Coronary Angioplasty in Women," *Circulation* 87 (1993): 720–27.

p. 105   "Once nearly twice as likely . . ." The older data—that women have nearly twice the risk of dying from bypass surgery—come from Steven S. Khan, et al., "Increased Mortality of Women in Coronary Artery Bypass Surgery: Evidence for Referral Bias," *Annals of Internal Medicine* 112.8 (1990): 561–67. Many cardiologists now say that centers such as the Mayo Clinic that operate on a lot of women are showing equally good results with men and women. If this is true, studies should soon be published reflecting this better outcome for women.

p. 105   "More than 70 percent of . . ." "Heart and Stroke Facts," p. 20.

p. 106   "In the summer of 1992 . . ." Stephen B. Hully, et al., "Health Policy on Blood Cholesterol," *Circulation* 86.3 (1992): 1028. The authors wrote that there *"is no as-*

sociation between high blood cholesterol and cardiovascular deaths in women" (emphasis in original). They added, "With the exception of those who already have coronary disease or other reasons for being at a comparable very high risk of CHD [cardiovascular disease] death, it no longer seems wise to screen for and treat high blood cholesterol in women."

p. 106   "The British journal ..." John R. Crouse III, "Gender, Lipoproteins, Diet, and Cardiovascular Risk," *Lancet* 1 (1989): 318–20.

p. 106   " 'If a low-fat diet ...' " John Crouse, personal interview, 28 May 1993. All subsequent quotes from Dr. Crouse are from this interview.

p. 108   " 'Exercise doesn't seem ...' " Trudy Bush, M.D., Johns Hopkins University, speaking at the session "Heart Disease," 1st Annual Congress on Women's Health, Washington D.C., 4 June 1993.

p. 108   "So far the studies ..." A few studies: Pamela A. Taylor and Ann Ward, "Women, High-Density Lipoprotein Cholesterol, and Exercise," *Archives of Internal Medicine* 153 (1993): 1178–84. E. Suter and B. Marti, "Little Effect of Long-Term Self-Monitored Exercise on Serum Lipid Levels in Middle-Aged Women," *Journal of Sports Medicine and Physical Fitness* 32 (1992): 400–11. Jane F. Owens, et al., "Can Physical Activity Mitigate the Effects of Aging in Middle-Aged Women?" *Circulation* 85.4 (1992): 1265–70.

p. 108   "In 1988 researchers ..." The Steering Committee of the Physicians' Health Study Research Group, "Preliminary Report: Findings from the Aspirin Component of the Ongoing Physicians' Health Study," *New England Journal of Medicine* 318.4 (1988): 262–64.

p. 108   " 'It's very difficult ...' " Pam Charney, personal interview, 19 July 1993.

pp. 108–109 "The researchers found ..." JoAnn E. Manson, et al., "A Prospective Study of Aspirin Use and Primary Prevention of Cardiovascular Disease in Women," *Journal of the American Medical Association* 266.4 (1991): 521–27.

p. 109   "The Harvard researchers had been ..." Fran Pollner, "MI Researchers Trying Again to Get Women's Study Funds," *Medical World News*, Jan. 1991, p. 13.

p. 109   "Another benefit-to-risk ..." Several studies have shown that moderate alcohol intake may help protect heart disease in women. Among them:

    • G. Razay, et al., "Alcohol Consumption and Its Relation to Cardiovascular Risk Factors in British Women," *British Medical Journal* 304 (1992): 80–83.
    • Rekha Garg, et al., "Alcohol Consumption and Risk of Ischemic Heart Disease in Women," *Archives of Internal Medicine* 153 (1993): 1211–16.
    • Meir J. Stampfer, et al., "A Prospective Study of Moderate Alcohol Consumption and the Risk of Coronary Disease and Stroke in Women," *New England Journal of Medicine* 319 (1988): 267–73.
    • Gerdi Weidner, et al., "Sex Differences in High Density Lipoprotein Cholesterol Among Low-Level Alcohol Consumers," *Circulation* 83 (1991): 176–80.

p. 109   "However, other studies ..." Walter C. Willett, et al., "Moderate Alcohol Consumption and the Risk of Breast Cancer," *New England Journal of Medicine* 316 (1987): 1174–80. Also, Arthur Schatzkin, et al., "Alcohol Consumption and Breast Cancer in the Epidemiologic Follow-up Study of the First National Health and Nutrition Examination Survey," *New England Journal of Medicine* 316 (1987): 1169–73.

p. 110   "A look at articles ..." Judith Hsia, George Washington University, speaking at the session "Heart Disease," 1st Annual Congress on Women's Health, Washington, D.C., 4 June 1993.

5: BREAST CANCER
Malignant Neglect

p. 111   "When Lorraine Pace ..." Lorraine Pace, personal interview, 12 Aug. 1993.

p. 112   "... at least 70 percent ..." "Breast Cancer, 1971–91: Prevention, Treatment, and Research" (Washington, D. C.: United States General Accounting Office, 1991), p. 4.

p. 112   "... the age at which risk ..." "Estimated Cases of Breast Cancer By Age, 1993," American Cancer Society, 1993. The ACS noted that an estimated 78.1 percent of breast cancers would occur in women fifty and older. Figures are based upon 1987–1989 SEER incidence rates and 1993 U.S. Census projections.

p. 112   "Pace is president . . ." Pace.

p. 112   " 'In 1960 one . . .' " American Cancer Society, 1994.

p. 112   ". . . one of 270 . . ." Fran Visco, president, National Breast Cancer Coalition, personal interview, 18 Aug. 1993.

p. 112   ". . . why up to 40 percent . . ." J. R. Harris, et al., "Breast Cancer," *New England Journal of Medicine* 327 (1992c): 473–80. Cited in *Strategies for Managing the Breast Cancer Research Program: A Report to the U.S. Army Medical Research and Development Command* (Washington, D. C.: National Academy Press, 1993), p. 10.

p. 113   "It's telling that . . ." American Cancer Society, *Cancer Facts & Figures—1994,* p. 10.

p. 113   " 'By the time . . .' " Susan Love, personal interview, 11 May 1992.

p. 113   "The technology misses . . ." National Cancer Institute.

p. 113   "And it has a false . . ." NCI. Also Judith Randal, "Mammoscam," *The New Republic,* Oct. 12, 1992, p. 14.

p. 113   "Susan Love hears . . ." Love.

p. 113   "In women ages fifty to sixty-nine . . ." S. Shapiro, et al., "Periodic screening for breast cancer—the health insurance plan project and its sequelae, 1963–1986," (Baltimore, MD: The Johns Hopkins University Press, 1988). See also L. H. Baker, "Breast cancer detection demonstration project: Five-year summary report," *Cancer* 32.4 (1982): 194–225; and L. Tabar, et al., "Reduction in mortality from breast cancer after mass screening with mammography," *Lancet* 8433 (1985): 829–32.

p. 113   "But even though . . ." "Estimated Cases of Breast Cancer by Age," 1993, American Cancer Society.

p. 113   "A 1992 Mammography . . ." Jacqueline A. Horton, et al., "Mammography Attitudes and Usage Study, 1992," *Women's Health Issues* 2.4 (1992): 184.

pp. 113–114 "According to the . . ." National Health Interview Survey, 1992.

p. 114   " 'We haven't educated . . .' " Barbara Rimer, personal interview, 27 April 1993.

p. 114   "Studies conducted in . . ." A review of the studies was reported at the International Workshop on Screening for Breast Cancer, National Cancer Institute, Bethesda, MD: 24–25 Feb. 1993.

The only major U. S. randomized trial of mammography, conducted in the sixties by the Health Insurance Plan of Greater New York, found a significant benefit for women over fifty but none for women in their forties. Nevertheless, in the seventies, the NCI and ACS launched the Breast Cancer Detection Demonstration Project to introduce mammography to women between the ages of forty and sixty-four. While the project found that mammography did pick up tumors at an earlier, and presumably more curable, stage, there was no control group with which to compare results. As a result of concerns that the high radiation doses would cause more cancer in young women than could be detected, women under fifty were eventually excluded from the study.

Then, in 1988, the NCI announced it would reinterpret the old HIP data. When researchers separated out women forty to forty-nine, they found a 25 percent reduction in deaths. Yet a closer look at the data revealed two troubling facts: first, the study did not have sufficient numbers of women under fifty, so the results were not statistically significant. What's more, most of the women were nearer fifty when they entered the study, and their tumors were detected not in their forties but in their fifties, making it likely that the results would have been the same had they waited until fifty to start mammography. Even so, the NCI, ACS, and ten other health agencies used this data to justify their recommendation that women in their forties get screened every one to two years.

Subsequent screening studies, conducted in Canada and Sweden, have failed to show a reduction in deaths in the younger age group. Critics say the Canadian study used outdated mammography equipment and had other flaws. One outspoken critic, Daniel Kopans, M.D., director of the Breast Imaging Center at Massachusetts General Hospital, says none of the screening studies have been specifically designed to answer the question about mammography in younger women.

The Canadian researchers, for instance, were looking for a 40 percent benefit in women under fifty, much greater than would be expected over five years, the period of time they were studying. "To show even a 25 to 30 percent benefit, which is more likely at five years, you'd need 450,000 women on the study," says Kopans. "They had 50,000 women."

Not only did the Canadian study fail to show a benefit, researchers found that the risk of dying of breast cancer was slightly higher in the screened group. Critics say this finding was a fluke.

p. 114   "What's more, false positives ..." Barbara Rimer, "Impact of Breast Cancer Screening," International Workshop on Screening for Breast Cancer, National Cancer Institute, Bethesda, MD: 24 Feb. 1993.

p. 114   "... all the unnecessary biopsies ..." Ruby Senie, personal interview, 8 May 1992. In an abstract presented at the 26th National Conference on Breast Cancer in Palm Desert, California, in May 1994, Martin Brown of the National Cancer Institute reported that the total number of follow-up procedures performed per cancer detected was inversely related to age. Women under forty had 127 procedures, including repeat mammography, ultrasound, needle aspiration, and biopsies. In contrast, women over seventy had only fifteen procedures.

p. 114   "But despite questions ..." Gerald Dodd, "American Cancer Society Guidelines from Past to Present," Workshop on Breast Cancer Detection in Younger Women: A Current Assessment, American Cancer Society, New York, 1 Feb. 1993.

p. 114   "But in late 1993 ..." "Note to Reporters and Editors," press release, National Cancer Institute, 14 Oct. 1993, p. 3.

p. 114   " 'The NCI is the ...' " Cindy Pearson, cited in Gina Kolata, "Panel Tells Cancer Institute to Stop Giving Advice on Mammograms," *New York Times*, 22 Oct. 1993, p. A 14.

p. 115   "Overall, in women ..." National Cancer Institute, 1994.

p. 115   " 'One reason we see ...' " Diana Godfrey, personal interview, 1 Sept. 1993.

p. 115   "In Washington, D.C. ..." Zora Brown, personal interview, 22 March 1993.

p. 115   "A recent review ..." Suzanne Haynes, personal interview, 25 Aug. 1993.

pp. 115–116 "Haynes found ..." Haynes.

p. 116   "One survey showed ..." Haynes.

p. 116   "On average, they get ..." Kristina Campbell, "1 in 3 Lesbians may get breast cancer, expert theorizes," *The Washington Blade*, 2 Oct. 1992, p. 23.

p. 116   "Susan Love ..." "Court Grants Parental Rights to Mother and Lesbian Lover," *New York Times*, 12 Sept. 1993, p. 42.

p. 116   "After performing a routine ..." Cass Brown, personal interview, 13 Oct. 1993.

p. 117   "Because the disease ..." Benjamin Hankey, Transcript of presentation at the conference, "Breast Cancer in Younger Women: Strategies for Future Research," National Cancer Institute, Bethesda, MD, 28 Jan. 1993, p. 20. According to data from the NCI's Surveillance, Epidemiology, and End Results Program (SEER), breast cancer occurs in .9 per 100,000 women between the ages of twenty and twenty-four. The rate is 26.7 for women thirty to thirty-four and 129.4 for women forty to forty-four. The highest incidence—of four hundred cases per 100,000—occurs in women sixty-five and older.

p. 117   "Although the incidence ..." Eliot Marshall, "Search for a Killer: Focus Shifts from Fat to Hormones," *Science* 259 (1993): 618–19.

p. 117   " 'It hasn't shown up ...' " Amy Langer, personal interview, 29 July 1991. The SEER program, the main source for data on cancer in Americans, was initiated by the NCI in 1973. Data reporting lags behind events by three years.

p. 117   "At the Marin ..." Amy Langer, Transcript of presentation, Breast Cancer in Younger Women, pp. 9–10.

p. 117   "The NCI estimates ..." Linda Anderson, National Cancer Institute, 1994.

p. 117   " 'Young women don't ...' " Langer, 29 July 1991.

pp. 117–118 "At an NCI ..." Kathy Albain, Transcript, Conference on Breast Cancer in Younger Women, 28 Jan. 1993, pp. 63–64. See also Joseph Crowe, Jr., et al., "Age Does Not Predict Breast Cancer Outcome," *Archives of Surgery* 129 (1994): 483. Crowe and his colleagues found that younger breast cancer patients generally have more aggressive and advanced disease compared to older patients.

p. 118   "Women under thirty . . ." Albain, p. 68; also Marie Swanson, Transcript of Conference on Breast Cancer in Younger Women, p. 203.

p. 118   "In a review of . . ." Swanson, p. 198.

p. 118   "Unable to draw . . ." Swanson, pp. 203–4.

p. 118   "Safety questions . . ." Carol Ann Rinzler, *Estrogen and Breast Cancer: A Warning to Women* (New York: Macmillan Publishing Company, 1993), p. 33.

The first study to show a link between the Pill and breast cancer was published in 1975 in the *Journal of the National Cancer Institute*. Ralph Paffenbarger, M.D., and Elfriede Fasal, M.D., then with the California State Department of Health, reported that women who had used the Pill for two to four years had almost twice the risk of breast cancer compared to women who had never been on OCs. In 1979, another study coauthored by Paffenbarger reported a higher risk for women who had used the Pill for more than a year.

That same year a study by Malcolm Pike, M.D., at the University of Southern California School of Medicine, found that OCs could prevent ovarian cancer. "By the end of the seventies," says Pike, "we had evidence that hormones could increase the risk of disease and tremendously decrease the risk of disease."

Pike was stumped. If the age at which a woman underwent her first full-term pregnancy was a strong risk factor for breast cancer (pregnancy hormones prior to age thirty were known to confer a protective effect on the breasts), Pike theorized, perhaps age might also play a role in the link between the Pill and breast cancer. In evaluating the medical records of 163 breast cancer patients under the age of thirty-five at diagnosis, he found that, indeed, young women who'd used the Pill prior to their first full-term pregnancy doubled their risk of premenopausal breast cancer. Use for more than eight years before a first full-term pregnancy tripled the risk.

But the CDC's large Cancer and Steroid Hormone (CASH) study did not support Pike's findings. Researchers analyzed data from 1980 to 1982 on 4,711 women with newly diagnosed breast cancer and 4,676 controls, all of whom were between the ages of twenty and fifty-four. The results, published in the *New England Journal of Medicine* in 1986, "showed no overall increase in the risk of breast cancer among women who used oral contraceptives as compared with women who never used them."

The Pill was deemed safe. But was it?

In the three years following the CASH analysis, five major studies from five different countries all supported Pike's findings. Why in the original CDC analysis, critics asked, had investigators adjusted for age rather than looking specifically to see if there were differences according to age—especially when other epidemiologists, using the same data set, were seeing an increased risk among younger women? In 1988, a new analysis of the CASH data was released. This one showed a fivefold risk of breast cancer among childless women who started taking the Pill before age twenty and who stayed on it for eight years. Another analysis, in 1991, found that the youngest women with the longest use were at the highest risk of getting breast cancer, while the oldest women with the longest use were at diminished risk. It was obvious how, if not adjusted for age, the results wiped each other out.

Taken as an aggregate, most studies suggested that oral contraceptive use in one's teens and twenties confers a 30 to 40 percent increased risk of developing breast cancer, and there may be a twofold increase for OC use of more than five to ten years.

p. 118   "Results of the most . . ." Emily White, et al., "Breast Cancer Among Young U. S. Women in Relation to Oral Contraceptive Use," *Journal of the National Cancer Institute* 86.7 (1994): 505, 511–13. The authors theorized that breast cells may be more susceptible to genetic damage between puberty and a first pregnancy, when the breasts are growing rapidly.

p. 119   "Danelle Butcher . . ." Danelle Butcher, personal interview, 9 Sept. 1993.

p. 119   "Cass Brown . . ." Brown.

p. 119   " 'The current situation . . .' " Malcolm Pike, personal interview, 21 Aug. 1993.

p. 119   "Margie Bernard . . ." Margie Bernard, personal interview, 11 Oct. 1993.

p. 121   ". . . among the 5 . . ." Barbara B. Biesecker, et al., "Genetic Counseling for Families with Inherited Susceptibility to Breast and Ovarian Cancer," *JAMA* 269.15 (1993): 1970.

p. 121   ". . . Tamoxifen Breast Cancer . . ." "Breast Cancer Prevention Trial Will Recruit 16,000 Women," press release, National Surgical Adjuvant Breast and Bowel Project (NSABP), 29 April 1992, p. 1.

p. 121   "To be conducted . . ." NSABP press release, pp. 1, 3, 7.

p. 121   "NCI head Samuel . . ." NSABP press release, p. 1.

p. 121   "A 'practical method'? . . ." Adriane Fugh-Berman, personal interview, 2 Dec. 1992.

p. 121   "Women who had taken . . ." Adriane Fugh-Berman and Samuel Epstein, "Tamoxifen: Disease prevention or disease substitution?" *The Lancet* 340 (1992): 1144.

pp. 121–122 " 'There's a certain . . .' " Fugh-Berman.

p. 122   "Originally tested . . ." Lawrence Wickerham, personal interview, 28 June 1993.

p. 122   "In a worldwide . . ." Early Breast Cancer Trialists' Collaborative Group, "Systemic treatment of early breast cancer by hormonal, cytotoxic, or immune therapy," *Lancet* 339.8784 (1992): 1.

p. 122   "On some tissue . . ." Susan G. Nayfield, et al., "Potential Role of Tamoxifen in Prevention of Brest Cancer," *Journal of the National Cancer Institute* 83.20 (1991): 1452–54.

p. 122   "Based on its . . ." NSABP press release, p. 2. Also Bernard Fisher, "Chemoprevention: Breast Cancer," in press.

p. 122   " 'If we can demonstrate . . .' " Wickerham.

p. 122   "As of early 1994 . . ." NSABP Operations Office, 1994.

p. 122   "According to the study . . ." NSABP. Also Fugh-Berman and Epstein, p. 1143.

p. 122   "Risk factors include . . ." "Questions and Answers: Breast Cancer Prevention Trial," NSABP (undated), see questions 4 and 5. Also Nayfield, pp. 1456–57.

p. 122   "Susan Granoff . . ." Susan Granoff, personal interview, 2 Dec. 1992.

p. 123   "At a congressional . . ." Human Resources and Intergovernmental Relations Subcommittee of the Committee on Government Operations, House of Representatives, Washington, D.C., 22 Oct. 1992.

p. 123   " 'I'm very concerned . . .' " Richard Love, personal interview, 17 Aug. 1993.

p. 123   "Love, who had . . ." Love.

p. 123   "In premenopausal women . . ." Love.

p. 123   "By the same token . . ." Love.

p. 123   "In the United Kingdom . . ." Stephanie Clark, "Prophylactic tamoxifen," *Lancet* 342 (1993): 168. Also Louis Smith, Medical Research Council toxicologist, personal interview, 5 May 1994.

p. 123   "The MRC is . . ." Smith.

pp. 123–124 "As of 1994 . . ." Jack Cuzick, Imperial Cancer Research Fund, personal interview, 5 May 1994.

p. 124   "In his grant . . ." Love.

p. 124   "NCI estimates . . ." NSABP Also Adriane Fugh-Berman, "The High Risks of Prevention," *The Nation*, 21 Dec. 1992, p. 772.

p. 124   "Love, however, did . . ." Richard R. Love, "The National Surgical Adjuvant Breast Project (NSABP) Breast Cancer Prevention Trial Revisited," *Cancer Epidemiology, Biomarkers and Prevention* 2 (1993): 403–07. See also Trudy L. Bush and Kathy J. Heizisouer, "Tamoxifen for the Primary Prevention of Breast Cancer: A Review and Critique of the Concept and Trial," *Epidemiologic Reviews* 15.1 (1993): 241. The authors noted that tamoxifen might cause sixty-nine cases of uterine and liver cancer and 13 life-threatening blood clots while preventing fifty-two cases of breast cancer and thirteen heart attacks. The net benefit, they wrote, would range from negative to "a small positive effect." They concluded: "The lack of significant benefit to participants may raise questions of whether the trial should continue as designed."

p. 124   " 'Even if major . . .' " Love, p. 406.

p. 124 " 'This is the first . . .' " Love.

p. 124 "Indeed in England . . ." Cuzick.

p. 124 "Sybil Fainberg . . ." Sybil Fainberg, personal interview, 15 Oct. 1993.

p. 125 "After a meeting . . ." Fainberg.

p. 125 "Meanwhile Fainberg had . . ." Fainberg.

p. 125 "Fugh-Berman says . . ." Fugh-Berman.

p. 125 "There 'has been . . .' " Adriane Fugh-Berman, Testimony before the Human Resources and Intergovernmental Relations Subcommittee of the Committee on Government Operations, 22 Oct. 1992.

p. 125 "Bernadine Healy has . . ." Warren E. Leary, "Questions Raised on Drug Used in Breast Cancer Study," *New York Times*, 23 Oct. 1992, p. A23.

p. 125 "Data from . . ." Bernard Fisher, et al., "Endometrial Cancer in Tamoxifen-Treated Breast Cancer Patients: Findings from the National Surgical Adjuvant Breast and Bowel Project (NSABP) B-14," *Journal of the National Cancer Institute* 86.7 (1994): 527. See also "NCI-Funded Study Evaluates Risk of Endometrial Cancer from Tamoxifen," press release, *National Cancer Institute*, released 18 Feb. 1994, revised 16 May 1994, p. 5.

p. 125 "Amazingly, Bernard Fisher . . ." Jeff Nesmith, "News of Cancer Deaths—Tamoxifen Link Delayed Six Weeks," *Atlanta Journal & Constitution*, 5 March 1994, p. E4. Also Jeff Nesmith, "Tamoxifen deaths kept in dark," *Atlanta Journal & Constitution*, 23 April 1994, p. E8. Nesmith described memorandums written by officials of Zeneca, saying that they had not been informed of the endometrial cancer deaths until December 1993.

pp. 125–126 "Admitting its inability . . ." Lawrence K. Altman, "U. S. Halts Recruitment of Cancer Patients for Studies, Pointing to Flaws in Oversight," *New York Times*, 30 March 1994: B8.

p. 126 "Under pressure from . . ." Altman.

p. 126 "Says Richard . . ." Nesmith, 5 March 1994.

p. 126 "In 1983 the NCI . . ." Ed Sondik, personal interview, 25 July 1991. Kara Smigel, "Women's Health Trial on Trial," *Journal of the National Cancer Institute* 83.5 (1991): 321. Also Susan Rennie, "Breast Cancer Prevention: Diet vs. Drugs," *Ms.*, May/June 1993, pp. 38–39.

p. 126 "But before the . . ." Sondik. Also William Insull, Jr. and Maureen M. Henderson, et al., "Results of a Randomized Feasibility Study of a Low-Fat Diet," *Archives of Internal Medicine* 150 (1990): 421–27. The study was conducted between 1985 and 1987.

p. 127 "Another feasibility . . ." Maureen Henderson, personal correspondence, 12 May 1994.

p. 127 "But to accurately detect . . ." Smigel, p. 321; Rennie, p. 39.

p. 127 "In spite of the . . ." Henderson.

p. 127 "According to Edward . . ." Sondik.

p. 127 "In recommending . . ." David Korn, personal correspondence to Samuel Broder, 11 Dec. 1989.

p. 127 "The trial 'could . . .' " Korn.

p. 127 "A third time . . ." Sondik. Smigel, pp. 321–23.

pp. 127–128 " 'There's not a shred . . .' " Quoted in Katharine Fong, "Government Ignores Women's Breasts," *SF Weekly* 13 March 1991, p. 9.

p. 128 "As David Korn . . ." Fong.

p. 128 ". . . the NIH had . . ." Alisa Solomon, "The Politics of Breast Cancer," *Village Voice*, 14 May 1991, p. 25.

p. 128 " 'Given the board's . . .' " Rennie, p. 40.

p. 128 "Sheila Swanson . . ." Solomon, p. 25.

p. 129 "Ironically, in April . . ." Rennie, p. 41.

p. 129 "Then a bomb . . ." Walter C. Willett, et al., "Dietary Fat and Fiber in Relation to Risk of Breast Cancer. An 8-year Follow-up," *JAMA* 268.15 (1992): 2037, 2040.

p. 129 " 'Diet is not . . .' " Walter Willett, conference on "Breast Cancer Research: Current Issues, Future Directions," sponsored by Emory University, the American Cancer Society, the CDC, and several other groups, Atlanta, GA, 27 April 1993.

p. 129   "Ross Prentice . . ." Rennie, p. 41.

p. 129   "What's more, some . . ." Marshall, p. 620.

p. 129   "Although the fat . . ." Susan Sieber, personal interview, 24 Aug. 1993.

p. 129   " 'It might not be . . .' " Sieber.

p. 130   "Lorraine Pace . . ." Pace.

p. 130   "Between 1983 and . . ." Gina Kolata, "L.I. Cancer Found to Be Explainable," *New York Times*, 19 Dec. 1992, p. 29.

p. 130   "Like Pace, Francine . . ." Francine Kritchek, personal interview, 16 Aug. 1993.

p. 130   "Kritchek and Quinn were   . . ." Kritchek.

p. 130   "The report found . . ." New York State Department of Health, "The Long Island Breast Cancer Study," Report Number 1, completed June 1988, released 1990. Also Susan Ferraro, "The Anguished Politics of Breast Cancer," *New York Times Magazine*, 15 Aug. 1993, p. 61.

p. 131   "Barbara Balaban, director . . ." Barbara Balaban, personal interview, 16 June 1993.

p. 131   ". . . 'screamed long and loud.' " Balaban.

p. 131   "In 1992 the CDC . . ." Centers for Disease Control and Prevention, "Breast Cancer on Long Island, New York," 17 Dec. 1992, pp. 1, 13.

p. 131   "A critic of the . . ." Devra Davis, Testimony at the Public Hearing on Breast Cancer and the Environment, sponsored by the New York City Commission on the Status of Women and the Women's Environment and Development Organization, New York City, 2 March 1993.

p. 131   "Davis asked . . ." Davis.

p. 132   "An obvious culprit . . ." "Breast Cancer and the Environment," a Greenpeace Report, 1992, pp. 6–7, 14.

p. 132   "During the mid-to-late . . ." Greenpeace, pp. 18, 20–21. According to the report, in 1985 an NCI analysis of the causes of death of 347 female chemists revealed breast cancer rates 63 percent higher than expected. In 1987, Walter Rogan, of the National Institute of Environmental Health Sciences (NIEHS), observed that DDT might mimic the activity of estrogen in breastfeeding women. And a 1989 study by the Environmental Protection Agency found that U.S. counties with toxic waste sites were 6.5 times more likely to have elevated breast cancer rates than counties without such sites.

          The experience in Israel—reported in 1990—lent further credence to these findings. Prior to 1976, when levels of DDT and other pesticides in Israel were up to 800 times greater than U. S. levels, Israel's breast cancer rates were among the highest in the world. In 1978, the Israeli government began an aggressive campaign to phase out several pesticides. By 1980, breast milk levels of DDT had fallen by 43 percent. Compared to what would have been expected based on worldwide increases, the breast cancer incidence in Israel fell by about 20 percent. The greatest reductions were among women under age forty-four, who had a 30 percent decline in mortality. These findings could not be explained by known risk factors.

p. 132   "Intrigued with the data . . ." Mary Wolff, personal interview, 29 June 1993.

p. 132   "Examining the breast . . . F. Y. Falck, M. S. Wolff, et al., "Pesticides and Polychlorinated Biphenyl Residues in Human Breast Lipids and their Relation to Breast Cancer," *Archives of Environmental Health* 47 (1992): 143–46.

p. 132   "Using these data . . ." Wolff.

p. 132   "Analyzing the blood . . ." Mary S. Wolff, et al., "Blood Levels of Organochlorine Residues and Risk of Breast Cancer," *Journal of the National Cancer Institute* 85.8 (1993): 648.

p. 132   " 'Too little is known . . .' " Wolff.

p. 133   " '. . . the NIH study section . . .' " Wolff.

p. 133   "Then came another . . ." Nancy Krieger, Mary S. Wolff, et al., "Breast Cancer and Serum Organochlorines: A Prospective Study Among White, Black, and Asian Women," *Journal of the National Cancer Institute* 86.8 (1994): 589. In the same issue, see also, Linda F. Anderson, "DDT and Breast Cancer: The Verdict Isn't In," pp. 576–77.

p. 133   "Several studies have reported . . ." Doris Delaney, Northeast Regional EMF Action

Network, Testimony at the Public Hearing on Breast Cancer and the Environment, 2 March 1993.

p. 133   "The first double-blind . . ." Scott Davis, Testimony, "Possible Environmental Influences on Breast Cancer, and Health Care Delivery and the Role of the Payor," President's Breast Cancer Panel, Special Commission on Breast Cancer, New York City, 29 April 1993.

p. 133   "The New York State . . ." James M. Melius, "Residence Near Industries and High Traffic Areas and the Risk of Breast Cancer on Long Island," New York State Department of Health, April 1994, pp. i, 4. See also, Diana Jean Schemo, "L.I. Breast Cancer Is Possibly Linked to Chemical Sites," *New York Times* 13 April 1994, p. A1.

p. 133   " 'The issue is . . .' " Devra Davis, Testimony, President's Breast Cancer Panel, Special Commission on Breast Cancer, New York City, 29 April 1993.

p. 134   "As a young surgeon . . ." Love, 2 Sept. 1993.

p. 134   "In 1988 Love . . ." Love.

p. 134   "Traveling the country . . ." Susan Love, *Dr. Susan Love's Breast Book* (Reading, MA: Addison-Wesley, 1991). The 2.6 million women living with breast cancer was compiled by the National Breast Cancer Coalition. In 1986, lung cancer overtook breast cancer as the leading cause of cancer mortality among women. In 1994, according to the American Cancer Society, lung cancer will claim the lives of an estimated 59,000 women. Smoking is responsible for most of the 70,000 or so new cases of lung cancer each year.

p. 134   "As Love recalls . . ." Cindy Kirshman, "Taking Care of Our Own: Rising Cancer Rates Prompt Lesbian Grass-Roots Health Projects," *The Advocate*, 23 April 1991, p. 58.

p. 134   "The year of Susan . . ." National Cancer Institute, Budget Office, 1994. The figure for the AIDS budget was supplied by the National Institute of Allergy and Infectious Diseases.

pp. 134–135   "Then, with the . . ." Sharon Green, personal interview, 6 Aug. 1993.

p. 135   "More than 100 women . . ." Green.

p. 135   "The coalition's first project . . ." Green.

p. 135   "Volunteers set out . . ." Green.

p. 135   "As a result of . . ." Green. Also Eliot Marshall, "The Politics of Breast Cancer," *Science* 259 (1993): 616.

p. 135   "Yet the National Cancer . . ." National Cancer Institute, 1994.

p. 135   "Indeed, a 1991 General . . ." U.S. General Accounting Office, *Breast Cancer, 1971–91: Prevention, Treatment, and Research* GAO/PEMD-92-12 (Washington, D.C.: 1991): 3, 5.

p. 135   "So the coalition . . ." Green.

p. 135   "They decided they needed . . ." Green.

p. 135   "As a result . . ." Green. Also *Strategies for Managing the Breast Cancer Research Program: A Report to the U. S. Army Medical Research and Development Command* (Washington, D.C.: Natural Academy Press, 1993), p. 5.

p. 135   "Although few people . . ." Susan Love, "Breast Cancer: What the Department of Defense Should Do with Its $210 Million," *JAMA* 269.18 (1993): 2417.

p. 135–136   "The money was used . . ." Love, p. 2417.

p. 136   "Meanwhile the NCI's . . ." Marshall, p. 616.

p. 136   "That the army . . ." Fran Visco, personal interview, 18 Aug. 1993.

p. 136   " 'We felt kind . . .' " Visco.

p. 136   "In a December 1992 . . ." Visco.

p. 136   "Their chutzpah . . ." Marshall, pp. 616–17.

p. 136   "But as Love . . ." Susan Love, personal interview, 2 Sept. 1993.

p. 136   "When the question . . ." Visco.

p. 136   " 'The scientific community . . .' " Visco.

p. 137   "Samuel Broder . . ." Confirmed by National Cancer Institute, Office of Cancer Communications.

p. 137   "Work-group head . . ." Sieber.

p. 137   " 'Dr. Broder . . .' " Sieber.

p. 137   "Broder, who is . . ." Marshall, p. 617.

p. 137   "By contrast, prostate . . ." Gina Kolata, "Weighing Spending on Breast Cancer," *New York Times*, 20 Oct. 1993, p. C14.

p. 137   "In late 1993 . . ." The President's Cancer Panel, Special Commission on Breast Cancer, "Breast Cancer: A National Strategy," 1993, p. 1.

p. 137   " 'The National . . .' " President's Cancer Panel, p. 1.

p. 137   "When breast cancer . . ." Ellen Crowley, personal interview, 20 Sept. 1993.

p. 137   "Breast cancer survivor . . ." Ellen Hobbs, personal interviews, 9 and 14 Sept. 1993. Also Sue Woodman, "Breast Cancer Cover-Up," *Allure*, Oct. 1991, p. 44.

p. 138   "Says Fran . . ." Fran Visco, "The Politics of Breast Cancer," Y-Me National Conference, Chicago, 23 July 1993.

6: AIDS

Women Are Not Immune

p. 139   "Mary Guinan . . ." Mary Guinan, personal interview, 30 Jan. 1993.

p. 139   "Across the country . . ." Judith Cohen, personal interview, 27 April 1993.

p. 140   "It didn't make . . ." Kathryn Anastos, personal interview, 4 April 1993.

p. 140   "In 1993 a total . . ." Centers for Disease Control and Prevention, *Morbidity and Mortality Weekly Report* (MMWR) 43.9 (1994): 155, 168.

p. 140   "Since 1992 . . ." MMWR, p. 168.

p. 140   "But even though . . ." MMWR, pp. 156, 168. In 1993, 6,056 of the 16,514 reported AIDS cases in women occurred as a result of heterosexual contact.

p. 140   "But even for those . . ." Howard L. Minkoff and Jack A. DeHovitz, "Care of Women Infected with the Human Immunodeficiency Virus," *JAMA* 266.16 (1991): 2253. The authors write, "Little is known about the course and consequences of human immunodeficiency virus (HIV) infection among women and about the appropriate standards for clinical care of HIV-infected women. What is known about HIV infection is derived principally from studies of individuals who, on the whole, differ from women not only in gender, but in race, income, and risk behavior. What is known about HIV disease in women has been derived principally from studies of pregnant women and has focused primarily on perinatal issues."

p. 141   ". . . most women with AIDS . . ." MMWR, p. 156. In 1993, 50 percent of the women with AIDS were black and 24 percent were Hispanic.

p. 141   ". . . although many more women . . ." "AZT Reduces Rate of Maternal Transmission of HIV," press release, National Institute of Allergy and Infectious Diseases, 21 Feb. 1994, p. 2. The press release notes that, as of 30 Sept. 1993, 4,906 AIDS cases in children under age thirteen had been reported to the CDC.

p. 141   "In June 1983 . . ." Rebecca Denison, personal interview, 5 Aug. 1993.

p. 141   "In a survey . . ." Bradley O. Boekeloo, et al., "Knowledge, Attitudes, and Practices of Obstetricians-Gynecologists Regarding the Prevention of Human Immunodeficiency Virus Infection," *Obstetrics & Gynecology* 81.1 (1993): 131–36.

p. 142   " 'This survey . . .' " Boekeloo, p. 135.

p. 142   "Wendi Alexis Modeste . . ." "Meeting on the Expansion of the AIDS Surveillance Case Definition," Summary Report, Centers for Disease Control and Prevention, 2 Sept. 1992: 18–19.

p. 142   "In a study of . . ." Ellie E. Schoenbaum and Mayris P. Webber, "The Underrecognition of HIV Infection in Women in an Inner-City Emergency Room," *American Journal of Public Health* 83.3 (1993): 363–68. HIV infection was three times more likely to be recognized among men than among women. HIV was completely unrecognized in women age twenty-five and under and forty-five and over. In contrast, among men it was recognized in all age groups.

p. 142   " 'There's a major . . .' " Leslie Laurence, "What Women Should Know," *Town & Country*, Dec. 1992, p. 147. Ellie Schoenbaum, personal interview, 16 Sept. 1992.

p. 142   "When Rebecca . . ." Denision. The following two paragraphs are from the same interview.

p. 143   "The New Jersey Women . . ." Marion Banzhaf, personal interview, 21 May 1993.

All subsequent quotes attributed to Banzhaf are from this interview. Figure for annual budget also from Banzhaf.

p. 143 "Gay Men's Health ..." Gay Men's Health Crisis, 1994.

p. 143 "When GMHC ..." GMHC.

p. 143 "Although GMHC ..." GMHC.

p. 143 "Early in the ..." R. Rothenberg, et al., "Survival with the Acquired Immunodeficiency Syndrome," *New England Journal of Medicine* 317 (1987): 1297–1302.

p. 143 "In a study at ..." Henry Sack, personal interview, 17 Sept. 1992. Also S. Szabo, L. H. Miller, Henry S. Sack, et al., "Gender Differences in the Natural History of HIV Infection," Abstract presented at the VIII International Conference on AIDS, Amsterdam, July 1992.

p. 144 " 'No recent data ...' " Anastos.

p. 144 " 'We don't know ...' " Mitchell Maiman, personal interview, 31 Aug. 1993.

p. 144 "While women are getting ..." Catherine A. Hankins and Margaret A. Handley, "HIV Disease and AIDS in Women: Current Knowledge and a Research Agenda," *Journal of Acquired Immune Deficiency Syndromes* 5.10 (1992): 957–71.

p. 144 "Women, for instance ..." Maiman.

p. 144 "In fact it was ..." Charles C. J. Carpenter, Kenneth H. Mayer, et al., "Human Immunodeficiency Virus Infection in North American Women: Experience with 200 Cases and a Review of the Literature," *HIV in American Women* 70.5 (1991): 307–24. Also Kenneth Mayer, personal interviews, 15 Sept. 1992 and 20 April 1993.

p. 144 "When Kathryn Anastos ..." Anastos.

p. 144 "There is concern ..." Tedd Ellerbrock, CDC, Division of HIV-AIDS, personal interview, 2 March 1993. Also Mitchell Maiman, et al., "Human Immunodeficiency Virus Infection and Cervical Neoplasia," *Gynecologic Oncology* 38 (1990): 377.

p. 145 "Tedd Ellerbrock ..." Ellerbrock. Also Mitchell Maiman, "Recurrent Cervical Intraepithelial Neoplasia in Human Immunodeficiency Virus-Seropositive Women," *Obstetrics & Gynecology* 82.2 (1993): 170.

p. 145 "Although research ..." Ellerbrock.

p. 145 "For instance, a woman. ..." Patricia Donovan, press briefing to announce the report *Testing Positive: Sexually Transmitted Disease and the Public Health Response*, Alan Guttmacher Institute, New York, 30 March 1993.

p. 145 "Adolescent girls ..." Penelope J. Hitchcock, chief, Sexually Transmitted Diseases Branch, National Institute of Allergy and Infectious Diseases, personal interviews, 7 and 27 April 1993.

p. 145 "For the last ..." *Testing Positive* (undated), p. 41.

p. 145 "For years ..." Cohen and Anastos.

p. 145 "Finally, in the summer ..." Caitlin Ryan, personal interview, 16 May 1993.

p. 145 "The meeting ..." National Conference on Women and HIV Infection, National Institute of Allergy and Infectious Diseases, Washington, D.C., 13–14 Dec. 1990.

p. 145 "A lesbian ..." Ryan.

p. 146 "The conference ..." Ryan. See also program, National Conference on Women and HIV Infection.

p. 146 "From the start ..." National Conference on Women and HIV Infection. The following few passages are from the same conference.

p. 146 " 'For years ...' " Ryan.

p. 147 "... the AIDS definition ..." "Meeting on the Expansion of the AIDS Surveillance Case Definition," Summary Report: 10. The AIDS surveillance case definition was developed in 1982 and included such conditions as pneumocystis carinii pneumonia, Kaposi's sarcoma, certain lymphomas, and cryptococcal meningitis.

p. 147 "For years activists ..." Theresa McGovern, personal interview, 20 May 1993. All subsequent quotes attributed to McGovern are from this interview.

p. 147 "The CDC had long ..." Confirmed by Ellerbrock.

p. 147 "But there was a paucity ..." Gena Corea, *The Invisible Epidemic: The Story of Women and AIDS* (New York: HarperCollins, 1992), p. 325, n1. Corea reports that by 1991 the government had spent $80 million studying the natural history of HIV in men. In contrast CDC had allocated only $4.5 million each for fiscal years 1991 and 1992 to conduct studies in women.

p. 147   "McGovern says . . ." McGovern.

p. 147   "McGovern was angry . . ." McGovern. The discussion of Social Security and
           Supplemental Security Income benefits is in the Third Amended Class Action
           Complaint, filed by nineteen New York State residents against Louis W.
           Sullivan, former Secretary of the Department of Health and Human Services, 7
           Dec. 1991.

p. 147   "In October 1990 . . ." McGovern.

p. 147   "One of the plaintiffs . . ." Third Amended Class Action Complaint, pp. 26–29.

p. 148   "She and other AIDS . . ." McGovern.

p. 148   "The CDC suggested . . ." James Buehler, "Meeting on the Expansion of the AIDS
           Surveillance Case Definition," Summary Report, p. 11.

p. 148   "On September . . ." "Meeting on the Expansion of the AIDS Surveillance Case
           Definition," Atlanta.

p. 148   "Marion Banzhaf . . ." Banzhaf. See also Summary Report, pp. 12–13.

p. 148   "The new definition . . ." "1993 Revised Classification System for HIV Infection
           and Expanded Surveillance Case Definition for AIDS Among Adolescents and
           Adults," Centers for Disease Control and Prevention, *Morbidity and Mortality
           Weekly Report* 41.RR-17 (1992).

pp. 148–149 "By the end . . ." "Impact of the Expanded AIDS Surveillance Case Definition on
           AIDS Case Reporting—United States, First Quarter, 1993," Centers for Disease
           Control and Prevention, *Morbidity and Mortality Weekly Report* 42.16 (1993): 308.
           From January through March 1993, 35,779 AIDS cases had been reported to
           CDC. Of these new cases, 21,582 (or 60 percent) were reported based on the med-
           ical conditions added to the definition in 1993.

p. 149   "Then in June . . ." Robert Pear, "U.S. Will Relax Disability Rules in H.I.V. Cases,"
           New York Times, 29 June 1993, pp. A1, B7.

p. 149   "The AIDS Clinical . . ." Mary Jane Walker, National Institute of Allergy and In-
           fectious Diseases, 1994. Also "Women and HIV Infection," press release, NIAID,
           April 1994, p. 3.

p. 149   "In 1994 the ACTG . . ." Mary Jane Walker, National Institute of Allergy and In-
           fectious Diseases, 10 May 1994.

p. 149   "As of April . . ." "Demographic Summary of ACTG Study Entries," AIDS Clinical
           Trials Group, 26 April 1994. Contains cumulative data through April 22, 1994.

p. 149   "Constance Wofsy . . ." Constance Wofsy, personal interview, 13 May 1993.

p. 149   "A closer look . . ." Iris L. Long, "Women's Access to Government-Sponsored
           AIDS/HIV Clinical Trials: Status Report, Critique and Recommendations," 27
           April 1993, p. 10.

p. 150   "But when the results . . ." James O. Kahn, et al., "A Controlled Trial Comparing
           Continued Zidovudine with Didanosine in Human Immunodeficiency Virus Infec-
           tion," *New England Journal of Medicine* 327.9 (1992): 583.

p. 150   "As Howard Minkoff . . ." Howard Minkoff, personal interview, 11 May 1993.

p. 150   "Studies suggest . . ." Fred J. Hellinger, "The Use of Health Services by Women
           with HIV Infection," *Health Services Research* 28.5 (1993): 543–61. Hellinger re-
           ported that a woman with AIDS is 20 percent less likely than a male IV drug user
           with AIDS of being hospitalized. That women with AIDS use fewer health services
           than men with AIDS "may simply reflect the fact that women have more childcare
           and other family-related responsibilities," wrote Hellinger. "Or to some extent, this
           may result from a situation where women are healthier than men . . . or where dis-
           crimination occurs against women with HIV infection."

p. 150   "Similarly Ruth Greenblatt . . ." Ruth Greenblatt, personal interview, 18 May
           1993. All subsequent Greenblatt quotes are from the same interview.

p. 151   "When Judith Feinberg . . ." Judith Feinberg, presentation at "AIDS Clinical Re-
           search and Care: Meeting the Challenges of an Epidemic in Flux," sponsored by
           Public Responsibility in Medicine and Research, 29–30 Oct. 1992.

p. 151   " 'If a clinic . . .' " Wofsy.

p. 151   " 'We often fail . . .' " Mary Young, personal interview, 17 Aug. 1993.

p. 152   "Indeed, shockingly . . ." Wofsy.

p. 152   " 'What was left . . .' " Young.

p. 152   "From the beginning . . ." Pamela Stratton, personal interviews, 16 April and 2 Sept. 1993.

p. 152   "At the ACTG . . ." Stratton.

p. 152   "Activists also objected . . ." Code of Federal Regulations, Part 46, "Protection of Human Subjects," Regulations 46.207 and 46.208, Department of Health and Human Services, National Institutes of Health, Office for Protection from Research Risks, Revised 18 June 1991: 13. For research directed toward pregnant women and fetuses in utero as subjects, the regulations require the informed consent of both the mother and the father, except that the father's consent can be waived if: "(1) his identity or whereabouts cannot reasonably be ascertained, (2) he is not reasonably available, or (3) the pregnancy resulted from rape." Many AIDS researchers get around these rules by simply asking the woman if her husband is reasonably available. If she says no, even if he's sitting in the next room, he's not considered available.
          In the case of pregnant women the father's consent is not required by law if the purpose of the research is to meet the health needs of the mother. The ACTG trial that is the subject of the next few paragraphs is not such a study.

p. 152   "But Johns Hopkins's . . ." Feinberg.

p. 153   "As of February . . ." "AZT Reduces Rate of Maternal Transmission of HIV," press release, National Institute of Allergy and Infectious Diseases, 21 Feb. 1994, p. 3.

p. 153   "An interim . . ." "Important Therapeutic Information on the Benefit of Zidovudine for the Prevention of the Transmission of HIV from Mother to Infant," *Clinical Alert*, National Institute of Allergy and Infectious Diseases, 22 Feb. 1994.

p. 153   " 'The resources . . .' " Anastos.

p. 153   "A few studies . . ." Hankins and Handley p. 963. See also transcript, "An Approved System for Continuing Medical Education," American College of Obstetricians and Gynecologists, 18.4: 5.

p. 153   "It is known . . ." Pamela Stratton, et al., "Human Immunodeficiency Virus Infection in Pregnant Women Under Care at AIDS Clinical Trials Centers in the United States," *Obstetrics & Gynecology* 79.3 (1992): 367.

p. 153   ". . . 33 percent of obstetricians . . ." State-of-the-art conference on azidothymidine therapy for early HIV infection, *American Journal of Medicine* 89 (1990): 335–44. Cited in Stratton, p. 367.

p. 153   "Pneumocystis carinii . . ." L. M. Koonin, et al., "Pregnancy-Associated Deaths due to AIDS in the United States, *JAMA* 261 (1989): 1306–1309. Cited in Stratton, p. 367.

p. 153   "Preventive pentamidine . . ." Howard Minkoff and Jonathan D. Moreno, "Drug Prophylaxis for Human Immunodeficiency Virus-Infected Pregnant Women: Ethical Considerations," *American Journal of Obstetrics and Gynecology* 163.4 (1990): 1111.

p. 153   "Noted Howard Minkoff . . ." Minkoff, p. 1111.

p. 153   "Minkoff and others . . ." Minkoff.

p. 154   ". . . only a 20 to 30 percent . . ." Anastos, Stratton.

p. 154   " 'For many HIV . . .' " Hortensia Amaro, "Reproductive Choice in the Age of AIDS: Policy and Counseling Issues," *Women and AIDS: Psychological Perspectives*, ed. Corinne Squire (London: Sage Publications, 1993), pp. 34–35.

p. 154   "Writes Amaro . . ." Amaro, p. 26.

p. 154   "In 1985 the CDC . . ." Centers for Disease Control, "Recommendations for Assisting in the Prevention of Perinatal Transmission of Human T-Lymphotropic Virus and Acquired Immunodeficiency Syndrome, *Morbidity and Mortality Weekly Report* 34.48 (1985): 725.

p. 154   "In 1987 the Surgeon . . ." *Report of the Surgeon General's Workshop on Children with HIV Infection and Their Families*, U. S. Department of Health & Human Services, DHHS Publication No. HRS-D-MC 87-1 (1987), p. 57.

p. 154   "That same year . . ." "Prevention of Human Immune Deficiency Virus Infection and Acquired Immune Deficiency Syndrome," ACOG Committee Statement, June 1987, p. 4. See also "Human Immunodeficiency Virus Infection: Physicians' Responsibilities," ACOG Committee Opinion, November 1993, p. 2. The updated report states: "An individual woman's reproductive choices should be respected regardless of her HIV status."

p. 154   "The attitude toward . . ." "Searching for Women: A Literature Review on Women, HIV, and AIDS in the United States," College of Public and Community Service at the University of Massachusetts, Boston, and the Multicultural AIDS Coalition, March 1992, pp. 129–30.

p. 155   " 'We're consultants . . .' " Anastos.

p. 155   ". . . federal funds . . ." Planned Parenthood, 1994.

p. 155   "One study in New York . . ." Corea, pp. 50–51.

p. 155   "A survey of . . ." Wendy Chavkin, "Drug Addiction and Pregnancy: Policy Crossroads," *American Journal of Public Health* 40 (1990): 483–87.

p. 156   "In one national . . ." "HIV Prevention Practices of Primary-Care Physicians—United States, 1992," CDC, *MMWR* 42.51 and 52 (1994): 989, 991.

p. 156   "In a review of one hundred . . ." Paula Schuman, presentation at Workshop A4, "The Morbidity/Mortality Gap: Is It Gender, or Unequal Access to Health Care?" AIDS Clinical Research and Care: Meeting the Challenges of an Epidemic in Flux, Public Responsibility in Medicine and Research, 29 Oct. 1992. All quotes attributed to Schuman are from this conference.

p. 156   "On Ward 86 . . ." Catherine Lyons, personal interview, 23 Aug. 1993.

p. 156   "When nurse practitioner . . ." Pat Kelly, personal interview, 30 June 1993.

p. 156   "Over at Bronx Lebanon . . ." Risa Denenberg, personal interview, 17 May 1993. All quotes attributed to Denenberg are from this interview.

p. 157   "Although these physicians . . ." Stratton.

p. 157   "Amazingly, of the ninety . . ." Stratton.

p. 157   " 'This is why . . .' " Stratton.

p. 158   "Frustrated by the lack . . ." Stratton.

p. 158   "The physicians agreed . . ." All information in this paragraph is from Stratton.

p. 158   "As an outcome . . ." Wofsy, 13 May 1993.

p. 158   "In 1992, the CDC . . ." "Women and HIV Infection," press release, National Institute of Allergy and Infectious Diseases, April 1994, p. 1.

p. 159   " 'If you're a lesbian . . .' " Amber Hollibaugh, personal interview, 28 July 1993. All subsequent quotes attributed to Hollibaugh are from this interview.

p. 159   "Constance Wofsy and . . ." Constance Wofsy, et al., "Isolation of AIDS-Associated Retrovirus from Vaginal Secretions of Women with Antibodies to the Virus," 1.8480 (1986): 527.

p. 159   "Cohen's research . . ." Rebecca M. Young, Gloria Weissman, and Judith B. Cohen, "Assessing Risk in the Absence of Information: HIV Risk Among Women Injection-Drug Users Who Have Sex with Women," *AIDS & Public Policy Journal* 7.3 (1992): 175–76.

p. 159   " 'But given the way . . .' " Cohen.

pp. 159–160 "In a review . . ." S. Y. Chu, et al., "Update: epidemiology of reported cases of AIDS in women who report sex only with other women, United States, 1980–1991," *AIDS* 6.5 (1992): 518–19.

p. 160   "Several unpublished . . ." Nancy Warren, et al., "Out of the Question: Obstacles to Research on HIV and Women Who Engage in Sexual Behaviors with Women," *SIECUS Report* 22.1 (1993): 13–16.

p. 160   "Applying these results . . ." Hollibaugh.

p. 160   "Currently, some two hundred . . ." Hollibaugh.

p. 160   "In April 1993 . . ." Mary Beth Caschetta, personal interview, 23 Aug. 1993. Subsequent Caschetta quotes from this interview.

p. 161   ". . . that 11.4 million women . . ." W. Baldwin and A. Campbell, "Reproductive Behavior and Women's Risk of AIDS." Paper presented at the NIMH/NIDA Workshop on "Women and AIDS: Promoting Healthy Behaviors," Bethesda, MD. Cited in Amaro, "Reproductive Choice in the Age of AIDS," p. 24.

p. 161   "After her fourth . . ." Marlena (pseudonym), personal interview, 30 June 1993.

p. 161   "In 1992, for the first . . ." CDC, "Update: Acquired Immunodeficiency Syndrome—United States, 1992," *MMWR* 42.28 (1993): 549–50.

p. 162   "In a paper . . ." Joseph Stokes, Lynda Doll, et al., "Female Sexual Partners of Bi-
             sexual Men: What They Don't Know Might Hurt Them," June 1993, pp. 5–6.
p. 162   "In the Latino . . ." "Behaviorally Bisexual Men and AIDS," Executive summary of a
             workshop sponsored by the Centers for Disease Control, 18–19 Oct. 1989, pp. 9–11.
p. 162   " 'How can women . . .' " Lynda Doll, personal interview, 28 May 1993.
p. 162   "Until the female . . ." Kim Painter, "Female condoms in stores soon," USA Today,
             15 April 1994, p. D1.
p. 162   "In a study . . ." "Poverty Preventing Many Haitian Women from Guarding Against
             AIDS, Study Shows," press release, University of North Carolina at Chapel Hill,
             no. 473, 25 Aug. 1993.
p. 163   ". . . 71 percent of respondents . . ." Joseph A. Catania, et al., "Prevalence of AIDS-
             Related Risk Factors and Condom Use in the United States," Science 258 (1992):
             1105.
p. 163   "Interestingly studies show . . ." Christopher J. Elias and Lori Heise, "The Devel-
             opment of Microbicides: A New Method of HIV Prevention for Women," The
             Population Council, Working Papers, no. 6, 1993, p. 45.
p. 163   "A number of studies . . ." CDC, "Update: Barrier Protection Against HIV Infec-
             tion and Other Sexually Transmitted Disease," MMWR 42.30 (1993): 590.
p. 163   "Only a handful . . ." Elias and Heise, p. 50.
p. 163   "Some suggest that . . ." Elias and Heise, pp. 50–51.
p. 163   "But another study . . ." Joan Kreiss, et al., "Efficacy of Nonoxynol 9 Contraceptive
             Sponge Use in Preventing Heterosexual Acquisition of HIV in Nairobi Prostitutes,"
             JAMA 268.4 (1992): 480–81.
p. 163   "Elias speculates . . ." Christopher Elias, personal interview, 26 Aug. 1993.
p. 163   "In 1992 . . ." Elias and Heise, pp. 54–55.
pp. 163–164 "Yet research . . ." Elias and Heise, p. 55.
p. 164   "In the meantime . . ." Anke Ehrhardt, personal interview, 15 Sept. 1992; Erica
             Gollub, personal interview, 16 Dec. 1992.
p. 164   "Since 1989 . . ." Ehrhardt.
p. 164   "The Population Council's . . ." Elias and Heise, PAV and 4.
p. 164   "In 1993 the National . . ." Mary Jane Walker, NIAID Office of Communications,
             10 May 1994.
p. 164   "At the same time . . ." World Health Organization, press release, 16 Nov. 1993.
p. 164   " 'Why have the needs . . .' " Elias and Heise, pp. 57–58.
p. 164   " 'We don't know . . .' " Elias.

7: SURGERY

The Unkindest Cut

pp.   " 'We learned in medical school . . .' " Wayne Burrows, personal interview, 23 April
166–167   1993.
p. 167   "Twenty-five years ago . . ." Medical World News, 23 Oct. 1970, cited in Gena
             Corea, The Hidden Malpractice, updated ed. (New York: Harper Colophon Books/
             Harper & Row, 1985), p. 14.
p. 167   "Approximately two tubal ligations . . ." "Facts in Brief: Contraceptive Use," Alan
             Guttmacher Institute, 15 March 1993.
p. 167   "Nearly fifteen million American women . . ." U. S. Bureau of the Census, Statis-
             tical Abstract of the United States: 1993, 113th ed. (Washington, D. C., 1993), p.
             127.
p. 167   "A list of the country's . . ." Edmund J. Graves, "National Hospital Discharge Sur-
             vey: Annual Summary, 1991," Vital and Health Statistics 13.114 (Hyattsville, MD:
             National Center for Health Statistics, 1993): 10.
p. 168   "Depending on which expert . . ." A 1991 Blue Cross and Blue Shield review of
             over nine thousand hospital cases concluded that 21.5 percent of hysterectomies
             were medically unjustified. At the other extreme, some feminist health advocates
             say that cancer—which is responsible for only about 10 percent of hysterec-
             tomies—is the only valid justification for the surgery.

p. 168   "And one-third to one-half . . ." This sentence is based on the current cesarean rate of 23.5 percent of births. The Centers for Disease Control claims that 15 percent is an ideal rate—a reduction of more than one-third. As always the government is conservative. Some gynecologists, including John M. Smith, author of *Women and Doctors* (New York: Atlantic Monthly Press, 1992), believes that half or more of cesareans in the United States are unnecessary (p. 136).

p. 168   "For instance, women have . . ." "Appendectomies Twice as Likely in Women," *Medical Aspects of Human Sexuality*, Dec. 1991, p. 31.

p. 168   "Women also lead the numbers . . ." "Warning: Your Shoes May Be Hazardous to Your Feet," press release, American Academy of Orthopaedic Surgeons, 19 October 1993.

p. 168   "Finally, women far outnumber men . . ." "1992 National Plastic Surgery Statistics" and "1992 Sex Distribution by Aesthetic Procedures," published by the American Society of Plastic & Reconstructive Surgeons, Inc. In 1992 there were a total of 338,968 aesthetic procedures for women, versus only 54,845 for men.

p. 169   "While nearly 25 percent . . ." "Cesarean Rates Vary," *Medical Tribune*, 7 May 1992.

p. 169   "Almost 40 percent of . . ." "Percent of Women with Intact Uteri by Age, United States: 1965–1987," National Hospital Discharge Survey, National Center for Health Statistics. Information on French women from Lynn Payer, *Medicine and Culture* (New York: Penguin Books, 1988), pp. 50–52.

p. 169   "Yet infant mortality rates . . ." Ingrid VanTuinen and Sidney M. Wolfe, *Unnecessary Cesarean Sections: Halting a National Epidemic* (Public Citizen's Health Research Group, 1992), p. 16. Also, Paul Lewis, "Japanese Live Longer, the U.N. Finds," *New York Times*, 26 April 1992, p. 12.

pp. 169–170 "Says John M. Smith . . ." *Women and Doctors* (New York: Atlantic Monthly Press, 1992), p. 19.

p. 170   " 'Physicians practice medicine . . .' " Joseph Gambone, personal interview, 7 January 1994. All subsequent quotes from Dr. Gambone in this chapter are from this interview.

p. 170   "A case in point is . . ." Elizabeth Rosenthal, "Doctors Time Therapies to Body Rhythms," *New York Times*, 2 Oct. 1990, pp. C1, C6.

p. 170   "Some recent research . . ." There have been more than half a dozen of these studies since 1991. For example, Ruby T. Senie, et al., "Timing of Breast Cancer Excision During the Menstrual Cycle Influences Duration of Disease-Free Survival," *Annals of Internal Medicine* 115 (1991): 337–42. Another article reporting on a separate study: Diana Swift, "Luteal Phase Best for Breast Surgery," *Medical Tribune*, 20 Jan. 1994.

p. 171   "The statistics on hysterectomy . . ." Graves, *Vital and Health Statistics*, p. 10.

p. 171   "More than one-third of women . . ." "Percent of Women with Intact Uteri by Age, United States: 1965–1987," National Hospital Discharge Survey, National Center for Health Statistics.

p. 171   " 'Many gynecologists feel . . .' " Smith, *Women and Doctors*, pp. 38–39.

p. 171   "Another gynecologist author . . ." Stanley West (with Paula Dranov), *The Hysterectomy Hoax* (New York: Doubleday, 1994), pp. 1–2.

p. 171   "Eighty to 85 percent of hysterectomies . . ." Joseph Gambone, personal interview, 7 Jan. 1994.

p. 171   "Before age fifty-five . . ." "Number of Hysterectomies by Age, Year and Diagnosis: United States 1965–1987," National Hospital Discharge Survey, National Center for Health Statistics.

p. 171   "After age fifty-five . . ." "Number of Hysterectomies . . . ," National Hospital Discharge Survey, NCHS.

p. 172   "But studies showed . . ." Joseph C. Gambone, et al., "Short-Term Outcome of Incidental Hysterectomy at the Time of Adnexectomy for Benign Disease," *Journal of Women's Health* 1.3 (1992): 197–200.

p. 172   "Women who have hysterectomies . . ." Gambone, *Journal of Women's Health* 1.3 (1992): 197–200.

p. 172   "Conversely, more than one-third . . ." "Number and Percent of Hysterectomies with and without a Bilateral Oopherectomy By Age, United States: 1985–87, National Hospital Discharge Survey, National Center for Health Statistics.

p. 172   "Alternative treatments . . ." Information on alternative treatments for noncancerous uterine conditions comes from a variety of sources, including the Iowa Foundation for Medical Care, "Hysterectomy: Justifying the Procedure," *IFMC News* 8.1:3; and "Hysterectomy Hesitation," *Harvard Health Letter*, Dec, p. 1993: 8; also Dr. Stanley West's book, *The Hysterectomy Hoax* (New York: Doubleday, 1994).

p. 172   "Fibroid tumors, the leading reason . . ." "Number of Hysterectomies by Age, Year and Diagnosis: United States, 1965–1987," National Hospital Discharge Survey, NCHS.

p. 173   "Less than 15 percent . . ." "Number of Hysterectomies . . . ," NHDS, NCHS.

p. 173   "As Dr. John Smith writes . . ." Smith, *Women and Doctors*, pp. 46–47.

p. 174   "Rates of hysterectomy . . ." Kristen Kjeruff, et al., "The Socioeconomic Correlates of Hysterectomies in the United States," *American Journal of Public Health* 83.1 (1993): 106–108. Also, Kristen H. Kjeruff, et al., "Hysterectomy and Race," *Obstetrics and Gynecology* 82.5 (1993): 757–64.

p. 174   "But it wasn't too long ago . . ." Deborah Larned, "The Epidemic in Unnecessary Hysterectomy," *Seizing Our Bodies*, ed. Claudia Dreifus (New York: Vintage Books, 1977), p. 202.

p. 174   "Swiss researchers looking at . . ." Gianfranco Domenighetti and Pierangelo Luraschi, "Hysterectomy and Sex of the Gynecologist" (letter), *New England Journal of Medicine* 313.23 (1985): 1482.

p. 174   "An American woman has . . ." Lynn Payer, *Medicine and Culture* (New York: Penguin Books, 1988), p. 125.

p. 174   "She writes . . ." *Medicine and Culture*, p. 22.

p. 175   "According to Payer . . ." *Medicine and Culture*, p. 52.

p. 175   "As if the sexual health . . ." A computer search of "MEDLINE," the National Library of Medicine's computerized data base, turned up a total of 618 articles on hysterectomies in 1993, but only 5 articles—all foreign—on subtotal hysterectomies.

p. 175   "A publicity packet . . ." Press packet from the United States Surgical Corporation, Norwalk, Conn., handed out to attendees at the 1st Annual Congress on Women's Health, Washington D.C., 3–4 June 1993.

p. 176   "In 1985 a landmark study . . ." Bernard Fisher, et al., "Five-Year Results of a Randomized Clinical Trial Comparing Total Mastectomy and Segmental Mastectomy with or Without Radiation in the Treatment of Breast Cancer," *New England Journal of Medicine* 312.11 (1985): 665–73.

pp. 176–177 "In spite of the growing . . ." DeAnn Lazovich, et al., "Underutilization of Breast-Conserving Surgery and Radiation Therapy Among Women with Stage I or II Breast Cancer," *Journal of the American Medical Association* 286.24 (1991): 3433–37.

p. 177   " 'Very often what a surgeon does . . .' " Susan Love, quoted in Gina Kolata, "Why Do So Many Women Have Breasts Removed Needlessly?" *New York Times*, 5 May 1993, p. C13.

p. 177   "In a 1984 article . . ." Kathryn M. Taylor, et al., "Physicians' Reasons for Not Entering Eligible Patients in a Randomized Clinical Trial of Surgery for Breast Cancer," *New England Journal of Medicine* 310.21 (1984): 1363–67.

p. 177   "Based on the medical evidence . . ." Dr. Sidney Salmon, director of the Arizona Cancer Center, quoted in Gina Kolata, "Why Do So Many Women Have Breasts Removed Needlessly?" *New York Times*, 5 May 1993, p. C13.

p. 177   "In one study . . ." Diana C. Farrow, et al., "Geographic Variation in the Treatment of Localized Breast Cancer," *New England Journal of Medicine* 326.17 (1992): 1097–1100.

p. 177   "For Medicare patients . . ." Ann Butler Nattinger, et al., "Geographic Variation in the Use of Breast-Conserving Treatment for Breast Cancer," *New England Journal of Medicine* 326.17 (1992): 1102–107.

p. 177   "The rate of surgery also varies . . ." *NEJM* 326.17 (1992): 1105.

p. 177   "According to Payer . . ." *Medicine and Culture*, p. 24.

p. 178   "In 1994 . . ." Lawrence K. Altman, "Researcher Falsified Data in Breast Cancer
            Study," *New York Times*, 14 March 1994, pp. A1, A9. The story was widely re-
            ported in the popular press for weeks afterwards.

p. 178   "The flawed information . . ." "Independent Analysis Reaffirms Results of Breast
            Cancer Study," press release, National Cancer Institute, 12 April 1994.

p. 178   "Scientists rushed to assure . . ." National Cancer Institute press release, 12 April
            1994, plus Lee-Feldstein, et al., "Treatment Differences and Other Prognostic Fac-
            tors Related to Breast Cancer Survival," *Journal of the American Medical Association*,
            271.15 (1994): 1163–68.

p. 179   " 'It's not an operation . . .' " Henry Lynch, quoted in Peter Korn, "Prophylactic
            Mastectomy Seen as Way to Cut Cancer Risk," *American Medical News*, 12 Oct.
            1992, p. 13.

p. 179   "It was November 1991 . . ." Diana St. James, personal interview, 1 May 1993.

p. 180   "Fewer than 10 percent . . ." Based on fact that Japan's cesarean rate is only 7 per-
            cent (with lower infant mortality than in the United States), and the American per-
            cent rate was 5.5 or lower until 1970.

p. 180   "One in four babies is now . . ." "Rate of Cesarean Delivery in the United States,
            1991," *Morbidity & Mortality Weekly Report* 42.15 (1993): 285–89.

p. 180   "Three-quarters will have . . ." "Doubt Cast on Surgical Child-Birth Procedure,"
            New York Times, 2 July 1992, p. A12. This article is a report on a Canadian study
            that was "published" in the inaugural issue (July 1, 1992) of *Online Journal of Cur-
            rent Clinical Trials*, a computer journal produced by the American Association for
            the Advancement of Science.

p. 180   "The rate of cesarean sections . . ." *MMWR* 42.15 (1993): 286.

p. 180   "The cesarean section rate quadrupled . . ." *MMWR* 42.15 (1993): 286.

pp. 180–181 "There are four main medical reasons . . ." *MMWR* 42.15 (1993): 287–88.

p. 181   "Studies have shown that . . ." Bruce L. Flamm, et al., "Vaginal Birth After Cesa-
            rean Delivery: Results of a 5-Year Multicenter Collaborative Study," *Obstetrics &
            Gynecology*, 76.5 (1990): 750–54. Also *MMWR* 42.15 (1993): 288.

p. 181   "It's been known . . ." Albert D. Haverkamp, et al., "A Controlled Trial of the Dif-
            ferential Effects of Intrapartum Fetal Monitoring," *American Journal of Obstetrics
            and Gynecology* 134.4 (1979): 399–412.

p. 181   "A 1989 bulletin to . . ." *Women and Doctors*, p. 135.

p. 181   "And even herpes outbreaks . . ." "C-Sections for Herpes: Too Many," *Health*,
            Sept.–Oct. 1993, pp. 28–29.

p. 181   "A 1993 study . . ." A. Russell Localio, et al., "Relationship Between Malpractice
            Claims and Cesarean Delivery," *Journal of the American Medical Association* 269.3
            (1993): 366–73.

pp. 181–182 "Another 1993 study found . . ." Jennifer S. Haas, et al., "The Effect of Health
            Coverage for Uninsured Pregnant Women on Maternal Health and the Use of Ce-
            sarean Section," *Journal of the American Medical Association* 270.1 (1993): 61–64.

p. 182   "Interestingly, the gender . . ." G. S. Berkowitz, et al., "Effect of Physician Charac-
            teristics on the Cesarean Birth Rate," *American Journal of Obstetrics and Gynecology*
            16.1 (1989): 146–49.

p. 182   "But older, more experienced . . ." Berkowitz, *American Journal of Obstetrics and
            Gynecology* 16.1 (1989): 146–49.

p. 182   "Cesarean sections are also more common . . ." J. F. Peipert and M. B. Bracken,
            "Maternal Age: An Independent Risk Factor for Cesarean Delivery," *Obstetrics
            & Gynecology* 81 (1993): 200–205. Also, Kiyoko M. Parrish, et al., "Effect of
            Changes in Maternal Age, Parity and Birth Weight Distribution on Primary Ce-
            sarean Delivery Rates," *Journal of the American Medical Association* 271.6
            (1994): 443–47.

p. 182   " 'Many times, a hospital staff . . .' " Patricia Burkhardt, personal interview, 20
            April 1993. The quote also appeared in Beth Weinhouse, "Is There a Right Time
            to Have a Baby?" *Glamour*, May 1994, p. 285.

p. 182   " 'Women are interesting people . . .' " John Goldkrand, quoted in Mary Lee
            Grisanti, "The Cesarean Epidemic," *New York*, 20 Feb. 1989, p. 58.

p. 183   "The United States has not only . . ." "Infant Mortality—United States, 1991," *Morbidity & Mortality Weekly Report* 42 (1993): 926–30.

p. 183   "In Japan, where . . ." Ingrid VanTuinen and Sidney M. Wolfe, *Unnecessary Cesarean Sections: Halting a National Epidemic* (Public Citizen's Health Research Group, 1992), p. 16.

p. 183   "In England, for example . . ." Pieter E. Treffers and Maria Pel, "The Rising Trend for Cesarean Birth," *British Medical Journal* 307 (1993): 1017.

p. 183   "The United States ranks twenty-fourth . . ." *MMWR* 42 (1993): 926–30 and *MMWR* 42.15 (1993): 285.

p. 183   "In Brazil women often . . ." "Minerva," *British Medical Journal* 306 (1993): 1280. Citing *Health Policy and Planning* 8 (1993): 33–42.

p. 183   "There are some signs . . ." *MMWR* 42.15 (1993): 286.

p. 183   "The less-than-2-percentage-point . . ." "Drop in C-Sections in 1991 Saves $322 Million," *The Female Patient*, May 1993.

p. 183   "In 1982 the American College . . . ." Bruce L. Flamm, "Cesarean Section: Update on America's Most Common Operation," ACOG Scientific Update, New York, 18 Feb. 1993.

p. 183   "Again in 1988 . . ." "Guidelines for Vaginal Delivery After a Previous Cesarean Birth," American College of Obstetricians and Gynecologists Committee Opinion No. 64, Oct. 1988.

p. 183   "A study at California hospitals . . ." Bruce L. Flamm, et al., "Vaginal Birth After Cesarean Delivery: Results of a 5-Year Multicenter Collaborative Study," *Obstetrics & Gynecology* 76.5 (1990): 750–54.

p. 183   "Yet in spite of . . ." *MMWR* 42.15 (1993): 286.

p. 183   "Repeat cesareans are still . . ." *MMWR* 42.15 (1993): 287.

p. 184   "While the rate . . ." *MMWR* 42.15 (1993): 286, 288.

p. 184   "Other experts feel . . ." *Unnecessary Cesarean Sections*, p. 9.

p. 184   "At Mt. Sinai Hospital . . ." Stephen A. Myers and Norbert Gleicher, "A Successful Program to Lower Cesarean Section Rates," *New England Journal of Medicine* 319.23 (1988): 1511–16. Plus *Unnecessary Cesarean Sections*, p. 44.

p. 184   "A Texas study . . ." John Kennell, et al., "Continuous Emotional Support During Labor in a U. S. Hospital," *Journal of the American Medical Association* 265.17 (1991): 2197–237.

p. 184   " 'The incentives are all . . .' " Sidney Wolfe, quoted in Mary Lee Grisanti, "The Cesarean Epidemic," *New York*, 29 Feb. 1989, p. 58.

p. 185   "The nearly universal use . . ." Harold Speert, *Obstetrics and Gynecology in America: A History* (Baltimore: Waverly Press, 1980), pp. 187–88.

p. 185   " 'I've been doing research into episiotomies . . .' " Nancy Fleming, personal interview, 29 April 1993.

p. 185   "One of the most recent studies . . ." "Doubt Cast on Surgical Child-Birth Procedure," *New York Times*, 2 July 1992, p. A12. A report of a Canadian study "published" in the inaugural issue (1 July 1992) of *Online Journal of Current Clinical Trials* by the American Association for the Advancement of Science. Another recent study with the same conclusion is by the Argentine Episiotomy Trial Collaborative Group: "Routine vs. Selective Episiotomy: A Randomised Controlled Trial," *Lancet* 342 (1993): 1517–18.

p. 186   "Studies conducted for . . ." "Mothers Who Use Nurse Midwives Have Fewer C-Sections, Episiotomies and Shorter Hospital Stays, Study Shows," press release, American Nurses Association, 16 Feb. 1993.

p. 187   "Information is still emerging . . ." "Who Has Implants? The Estimates Vary," *New York Times*, 29 Jan. 1992, p. C12.

pp. 187–188 "One surgeon likened . . ." Sandra Blakeslee, "The True Story Behind Breast Implants," *Glamour*, Aug. 1991, p. 186.

p. 188   " 'One of the petitions . . .' " Jane Zones, personal interview, 2 Feb. 1994.

p. 188   "The silicone gel . . ." Andrew Purvis, "A Strike Against Silicone," *Time*, 20 Jan. 1992, p. 40.

p. 188   "The polyurethane foam used to cover . . ." Nicholas Regush, "Toxic Breasts," *Mother Jones*, Jan.–Feb., 1992, p. 29.

p. 188   " 'My eyes popped out when Powell . . .' " Ed Griffiths, quoted in "Toxic Breasts,"
              Mother Jones, Jan.–Feb. 1992, p. 29.

p. 188   "Manufacturers were free . . ." Sandra Blakeslee, "The True Story Behind Breast
              Implants," *Glamour*, Aug. 1991, p. 188.

p. 188   "The most common complication . . ." J. Arthur Jensen and Melvin J. Silverstein,
              " 'Doctor, Should I Have My Breast Implants Removed?' " *Emergency Medicine*
              25.16 (1993): 20.

p. 189   "Dow Corning, the leading . . ." Min Kyung Kim, "After 30 Years, a Major Mich-
              igan Multi-Study Report Gives Silicon-Breast Implants a Clean Bill of Health,"
              Medical Tribune, Aug. 1991, pp. 12–14.

p. 189   " 'In the package insert . . .' " Sybil Goldrich, personal interview, 3 Feb. 1994. All
              subsequent quotes from Ms. Goldrich come from this interview.

p. 189   "In the 1980s . . ." Melvin J. Silverstein, et al., "Breast Cancer in Women After
              Augmentation Mammoplasty," *Archives of Surgery* 123 (1988): 681–85. Also, Neal
              Handel, et al., "Factors Affecting Mammographic Visualization of the Breast After
              Augmentation Mammoplasty," *Journal of the American Medical Association* 268.14
              (1992): 1913–17.

p. 189   "There was some evidence . . ." *Mother Jones*, p. 30.

p. 189   "Then it was found . . ." *Mother Jones*, pp. 26, 29. Also Philip J. Hilts, "Studies
              Confirm Potential Cancer Risk from Coated Breast Implants," *New York Times*, 25
              Sept. 1993, p. 10. Only two of the recently available implants—the Meme and the
              Replicon, both manufactured by Bristol-Myers Squibb—had a polyurethane foam
              covering that could potentially release 2-toluene diamine.

p. 189   " 'It's like somebody playing . . .' " Jane Gross, "What Now? Many Ask After Im-
              plant Decision," *New York Times*, 8 Jan. 1992, p. A16.

p. 189   "Radiation can cause . . ." Neal Handel, et al., "Conservation Therapy for Breast
              Cancer Following Augmentation Mammoplasty," *Plastic and Reconstructive Surgery*
              87.5 (1991): 873–78.

p. 189   "Some women reported . . ." E. Jane McCarthy, et al., "A Descriptive Analysis of
              Physical Complaints from Women with Silicone Breast Implants," *Journal of Wom-
              en's Health* 2.2 (1993): 111–15. Also, Jean McCann, "Silicone Implants Linked to
              Memory Loss, Sjögren's," *Medical Tribune*, 4 Nov. 1993, p. 11.

p. 190   "Now doctors suspect . . ." Marjorie Shaffer, "Sjögren's-like Syndrome Linked to
              Breast Implants," *Medical World News*, May 1993, p. 52.

p. 190   "One woman described the mess . . ." Jane Gross, "Recipients of Breast Implants
              Split on Need for U.S. Controls, *New York Times*, 5 Nov. 1991, p. A18.

p. 190   "And after having implants removed . . ." " 'Doctor, Should I Have . . . ,' " *Emer-
              gency Medicine* 25.16 (1993): 30.

p. 190   "Dow Corning took out newspaper ads . . ." For example ads appeared in *The New
              York Times* on 12 Nov. 1991 and 17 Dec. 1991.

p. 190   "Although some of that research . . ." Philip J. Hilts, "Breast Implants Are Imper-
              iled as U.S. Rejects Safety Data," *New York Times*, 14 Nov. 1991, pp. A1, A21.

p. 190   "One of these ads appeared . . ." "Woman Wins Implant Suit," *New York Times*, 17
              Dec. 1991, p. A16.

p. 190   "That same month . . ." Philip J. Hilts, "Breast Implant Maker Accused on Data,"
              New York Times, 21 Dec. 1991, p. 8.

p. 190   "In April 1994 . . ." Sandra Blakeslee, "Lawyers Say Dow Study Saw Implant Dan-
              ger," *New York Times*, 7 April 1994, pp. A1, A11.

pp. 190–191   "The FDA charged . . ." Philip J. Hilts, "Breast Implant Maker Is Accused of Mis-
              leading Telephone Callers," *New York Times*, 31 Dec. 1991, p. A12.

p. 191   "In early 1992 the FDA . . ." "FDA Calls for Moratorium on Use of Silicone Gel
              Breast Implants," *Medical Tribune*, 30 Jan. 1992. And Philip J. Hilts, "F.D.A.
              Seeks Halt in Breast Implants Made of Silicone," *New York Times*, 7 Jan. 1992, pp.
              A1, C5.

p. 191   "While professional surgeons' . . ." *Medical Tribune*, 30 Jan. 1992. And Felicity
              Barringer, "Many Surgeons Reassure Their Patients on Implants," *New York Times*,
              29 Jan. 1992, pp. C1, C12.

p. 191   "Dow continued to insist . . ." Philip J. Hilts, "Maker of Silicone Breast Implants

Say Data Show Them to Be Safe," *New York Times*, 14 Jan. 1992, pp. A1, A19. And Philip J. Hilts, "Biggest Maker of Breast Implants Is Said to Be Abandoning Market," *New York Times*, 19 March 1992, pp. A1, B11.

p. 191   "Said FDA commissioner David Kessler . . ." "FDA Puts Strict Limits on Silicone," *Medical Tribune*, 7 May 1992.

p. 191   "Now hundreds of lawyers . . ." David Margolick, "At the Bar," *New York Times*, 31 July 1992, p. B7. And Gina Kolata, "3 Companies in Landmark Accord on Lawsuits Over Breast Implants," *New York Times*, 24 March 1994, pp. A1, B10. And Gina Kolata, "Details of Implant Settlement Announced by Federal Judge," *New York Times*, 5 April 1994, p. A10.

p. 191   "In late 1993 the . . ." American Medical Association Council on Scientific Affairs, "Silicone Gel Breast Implants," *Journal of the American Medical Association* 270.21: 2602–606.

p. 191   "The article appeared . . ." Jeremiah J. Levine and Norman T. Ilowite, "Sclerodermalike Esophageal Disease in Children Breast-fed by Mothers with Silicone Breast Implants," *Journal of the American Medical Association* 271.3 (1994): 213–16.

p. 191   "The author of the *JAMA* article . . ." "Silicone Gel Breast Implants," *JAMA* 270.21: 2602.

p. 191   "Referring to the journal's emphasis . . ." Jane Zones, personal interview, 2 Feb. 1994.

p. 192   "In France . . ." Lynn Payer, *Medicine and Culture* (New York: Penguin Books, 1988), p. 55.

p. 192   " 'Many breasts reduced . . .' " *Medicine and Culture*, p. 55.

p. 192   "Face-lifts are also . . ." *Medicine and Culture*, p. 55.

p. 192   "Marketed as a quick and easy . . ." Robin Marantz Henig, "The High Cost of Thinness," *New York Times Magazine*, 28 Feb. 1988, pp. 41–42.

p. 192   "Naomi Wolf, author of . . ." Naomi Wolf, *The Beauty Myth* (New York: Anchor Books/Doubleday, 1991), pp. 261–62.

p. 192   "Worst of all . . ." "Liposuction: One Year Later," *Health*, March/April 1994, pp. 20, 24.

8: REPRODUCTIVE HEALTH

Fertile Ground for Bias

p. 193   " 'In that one sentence . . .' " Sally Faith Dorfman, personal interview, 21 Feb. 1994.

p. 194   "According to The Alan Guttmacher Institute . . ." Jacqueline Darroch Forrest (vice president for research, The Alan Guttmacher Institute), "Timing of Reproductive Life Stages," *Obstetrics and Gynecology*, 82.1 (1993): 109–10.

p. 194   " 'We are a nation . . .' " Ron Wyden, letter, *New York Times*, 16 Jan. 1992, p. A22.

p. 194   "Sterilization is now the most commonly . . ." "Facts in Brief: Contraceptive Use" (New York and Washington: The Alan Guttmacher Institute, 13 March 1993).

p. 194   "A 1992 report by the . . ." Jessica Townsend, ed., *Strengthening Research in Academic OB/GYN Departments*, Institute of Medicine (Washington, D.C.: National Academy Press, 1992), p. 166.

p. 194   "And reliance on female . . ." William D. Mosher, "Contraceptive Practice in the United States, 1982–1988," *Family Planning Perspectives* 22.5 (1990): 200.

p. 194   " 'Women in Bangladesh . . .' " Statements made by David Grimes in his talk, "New Developments in Contraception," at the annual meeting of the American College of Obstetricians and Gynecologists, 27–30 April 1992. Although Dr. Grimes made his remarks at a time when Reagan/Bush politics were severely hampering funding for contraceptive research, when phoned in April 1994, he said he still stood by his comments. Even with the additions of the Norplant implant, Depo-Provera, and the female condom, women in the United States are still denied oral contraceptives and IUDs that are available elsewhere in the world. And contraceptive research is still not a national priority.

p. 194   "*Time* magazine reported . . ." Philip Elmer-DeWitt, "A Bitter Pill to Swallow," *Time*, 26 Feb. 1990, p. 44.

pp. 194–195 "Said Carl Djerassi ..." Elmer-DeWitt, *Time*, 26 Feb. 1990, p. 44.

p. 195   "Currently only two ..." According to The Alan Guttmacher Institute, while sev-
              eral smaller companies are conducting contraceptive research, only two large phar-
              maceutical companies—Ortho Pharmaceutical Corporation and Gynopharma
              Inc.—have been conducting contraceptive research as of April 1994.

p. 195   "It takes an estimated ..." Elmer-DeWitt, *Time*, 26 Feb. 1990, p. 44.

p. 195   "The birth control pill ..." Gena Corea, *The Hidden Malpractice* (New York:
              Harper Colophon Books, updated ed., 1985), p. 13.

p. 195   "Research into new male contraceptives ..." Florence P. Haseltine, M.D., director
              of the Center for Population Research at the National Institute of Child Health and
              Human Development, personal interview, 29 June 1990.

p. 196   " 'There's no data yet ...' " Gary Hodgen, speaking at the National Health Coun-
              cil's conference, "Health for Women in the 21st Century," Washington, D.C., 2
              June 1993.

p. 196   "But according to the Institute of Medicine ..." Townsend, ed., *Strengthening Re-
              search in Academic OB/GYN Departments*, p. 20.

p. 197   "Says the report ..." Townsend, ed., *Strengthening Research in Academic OB/GYN
              Departments*, p. 167.

p. 197   "One study found ..." Carolyn Westhoff, et al., "Residency Training in Contracep-
              tion, Sterilization, and Abortion," *Obstetrics and Gynecology* 81.2 (1993): 312.

p. 197   "... nearly half of the physicians ..." "Experts Say That IUDs Are Safe but
              Largely Ignored," *Medical World News* 35.2 (1994): 13.

p. 197   "Many physicians also don't know ..." James Trussell, et al., "Emergency Contra-
              ceptive Pills: A Simple Proposal to Reduce Unintended Pregnancies," *Family Plan-
              ning Perspectives*, Nov.–Dec. 1992.

p. 197   "With the lack of acceptable contraceptive ..." "Facts in Brief: Abortion in the
              United States," The Alan Guttmacher Institute, 1991.

p. 198   " 'Most women say ...' " From Elizabeth Karlin's talk, "Abortion," at the annual
              meeting of the American Medical Women's Association, New York, 5 Nov. 1993.

p. 199   "*Roe* v. *Wade* established ..." Information on abortion court decisions was com-
              piled from a variety of sources, including "A Woman's Right to Choose After
              Planned Parenthood v. *Casey*," published by the Center for Reproductive Law and
              Policy, 23 Dec. 1993.

p. 199   " 'We talk about abortion on demand ...' " Lynn Paltrow, personal interview, 8
              March 1994.

p. 199   "Currently 83 percent of the nation's counties ..." David A. Grimes, "Graduate
              Education—Clinicians Who Provide Abortions: The Thinning Ranks," *Obstetrics
              and Gynecology* 80.4 (1992): 719.

p. 199   "Seventy of the country's ..." "70 U. S. Metropolitan Areas Have No Abortion
              Provider," press release, Guttmacher Institute, 21 May 1992. Citing data from
              Abortion Factbook, 1992 Edition: Readings, Trends, and State and Local Data to 1988
              (New York: The Alan Guttmacher Institute).

p. 199   "Twenty-five states ..." "State Laws on Abortion," Guttmacher Institute, 1 March
              1994.

p. 199   "Seven states currently have waiting periods ..." Guttmacher Institute, April 1994.

p. 199   "Lynn Paltrow tells ..." Personal interview, 8 March 1994.

p. 200   "Well into 1994 ..." Robert Pear, "6 or More States to Flout New Federal Law on
              Paying for Incest or Rape Abortions," *New York Times*, 1 April 1994, p. A20.

p. 200   " 'We're beginning to see a trend ...' " Kathryn Kolbert, personal interview, 4
              March 1994.

p. 200   "Only 12 percent of the nation's ..." "Fewer Medical Programs Offer Abortion
              Training," *Medical Tribune*, 7 May 1992.

p. 200   "... and nearly one-third do not offer ..." Carolyn Westhoff, et al., "Residency
              Training in Contraception, Sterilization, and Abortion," *Obstetrics and Gynecology*
              81.2 (1993): 312.

p. 200   "Between 1985 and 1991 ..." *Medical Tribune*, 7 May 1992.

p. 200   "Since 1982 ..." The Alan Guttmacher Institute, cited in Luba Vikhanski, "Few
              Residents Trained in Abortion Procedures," *Medical Tribune*, 24 Dec. 1992.

p. 200   "Yet the 1.6 million abortions . . ." "Facts in Brief: Abortion in the United States,"
            Guttmacher Institute, 1991.

p. 200   "When the Feminist Women's Health Center . . ." Lisa Belkin, "Planned Parenthood
            Starting to Train Doctors in Abortion," *New York Times*, 19 June 1993, p. 1.

p. 201   "And only 13 percent . . ." "Issue Paper: Hospitals Have Essential Roles in Abortion
            Services," National Abortion Federation, Washington, D. C., 1992.

p. 201   "In announcing the program . . ." Belkin, *New York Times*, 19 June 1993.

p. 201   " 'The vast majority . . .' " Dr. Rosenfield spoke at a conference titled, "Meeting the
            Health Care Needs of Women: Developing a Funders' Agenda," sponsored by the Na-
            tional Conference on Philanthropy and Women's Health, New York, 22 Jan. 1992.

p. 201   "Although a 1985 survey of ACOG members . . ." "Abortion Attitudes: Little
            Change in 14 Years," press release, ACOG, 21 August 1985.

pp. 201–202 "Said ACOG president . . ." Diane M. Gianelli, "ACOG Backs Training
            Nonphysicians for Abortions, *American Medical News*, 24–31 Jan. 1994, p. 3.

p. 202   "While physicians' assistants . . ." National Abortion Federation, Washington,
            D.C., April 1994.

p. 202   " 'There's a deterrent effect . . .' " Ann Allen, personal interview, 8 March 1994.

p. 202   "As columnist Anna Quindlen wrote . . ." "Beyond Doctors," *New York Times*, 21
            April 1993, p. A15.

p. 202   "Wrote a disgusted Quindlen . . ." "At the Clinics," *New York Times*, 5 April 1992,
            section 4, p. 17.

p. 203   "At a Chicago . . ." Connie (pseudonym), personal interview, 29 Jan. 1993. All
            quotes attributed to Connie are from this interview.

p. 203   "A 1991 cover . . ." Philip Elmer-DeWitt, "Making Babies," *Time*, 30 Sept. 1991,
            pp. 56–63.

p. 204   " 'The urge to . . .' " Zev Rosenwaks, personal interview, 17 March 1994.

p. 204   " 'No one has . . .' " Terry Stoller, personal interview, 1 April 1994.

p. 204   ". . . the take-home baby . . ." "Assisted reproductive technology in the United
            States and Canada: 1991 results from the Society for Assisted Reproductive Tech-
            nology generated from The American Fertility Society Registry," *Fertility and Steril-
            ity* 59.5 (1993): 956. See article for rates for ZIFT and GIFT.

p. 204   "Zygote intrafallopian . . ." "Glossary of Medical Terms Relevant to Infertility," IVF
            America (undated).

p. 204   "Specialists may set . . ." Alan H. DeCherney, transcript, hearing before a Sub-
            comittee of the Committee on Government Operations, House of Representatives,
            "Medical and Social Choices for Infertile Couples and the Federal Role in Preven-
            tion and Treatment," 14 July 1988, pp. 76–77.

p. 205   "There's nothing to stop . . ." Janice G. Raymond, *Women as Wombs: Reproductive
            Technologies and the Battle Over Women's Freedom* (San Francisco: HarperSan
            Francisco, 1993), pp. 9–10.

p. 205   ". . . most clinics' tallies . . ." American Fertility Society, 1993.

p. 205   ". . . the best epidemiological . . ." Summary Report, "Consultation on the Place of
            In Vitro Fertilization in Infertility Care," World Health Organization, Copenhagen,
            18–22 June 1990, p. 3.

p. 205   " 'That's why . . .' " A woman who wished to remain anonymous, personal inter-
            view, 28 Jan. 1993.

p. 205   " 'If a couple . . .' " Patricia McShane, personal interview, 21 March 1994.

p. 205   "Soon the treatments . . ." McShane. McShane described all the fertility procedures
            in this chapter.

p. 206   "Ellen, a New York . . ." Ellen (a pseudonym), personal interview, 28 Jan. 1993.

p. 206   " 'My second IVF attempt . . .' " Stoller.

p. 206   "Given that the . . ." McShane.

p. 206   "In one study . . ." Jennifer Downey, "Infertility and the New Reproductive Tech-
            nologies," *Psychological Aspects of Women's Health Care*, eds. Donna E. Stewart and
            Nada L. Stotland (Washington, D.C.: American Psychiatric Press 1993), p. 194.
            Downey was referring to an abstract by W. R. Keye, et al., "Psychosexual Responses
            to Infertility: Differences Between Infertile Men and Women," *Fertility and Sterility*
            36 (1981): 426.

p. 206   "Few studies ..." McShane.

p. 206   "Applying the same ..." Margaret Carlson, "Old Enough to Be Your Mother," *Time*, 10 Jan. 1994, p. 41.

p. 207   "As Margaret Carlson ..." Carlson.

p. 207   "So far only ..." Maria Bustillo, personal interview, 4 May 1994.

p. 207   "Studies do show ..." C. R. Newton, et al., "Psychological Assessment and Follow-up After In Vitro Fertilization: Assessing the Impact of Failure," *Fertility and Sterility* 54 (1990): 879–86. Cited in Downey, p. 195.

p. 207   " 'Intellectually you know ...' " Pamela Loew, cited in Elmer-DeWitt, *Time*, p. 63.

p. 207   " 'When I left ...' " Ellen.

p. 207   "In her book ..." Raymond, pp. ix, xxv.

p. 207   "In an interview ..." Janice Raymond, personal interview, 15 Aug. 1993.

p. 208   " 'Adventure and adventurism ...' " Raymond.

p. 208   "The real kicker ..." American Fertility Society, 1993.

p. 208   "An estimated ..." William D. Mosher and William F. Pratt, "Fecundity and Infertility in the United States, 1965–88," Advance Data, Vital and Health Statistics of the National Center for Health Statistics, no. 192, 4 Dec. 1990.

p. 208   "The tendency to ..." Mosher and Pratt, p. 3. The number of infertile women between the ages of thirty-five and forty-four, 166,000, or more than one-third increased by/between 1982 and 1988, the last year for which data are available. During that same period the number of women between thirty-five and forty-four increased by more than three million. "In some popular descriptions of infertility," write the authors, "it has been suggested ... that there is an 'epidemic' of infertility in the United States. The findings of this report indicate that these perceptions are inaccurate, but the increased use of infertility services, the increased number of childless older women with impaired fecundity, and other factors ... may help to account for the perception that infertility is increasing or that it is more common than it actually is."

p. 208   "... there were 1.35 million ..." Mosher and Pratt, p. 6.

p. 208   "... up from 600,000 ..." "Infertility: Medical and Social Choices," U.S. Congress, Office of Technology Assessment, May 1988, p. 5.

p. 208   "Couples spend ..." "Infertility in America: Why Is the Federal Government Ignoring a Major Health Problem?" 8th Report by the Committee on Government Operations, 1 Dec. 1989, p. 3.

p. 208   "The number of ..." Joyce Zeitz, American Fertility Society, 1994.

p. 208   "France boasts ..." Raymond, p. 8.

p. 209   "As Janice Raymond ..." Raymond, p. 9.

p. 209   " 'The rapid proliferation ...' " Summary Report, World Health Organization, p. 2.

p. 209   "Even though there are ..." Jeffrey May, associate professor of obstetrics and gynecology, University of Kansas, personal interview, 15 Aug. 1993.

p. 209   " 'The bulk of ...' " WHO, p. 3.

p. 209   "Only twenty-eight of the ..." American Fertility Society, 1994.

p. 209   "If women were ..." Florence Haseltine, personal interview, 28 March 1994. All of Haseltine's quotes are from this interview.

p. 209   "Yet how many women ..." WHO, p. 3.

p. 210   "Birth defects ..." Michael P. Steinkampf, personal interview, 21 March 1993.

p. 210   " 'DES-exposed women ...' " Michael P. Steinkampf, "Infertility Treatment Complications: The Next Front-Page Scandal?" (unpublished paper), p. 7.

p. 210   "Up to 60 percent ..." Steinkampf, p. 2.

p. 210   "In the severe form ..." Steinkampf, p. 2.

p. 210   "But women who ..." Robert Spirtas, et al, "Fertility Drugs and Ovarian Cancer: Red Alert or Red Herring?, *Fertility and Sterility* 59.2 (1993): 291.

p. 210   "... a disease that kills ..." American Cancer Society, Cancer Facts & Figures, 1994, p. 16.

p. 210   "Compiling data from ..." Alice Whittemore, "Characteristics Relating to Ovarian Cancer Risk: Collaborative Analysis of 12 U.S. Case-Control Studies," *American Journal of Epidemiology* 136.10 (1992): 1188.

p. 210   "Women who had used ..." Whittemore.

p. 211   "As fertility clinics . . ." Joyce Zeitz, American Fertility Society, 22 Jan. 1993.

p. 211   " 'It was a limited . . .' " Rosenwaks.

p. 211   "Whittemore openly . . ." Alice Whittemore, personal interview, 22 Jan. 1993.

p. 211   " 'Most clinicians haven't . . .' " Carolyn Westhoff, personal interview, 17 March 1994.

p. 211   "According to the . . ." Robert Spirtas, et al., p. 291.

p. 211   "Whittemore's results . . ." Spirtas, pp. 291–92. All facts in this paragraph are from the Spirtas study.

p. 211   "Around the same time . . ." Robert Spirtas, National Institute of Child Health and Human Development, phone conversation, 12 May 1994.

p. 211   " 'On the most . . .' " Westhoff.

p. 212   " 'There is no . . .' " Maria Bustillo, personal interview, 15 Aug. 1993.

p. 212   ". . . an 'experimental' treatment." WHO, 1–3.

p. 212   "Women may be surprised . . ." Confirmed by Michael McClure, M.D., chief of the Reproductive Sciences Branch, NICHD, 5 July 1994. See also "Infertility in America," p. 6.

p. 212   "The institute has . . ." "Infertility in America," pp. 6–7, 13–19. Quote is on p. 7.

pp. 212–213 "The ban on human . . ." Congressional Caucus for Women's Issues, "Update on Women and Family Issues in Congress," 13.1 (1993): 1, 11.

p. 213   "In 1993, President . . ." Congressional Caucus 1, 11. Also confirmed by Steve Kaufman, M.D., a medical officer at the National Institute of Child Health and Human Development.

p. 213   "Florence Haseltine . . ." Haseltine.

p. 213   "IVF averages . . ." Zeitz.

p. 213   "Infertile couples . . ." "Infertility in America," p. 19.

p. 213   "The bulk of funding . . ." Bustillo, 4 May 1994.

p. 213   ". . . Serono Laboratories . . ." See booklets, "Insights Into Fertility" and "Serono Symposia, USA Events and Publications," by Serono Symposia, USA.

p. 213   "There would be . . ." Patricia Donovan, *Testing Positive: Sexually Transmitted Disease and the Public Health Response*, The Alan Guttmacher Institute, 1993, p. 11.

p. 213   "The twelve million . . ." Donovan, p. 4.

p. 213   ". . . one national survey . . ." "Women & Sexually Transmitted Diseases: The Dangers of Denial," The Campaign for Women's Health and the American Medical Women's Association, Feb. 1994, pp. 5–6. The survey found that 84 percent of American women were not worried about getting an STD.

p. 213   "The bulk of . . ." Donovan, p. 41.

p. 214   "At one overburdened . . ." Lisa Kaeser, personal interview, 17 Feb. 1994.

p. 214   ". . . many primary care . . ." Donovan, p. 38.

p. 214   ". . . a paltry $90 million . . ." Centers for Disease Control and Prevention, 1994.

p. 214   "A Guttmacher . . ." Donovan, pp. 32, 39.

p. 214   "As far back . . ." "Infertility in America," p. 10.

p. 214   "The CDC has . . ." "Infertility in America," p. 11.

p. 214   "When Planned Parenthood's . . ." Barb Sturbaum, Planned Parenthood of Southern Indiana, confirmed 19 May 1994.

p. 214   "A 1986 California . . ." Donovan, pp. 43–44.

p. 215   "The Centers for . . ." CDC, 1994.

p. 215   "And the American Medical . . ." Dorfman.

9: FROM MIDLIFE TO THE MATURE YEARS

The Medicalization of Aging

p. 216   " 'To many women . . .' David R. Reuben, *Everything you always wanted to know about sex but were afraid to ask* (New York; David McKay Company, Inc., 1969), p. 293.

p. 216   ". . . 'by extension menopause . . .' " Emily E. Martin, *The Woman in the Body: A Cultural Analysis of Reproduction*, 1987. Cited in *Proceedings, 8th Conference, Society for Menstrual Cycle Research*, eds. Ann M. Voda, Ph.D., and Rosemary Conover, Ph.D. (The Society for Menstrual Cycle Research, May 1991), p. 197.

p. 216   "As Dr. David Reuben wrote . . ." Reuben, p. 292.

pp. 216–217 "... 'red-faced, emotionally labile ...' " L. Martin, *Health Care of Women* (Philadelphia: J. B. Lippincott Co., 1978), pp. 41–48.

p. 217   "... 'a pair of ovaries ...' " Germaine Greer, *The Change* (New York: Alfred A. Knopf, 1992), p. 41.

p. 217   " 'There's been a focus ...' " Diana Taylor, personal interview, 18 Aug. 1993.

p. 217   "... 'the chemistry of women ...' " Margaret Lock, *Encounters with Aging: Mythologies of Menopause in Japan and North America* (Berkeley: University of California Press, 1993), p. xxxiii.

p. 217   " 'Menopause is only ...' " Taylor.

pp. 217–218 " 'Menopause is a universal phenomenon ...' " "Menopause Research," Information sheet, National Institute on Aging, undated.

p. 218   "Considering that in the next two decades ..." Andrew A. Skolnick, "At Third Meeting, Menopause Experts Make the Most of Insufficient Data," *Journal of the American Medical Association* 268.18 (1992): 2483.

p. 218   " 'Medicine's sudden interest ...' " Skolnick.

p. 218   "At the NIH ..." "Workshop on Menopause: Current Knowledge and Recommendations for Research," sponsored by the National Institute on Aging, National Center for Nursing Research, Office of Research on Women's Health and North American Menopause Society, Bethesda, MD, 22–24 March 1993.

p. 218   " 'When women are told ...' " Brenda Weiss, personal interview, 5 Aug. 1993.

pp. 218–219 "The medical community's ..." Robert A. Wilson, *Feminine Forever* (New York: David McKay, 1966), p. 18.

p. 219   "Much as diabetics ..." Carol Ann Rinzler, *Estrogen and Breast Cancer: A Warning to Women* (New York: Macmillan Publishing, 1993), pp. 45–46.

p. 219   "Wilson, who viewed ..." Greer, p. 164.

p. 219   "Wilson based his ..." Nancy Sommers and James Ridgeway, "Can a Woman Be Feminine Forever?" *The New Republic*, 19 March 1966, pp. 15–16.

p. 219   "In it he ..." Wilson, p. 116.

p. 219   "No one seemed ..." Sommers and Ridgeway, p. 16.

p. 219   "In his book ..." Wilson, p. 44.

p. 219   " 'The outward signs ...' " Wilson, p. 16.

p. 219   "By 1975 ..." B. Stadel and N. Weiss, "Characteristics of Menopausal Women: A Survey of King and Pierce Counties in Washington, 1973–1974," *Journal of Epidemiology* 102 (1975): 215. Also National Women's Health Network, 1989.

pp. 219–220 "Between 1975 and 1976 ..." Donald C. Smith, Ross Prentice, et al., "Association of Exogenous Estrogen and Endometrial Carcinoma," *New England Journal of Medicine* 293.23 (1975): 1164. Harry K. Ziel and William D. Finkle, "Increased Risk of Endometrial Carcinoma Among Users of Conjugated Estrogens," *New England Journal of Medicine* 293.23 (1975): 1167. Noel S. Weiss, et al., "Increasing Incidence of Endometrial Cancer in the United States, *New England Journal of Medicine* 294.23 (1976): 1259. Thomas M. Mack, Malcolm C. Pike, et al., "Estrogens and Endometrial Cancer in a Retirement Community," *New England Journal of Medicine* 294.23 (1976): 1262.

p. 220   "Two weeks after ..." National Women's Health Network, 1994.

p. 220   "Estrogen prescriptions dropped ..." Kathleen MacPherson, "Hormone Replacement Therapy for Menopause: A Contrast Between Medical and Women's Health Movement Perspectives." In *Proceedings of the 8th Conference of Menstrual Cycle Research*, p. 198.

p. 220   "Given the known ..." Isaac Schiff, "Treatment Issues in the Menopausal Woman," Plenary Session III: The Menopausal Woman, 1st Annual Congress on Women's Health, Washington, D. C., 4 June 1993.

p. 220   "Ninety percent ..." Schiff.

p. 221   "... odds ratios are ..." U. S. Congress, Office of Technology Assessment, *The Menopause, Hormone Therapy, and Women's Health*, OTA-BP-BA-88 (Washington, D.C.: U.S. Government Printing Office, May 1992), pp. 40–41.

p. 221   "The American College ..." "Hormone Replacement Therapy," American College of Obstetricians and Gynecologists Technical Bulletin, April 1992, p. 6.

p. 221   "The bone-thinning disorder . . ." Robert Lindsay, *Osteoporosis: A Guide to Diagnosis, Prevention and Treatment* (New York; Raven, 1992), p. 1.

p. 221   ". . . a woman's bone density declines . . ." Bruce Ettinger and Deborah Grady, "The Waning Effect of Postmenopausal Estrogen Therapy on Osteoporosis," *New England Journal of Medicine* 329.16 (1993): 1192.

pp. 221–222 "If osteoporosis is billed . . ." J. C. Stevenson, et al., "Effects of Transdermal Versus Oral Hormone Replacement Therapy on Bone Density in Spine and Proximal Femur in Postmenopausal Women," *Lancet* 336 (1990): 265–69.

p. 222   ". . . a 1993 Boston study . . ." David T. Felson, et al., "The Effect of Postmenopausal Estrogen Therapy on Bone Density in Elderly Women," *New England Journal of Medicine* 329.16 (1993): 1141–46.

p. 222   "When estrogen is stopped . . ." Ettinger and Grady, p. 1192.

p. 222   "One option . . ." Ettinger and Grady, p. 1192.

p. 222   "Because these studies . . ." Sonja M. McKinlay, "Summary of Current Knowledge Concerning Menopause and Potentially Related Pathologies, 1993," Paper presented at workshop on Menopause: Current Knowledge and Recommendations for Research, Bethesda, MD, 23 March 1993.

p. 222   "Such techniques as . . ." "Clinical Indications for Bone Mass Measurements," a report from the Scientific Advisory Board of the National Osteoporosis Foundation, *Journal of Bone and Mineral Research* 4.2 (1989): 3. Also National Osteoporosis Foundation, 1994.

p. 222   ". . . Medicare considers some . . ." Sandra Raymond, executive director, National Osteoporosis Foundation, personal interview, 30 Dec. 1992.

p. 223   "A 1989 study . . ." Raymond.

p. 223   " 'If you're a . . .' " Ethel Siris, personal interview, 11 Aug. 1992.

p. 223   "A magazine ad . . ." Estraderm, Ciba-Geigy Corporation, in *McCall's*, Aug. 1992.

p. 223   "The 1991 Nurses' Health Study . . ." Meir J. Stampfer, et al., "Postmenopausal Estrogen Therapy and Cardiovascular Disease: Ten-Year Follow-up from the Nurses' Health Study, *New England Journal of Medicine* 325.11 (1991): 756.

p. 224   " 'I tried to find . . .' " Jane Porcino, personal interview, 23 Aug. 1993.

p. 224   " '. . . most of us believe . . .' " William Harlan, personal interview, 4 May 1994.

p. 224   " '. . . we're dealing with . . .' " Skolnick.

p. 224   "Some studies suggest . . ." Skolnick, p. 2485 Also Harlan.

pp. 224–225 "Of sixteen prospective . . ." David Barad, M.D., "Hormone Replacement: An Overview of Risks, Benefits, Indications and Contraindications," Controversies in Gynecologic Oncology, Department of Obstetrics and Gynecology, Albert Einstein College of Medicine–Montefiore Medical Center, New York, 1 Nov. 1992.

p. 225   " 'To think of estrogen . . .' " Taylor.

p. 225   "Even William Harlan . . ." Harlan.

p. 225   "A review of the studies . . ." Karen K. Steinberg, et al., "A Meta-analysis of the Effect of Estrogen Replacement Therapy on the Risk of Breast Cancer," *Journal of the American Medical Association* 265.15 (1991): 1985.

p. 225   "Of six studies . . ." Lila Wallis, M.D., "Hormone Replacement Therapy," Advanced Curriculum on Women's Health, American Medical Women's Association, New York, 31 Oct. 1993.

p. 225   " 'Despite more than 50 . . .' " Skolnick, p. 2483.

pp. 225–226 " 'I honestly don't . . .' " Trudy Bush, "Balancing Risks: Postmenopausal Hormone Therapy," Breast Cancer Research: Current Issues—Future Directions, Emory University, American Cancer Society, Centers for Disease Control and Prevention, National Cancer Institute, International Life Sciences Institute, Atlanta, 28 April 1993.

p. 226   " 'If you go back . . .' " Bush.

p. 226   " 'There aren't any data . . .' " Peter Hickox, personal interview, 20 Sept. 1993.

p. 226   ". . . 'there is physician fear . . .' " Hickox.

p. 227   "Many women are . . ." Deborah Anderson, personal interview, 5 Nov. 1993.

p. 227   " 'Drugs that rapidly . . .' " Susan Bewley, *Lancet* 339 (1992): 290–91.

p. 227   " 'I believe . . .' " Howard Judd, personal interview, 15 Oct. 1993.

p. 227   "Despite Bewley's . . ." Susan Bewley, correspondence to Ann Voda, 3 May 1993.

pp. 227–228 "In 1992 Wyeth-Ayerst spent . . ." *Advertising Age*, in Karen Stabiner, "In the Menopause Market, a Gold Mine of Ads," *New York Times*, 4 April 1994, p. D6.

p. 228   "Ciba-Geigy has been . . ." Doug Arbesfeld, Ciba-Geigy, personal interview, 10 Aug. 1993.

p. 228   "Ciba-Geigy has also sent . . ." National Women's Health Network, 1991.

p. 228   ". . . told a congressional hearing . . ." Cynthia Pearson, "Women at Midlife: Consumers of Second-Rate Health Care?" Testimony Before the Subcommittee on Housing and Consumer Interests, Select Committee on Aging, House of Representatives, Washington, D.C., 30 May 1991.

p. 228   "In 1993 Wyeth-Ayerst . . ." Audrey Ashby, Wyeth-Ayerst Laboratories, 2 May 1994. Also "NIH Receives Donation from Wyeth-Ayerst to Launch Large-Scale Women's Health Studies," National Institutes of Health, 13 April 1993.

p. 228   " 'They realize the potential . . .' " Nancy Reame, personal interview, 8 July 1993.

p. 228   "In 1990 U.S. . . ." Office of Technology Assessment (OTA), *The Menopause, Hormone Therapy, and Women's Health*, p. 106.

p. 228   ". . . and in 1992 . . ." "Top 200 Survey," *American Druggist*, 209.4 (1994): 27–28. p. 106.

p. 228   ". . . only 15 percent . . ." OTA, p. 104.

p. 229   " 'The problem is . . .' " Lewis Kuller, Workshop on Menopause, 24 March 1993.

p. 229   "As one sixty-six-year-old . . ." New York City woman who asked to remain anonymous, personal interview, 29 Nov. 1993.

p. 229   "Just how confusing . . ." Marilyn Rothert, "Women at Midlife: Consumers of Second-Rate Health Care?" testimony before the Subcommittee on Housing and Consumer Interests, Select Committee on Aging, House of Representatives, Washington, D.C., 30 May 1991.

p. 229   " 'I can't go to . . .' " Sheryl Sherman, personal interview, 14 Sept. 1993.

p. 229   "Brenda Weiss remembers . . ." Brenda Weiss, personal interview, 5 Aug. 1993.

pp. 229–230 " 'We're all in our forties . . .' " Karen Johnson, personal interview, 13 Sept. 1993.

p. 230   ". . . 'We can't expect women . . .' " Teri Randall, *Journal of the American Medical Association* 270.14 (1993): 1664.

p. 230   " 'A physician can't say . . .' " Judd.

p. 230   "In one San Diego clinic . . ." Sheryl Stark Sherman, "Gender, Health, and Responsible Research," *Clinics in Geriatric Medicine* 9.1 (1993): 266.

p. 230   "Another survey . . ." Sherman.

p. 230   " 'If you get six . . .' " Congresswoman Patricia Schroeder, "Menopause," *Newsweek*, 25 May 1992, p. 71.

p. 230   "Women want an unbiased . . ." Phyllis Kernoff Mansfield and Ann M. Voda, "From Edith Bunker to the 6:00 News: How and What Midlife Women Learn About Menopause," in Ellen Cole, Esther D. Rothblum, Nancy D. Davis, eds., *Women and Therapy: Faces of Women and Aging* (New York: The Haworth Press, 1993), pp. 89–104.

p. 231   "A 1993 Gallup . . ." "Women's Information About Menopause is Limited," North American Menopause Society, 4 Sept. 1993. Results of a Gallup survey of 833 women between the ages of forty-five and sixty.

p. 231   ". . . female doctors were more . . ." Gail A. Greendale, et al., "Estrogen and Progestin Therapy to Prevent Osteoporosis: Attitudes and Practices of General Internists and Gynecologists," *Journal of General Internal Medicine* 5 (1990): 464.

p. 231   " 'What women want . . .' " Ruth Jacobowitz, personal interview, 11 Aug. 1993.

p. 231   "Studies by Robert Freedman . . ." Robert Freedman and Suzanne Woodward, "Behavioral Treatment of Menopausal Hot Flushes: Evaluation by Ambulatory Monitoring," *American Journal of Obstetrics and Gynecology* 167.2 (1992): 436–39.

p. 231   "Studies suggest that . . ." Barbara Sherwin and Morrie Gelfand, "Sex Steroids and Affect in the Surgical Menopause: A Double-Blind, Cross-Over Study," *Psychoneuroendocrinology*, 10.3 (1985): 325–35. Also Barbara Sherwin, North American Menopause Society Annual Meeting, San Diego, 3 Sept. 1993.

p. 232   " 'Of the women . . .' " Morrie Gelfand, personal interview, 12 Oct. 1993.

p. 232   "In studies at McGill . . ." Gelfand.

p. 232   "The FDA's . . ." Jean Fourcroy, comment during talk on "Sexuality in the Repro-ductive and Post Menopause Years," by June LaValleur, Advanced Curriculum on Women's Health, American Medical Women's Association, New York, 30 Oct. 1993.

p. 232   ". . . that nineteenth-century . . ." Sheryl A. Kingsberg, Ph.D., "Psychobiologic and Sexual Aspects of Menopause," paper presented at the 101st Annual Convention of the American Psychological Association, Toronto, Canada, Aug. 1993.

p. 232   "Small, uncontrolled . . ." Greer, pp. 239–40.

p. 233   ". . . the brain, like a woman's . . ." Bruce McEwen, "Estradiol and Progesterone Regulate Neuronal Structure and Synaptic Connectivity," Workshop on Meno-pause: Current Knowledge and Recommendations for Research, paper presented at workshop on menopause, Bethesda, MD, 22 March 1993.

p. 233   "Research at McGill . . ." Barbara Sherwin, personal interview, 21 March 1994.

p. 233   " 'Typically, women go . . .' " Gillian Ford, personal interviews, 13 Oct. 1993 and 22 Feb. 1994.

p. 233   "Adult children may be . . ." Sheryl Kingsberg, assistant professor of psychology, de-partment of reproductive biology, Case Western Reserve, personal interview, 27 Aug. 1993.

pp. 233–234 " 'The culture has managed . . .' " Margaret Morganroth Gullette, "What, Meno-pause Again?," *Ms.* July–Aug. 1993, p. 36.

p. 234   ". . . menopause 'is on its way . . .' " Gullette.

p. 234   "Difficulties with menopause . . ." Marcha Flint, personal interview, 17 Sept. 1993.

p. 234   "Women currently constitute . . ." Task Force on Older Women's Health, "Older Women's Health," *Journal of the American Geriatrics Society* 41.6 (1993): 680. See also Report of the National Institutes of Health: "Opportunities for Research on Women's Health," Sept. 1992, p. 123.

p. 234   "By the year 2020 . . ." Panel on Statistics for an Aging Population, *The Aging Pop-ulation in the 21st Century: Statistics for Health Policy,* Washington, D.C.: National Academy Press, 1988. Cited in Report of the National Institutes of Health: *Oppor-tunities for Research on Women's Health,* p. 9.

pp. 234–235 " 'Women survive through . . .' " Report of the National Institutes of Health: *Op-portunities for Research on Women's Health,* p. 123.

p. 235   "Yet, the report . . ." Report of the National Institutes of Health: *Opportunities for Research on Women's Health,* p. 124.

p. 235   "In 1992, 270 fellowships . . ." David H. Solomon, "Women in Geriatrics," *Journal of the American Geriatrics Society* 41.7 (1993): 779.

p. 235   "A paltry eight . . ." Robert Butler, chairman of the Department of Geriatrics, Mount Sinai School of Medicine, personal interview, 14 Sept. 1993.

p. 235   " 'Physicians don't . . .' " Mildred Seltzer, personal interview, 27 Aug. 1993.

p. 235   "Elderly women are less . . ." "Critical Condition: Midlife and Older Women in America's Health Care System, 1992 Mother's Day Report," Older Women's League, p. 4.

pp. 235–236 " 'They enter the netherworld . . .' " Myrna Lewis, personal interview, 17 Sept. 1993.

p. 236   "One of the largest . . ." E. Jeffrey Metter, medical director, Baltimore Longitudinal Study on Aging, personal interview, 13 Oct. 1993.

p. 236   "Myrna Lewis was . . ." Lewis.

p. 236   "One accomplishment . . ." Nathan W. Shock, et al., *Normal Human Aging, The Baltimore Longitudinal Study* (Washington, D.C.: U.S. Department of Public Health, Nov. 1984).

p. 236   ". . . 'years of information . . .' " Anne Colston Wentz, transcript of testimony be-fore the Subcommittee on Housing and Consumer Interests, Select Committee on Aging, House of Representatives, 24 July 1990, p. 32.

p. 236   "Testifying before . . ." Subcommittee on Housing and Consumer Interests, p. 122.

pp. 236–237 " 'Considering that . . .' " Seltzer.

p. 237   "Work by Janice . . ." Janice Kiecolt-Glaser, personal interview, 11 Feb. 1994.

p. 237   "Caregiving also places . . ." Linda K. George, "Social Factors and Depression in Late Life," *Diagnosis and Treatment of Depression in Late Life: Results of the NIH*

Consensus Development Conference, eds. L. S. Schneider, C. F. Reynolds, B. D. Lebowitz, A. F. Friedhoff (Washington, D.C.: American Psychiatric Press, 1994), pp. 139–40

p. 237   "At least one-third . . ." George.

p. 237   " 'It turns out . . .' " William Hazzard, personal interview, 26 Aug. 1993.

p. 237   " 'These illnesses . . .' " Christine Cassel, Plenary Session IV, "Aging in a New Millennium," Health for Women in the 21st Century, The National Health Council, Washington, D.C., 2 June 1993.

p. 238   "Although some 37 . . ." Older Women's League, *Critical Condition: Midlife and Older Women in America's Health Care System*, 1992, p. 3. Also *Opportunities for Research on Women's Health*, p. 124.

p. 238   "After reviewing data . . ." J. Andrew Fantl, personal interview, 2 Sept. 1993.

p. 238   "Fantl tells . . ." Fantl.

p. 238   "In a study . . ." Fantl.

p. 238   "When urogynecologist . . ." Peggy Norton, personal interview, 8 Aug. 1992.

p. 238   " 'Incontinence is not . . .' " Fantl.

p. 238   "That female urinary . . ." Fantl.

p. 238   " 'There are six . . .' " Fantl.

p. 239   "When the subject . . ." June LaValleur, "Sexuality in the Reproductive and Post Menopause Years," Advanced Curriculum on Women's Health, American Medical Women's Association, New York, 30 Oct. 1993. All of LaValleur's quotes are from this conference.

p. 239   "Only three of . . ." Cited in Betty Friedan, *The Fountain of Age* (New York: Simon & Schuster, 1993), p. 259.

p. 239   "Yet studies suggest . . ." LaValleur.

p. 239   " 'Older women can . . .' " Sheryl Kingsberg, personal interview, 27 Aug. 1993.

p. 240   "When a woman's . . ." Friedan, p. 262.

p. 240   " 'Aging is not . . .' " Hazzard.

p. 240   "Between the ages . . ." Older Women's League, p. 5.

p. 240   "In 1993 . . ." Health Care Financing Administration, 1994.

p. 240   "Women make up three-fourths . . ." Older Women's League, p. 8. Also, Suzanne R. Kunkel, assistant director of Scripps Gerontology Center at Miami University, Oxford, Ohio, made the same point in a personal interview, 27 Aug. 1993.

p. 240   "Says Mary Harding . . ." Mary Harding (a pseudonym), personal interview, 26 Jan. 1994.

p. 241   "As Nena O'Neill . . ." Nena O'Neill, personal interview, 21 Jan. 1994.

p. 241   "How else to explain . . ." Hazel Johnson's experiences were related by her daughter, Sylvia Eggleston-Wehr, in a personal interview, 28 Jan. 1994.

pp. 241–242 "Marjorie Pearson . . ." Marjorie Pearson, personal interview, 8 Sept. 1993. See also Marjorie Pearson, et al., "Differences in Quality of Care for Hospitalized Elderly Men and Women," *Journal of the American Medical Association* 268.14 (1992): 1883–89.

p. 242   "If a woman is seeing . . ." Mary C. Ciotti, "Screening for Gynecologic and Colorectal Cancer: Is It Adequate?" *Women's Health Issues* 2.2 (1992): 83–84.

p. 242   "In one study, 15 . . ." Ciotti, p. 84.

p. 242   " 'The most famous . . .' " Butler.

p. 242   "An Atlanta woman . . ." Gail Poulton, conversation, 5 Aug. 1993.

p. 242   "But women sixty-five . . ." Marianne C. Fahs, Jeanne Mandelblatt, et al., "Cost Effectiveness of Cervical Cancer Screening for the Elderly," *Annals of Internal Medicine* 117.6 (1992): 520.

p. 242   "The National Cancer . . ." National Cancer Institute, 1994.

p. 242   "The American Cancer . . ." Fahs, p. 520.

p. 243   " 'Women develop . . .' " Anthony Miller, personal interview, 10 Sept. 1993. See also Anthony Miller, "The Cost Effectiveness of Cervical Cancer Screening," *Annals of Internal Medicine* 117.6 (1992): 529–30.

p. 243   "The United States . . ." Fahs, p. 520.

p. 243   "As some of the major . . ." Marianne Fahs, personal interview, 9 Sept. 1993.

p. 243   "Medicare's new guidelines . . ." Fahs.

p. 243   "A subsequent . . ." Marianne C. Fahs, Jeanne Mandelblatt, et al., "Cost Effectiveness of Cervical Cancer Screening for the Elderly," pp. 520–27.
p. 243   "And they receive . . ." Rebecca Silliman, personal interview, 21 May 1993.
p. 244   "Kathleen Brenneman . . ." Kathleen Brenneman, transcript of testimony before the
            Subcommittee on Housing and Consumer Interests, Select Committee on Aging,
            House of Representatives, 24 July 1990, pp. 24–25.
p. 244   "In general older . . ." Silliman.
p. 244   "In 1986 . . ." Rebecca A. Silliman, et al., "Breast Cancer Care in Old Age: What
            We Know, Don't Know, and Do," *Journal of the National Cancer Institute* 85.3
            (1993): 194.
p. 244   " 'There are many . . .' " Silliman.
p. 244   "It is known . . ." Silliman, et al., p. 195.
p. 244   "For instance, a study . . ." Silliman, et al., p. 194.
p. 245   " 'It is well . . .' " Silliman, et al., p. 194.
p. 245   "Older women take . . . Mary S. Harper, Symposium, "Older Women's Health and
            Mental Health: Research Directions and Funding," Conference on Psychosocial and
            Behavioral Factors in Women's Health: Creating an Agenda for the 21st Century,"
            American Psychological Association, Washington, D.C., 14 May 1994.
p. 245   "Although 64 percent . . ." Jerry Gurwitz, et al., "The Exclusion of the Elderly and
            Women from Clinical Trials in Acute Myocardial Infarction," *Journal of the American Medical Association* 268.11 (1992): 1417–22. The data in this paragraph and
            subsequent Gurwitz quotes are all from the *JAMA* study.
p. 246   "It is known . . ." Bruce Pollock, geriatric psychopharmacologist, personal interview, 28 Jan. 1994. See also Karon Dawkins and William Z. Potter, "Gender Differences in Pharmacokinetics and Pharmacodynamics of Psychotropics: Focus on
            Women," *Psychopharmacology Bulletin* 27.4 (1991): 418.
p. 246   "Antipsychotics . . ." Kimberly A. Yonkers, et al., "Gender Differences in Pharmacokinetics and Pharmacodynamics of Psychotropic Medication," *American Journal
            of Psychiatry* 149.5 (1992): 589.
p. 246   " 'At best . . .' " Pollock.
p. 246   "Antidepressants also . . ." Yonkers, p. 592.
p. 246   "Research conducted in . . ." Wayne A. Ray, Marie R. Griffin, and Ronald I. Shorr,
            commentary, submitted to the Joint Hearing before the Subcommittee on Regulation, Business Opportunities and Energy, Committee on Small Business, Select
            Committee on Aging, House of Representatives, 28 April 1992, p. 257.
p. 247   "A 1989 study . . ." W. Harrison, et al., *Journal of Clinical Psychiatry* 50 (1989): 64.
            Cited in testimony by Philip Hansten, professor of pharmacy, University of Washington, Seattle, before the Joint Hearing before the Subcommittee on Regulation,
            28 April 1992, pp. 267–70.
p. 247   " 'One of the things . . .' " Metter.
p. 247   "Researchers at the Yale . . ." Lisa F. Berkman, codirector of the Yale Health and
            Aging Project, personal interview, 30 Aug. 1993.
p. 248   "If aging is . . ." Friedan, p. 85.
p. 248   " 'There's a massive . . .' " Lewis.

10: "IT'S ALL IN YOUR HEAD"
Misunderstanding Women's Complaints

p. 249   "Somatization, as this . . ." J. W. Pennebaker, et al., "Lack of Control as a Determinant of Perceived Physical Symptoms," *Journal of Personal Social Psychology* 35
            (1977): 167–74.
p. 249   "But it's equally . . ." Donna Stewart, personal interview, 15 April 1994. See also
            Alison C. Mawle, et al., "Is Chronic Fatigue Syndrome an Infectious Disease?" *Infectious Agents and Disease* 2.5 (1994): 339.
p. 249   "In terms of . . ." Mawle, p. 339.
p. 250   "Given the long . . ." Edward Shorter, *From Paralysis to Fatigue: A History of Psychosomatic Illness in the Modern Era* (New York: The Free Press, 1992), p. x.
p. 250   " 'The unconscious . . .' " Shorter, p. x.
p. 250   "The French . . ." Donna E. Stewart, "Emotional Disorders Misdiagnosed as Phys-

ical Illness: Environmental Hypersensitivity, Candidiasis Hypersensitivity, and Chronic Fatigue Syndrome," *International Journal of Mental Health* 19.3 (1990): 57.

p. 250   "The British . . ." Ridgely Ochs, "Chronic Fatigue Puzzle," *Newsday*, 24 Nov. 1992, p. 52.

p. 250   "People in Western . . ." Stewart, p. 58.

p. 250   " 'Patients want . . .' " Shorter, p. 1.

p. 251   "Such a dynamic . . ." Stewart. Also Alison Mawle, personal interview, 24 Jan. 1994.

p. 251   " 'These are very . . ." Nortin Hadler, "Does Fibromyalgia Exist?" Seminar in Advance Rheumatology, New York University, New York, 18 March 1993.

p. 251   " 'The perception among . . .' " Stewart.

p. 251   "For instance, neurasthenia . . ." Shorter, pp. 220–32.

pp. 251–252 "While the diagnosis . . ." Shorter, pp. 307–308.

p. 252   "A decade later . . ." Shorter, p. 309.

p. 252   ". . . 'a disease of fashion . . .' " Shorter, pp. 309–10.

p. 252   "In 1984 . . ." Shorter, p. 310.

p. 252   "At the same . . ." Stewart.

p. 252   "So in 1988 . . ." Gary P. Holmes, et al., "Chronic Fatigue Syndrome: A Working Case Definition," *Annals of Internal Medicine* 108.3 (1988): 387–89.

p. 253   "People with CFS . . ." Stewart.

p. 253   "A study by . . ." Donna E. Stewart, "The Changing Faces of Somatization," *Psychosomatics* 31.2 (1990): 153–58.

p. 253   "Interestingly women . . ." Stewart.

p. 253   "In an attempt . . ." Peter J. Schmidt, et al., "Lack of Effect of Induced Menses on Symptoms in Women with Premenstrual Syndrome," *New England Journal of Medicine* 324.17 (1991): 1174–79.

p. 253   "A study by . . ." Sheryle J. Gallant, et al., "Using Daily Ratings to Confirm Premenstrual Syndrome/Late Luteal Phase Dysphoric Disorder. Part II. What Makes a 'Real' Difference?" *Psychosomatic Medicine* 54 (1992): 169–70, 177.

p. 254   " 'There are very . . .' " Nada Stotland, personal interview, 17 Feb. 1994.

p. 254   "In the Middle . . ." Alice J. Dan and Lisa Monagle, "Sociocultural Influences on Women's Experiences of Premenstrual Symptoms," in Judith H. Gold and Sally K. Severino, eds., *Premenstrual Dysphorias: Myths and Realities* (Washington, D.C.: American Psychiatric Press, 1994), pp. 207–208.

p. 254   "In contrast . . ." Late Luteal Phase Dysphoric Disorder Work Group, DSM-IV Literature Review, American Psychiatric Association, "Late Luteal Phase Dysphoric Disorder," unpublished, undated, p. 63.

p. 254   " 'It's part of . . .' " Stotland.

p. 254   " 'The weight of never . . .' " Prodigy Services, Medical Support Bulletin Board, 13 Nov. 1993.

p. 255   " 'If the perfunctory . . .' " Stewart.

p. 255   "Those who persevere . . ." Nelson M. Gantz and Gary P. Holmes, "Treatment of Patients with Chronic Fatigue Syndrome," *Drugs* 38.6 (1989): 856–60. Also Stewart, "Emotional Disorders Misdiagnosed . . . ," pp. 60–63.

p. 255   "One woman suffering . . ." Prodigy Services, Medical Support Bulletin Board, 11 Jan. 1994.

p. 255   "Stewart has seen . . ." Stewart.

p. 255   "In her job . . ." Alisha Ali, personal interview, 13 April 1994.

p. 255   "Not surprisingly . . ." M. S. Zoccolillo and C. R. Cloninger, "Excess medical care of women with somatization disorder," *Southern Medical Journal* 79.5 (1986): 532–35.

p. 256   "Gerald Weissmann . . ." Gerald Weissmann, panel discussion, session on fibromyalgia, Seminar in Advanced Rheumatology, New York, 18 March 1993.

p. 256   "When told of . . ." Stewart.

p. 256   "In the same vein . . ." Stewart, "Emotional Disorders Misdiagnosed . . . ," pp. 60–61.

p. 256   "The same holds . . ." Stewart, p. 59.

p. 256   "Writes Stewart . . ." D. E. Stewart, "Environmental Hypersensitivity Disorder, To-
            tal Allergy and 20th Century Disease: A Critical Review," *Canadian Family Physi-*
            cian 33 (1987): 409.

p. 256   "In one of . . ." Stewart, "The Changing Faces of Somatization," p. 157.

p. 257   "Donna Stewart . . ." Stewart.

p. 257   " 'These people . . .' " Stewart.

p. 257   "One of Stewart's patients . . ." Stewart.

p. 257   "For instance one study . . ." M. J. Kruesi, et al., "Psychiatric Diagnoses in Patients
            Who Have Chronic Fatigue Syndrome," *Journal of Clinical Psychiatry* 50.2 (1989):
            53–56.

p. 257   "Another study found . . ." P. Manu, et al., "The Mental Health of Patients with
            a Chief Complaint of Chronic Fatigue: A Prospective Evaluation and Follow-up,"
            Archives of Internal Medicine 148 (1988): 2213–17. All of Manu's patients, however,
            did not meet diagnostic criteria for chronic fatigue syndrome. See also Paul J.
            Goodnick and Nancy G. Klimas, eds., *Chronic Fatigue and Related Immune Defi-*
            ciency Syndromes (Washington, D.C.: American Psychiatric Press, Inc., 1993), p. 76.
            In a 1990 follow-up, Manu identified twenty-six of one hundred patients with
            chronic fatigue syndrome. Seventy-seven percent of the CFS sample had active psy-
            chiatric disorders.

p. 257   " 'Having a physical . . .' " Stewart.

p. 258   ". . . 'the language of . . .' " Stewart.

p. 258   " 'If you really . . .' " Stewart.

p. 258   "A 41-year-old . . ." Stewart, "Environmental Hypersensitivity Disorder . . . ,"
            p. 406. All references to this case are from the same page.

p. 259   "One study found . . ." Barbara Bernstein and Robert Kane, "Physician's Attitudes
            Toward Female Patients," *Medical Care* XIX.6 (1981): 600.

p. 259   "Perhaps not surprisingly . . ." *The Commonwealth Fund Women's Health Survey*
            (New York: Louis Harris and Associates, Inc., 1993), p. 7.

p. 259   "Shortly after . . ." Patricia Niemin, personal interview, 8 Feb. 1994. All references
            to Niemin are from this interview.

p. 261   " 'When women have . . .' " Ann Turkel, "Abuse in the Physician/Patient Relation-
            ship," Panel 1: Ethical Dilemmas in Patient Care, Issues in Medical Ethics from
            Women's Perspective, National Council on Women's Health, New York, 21 Nov.
            1992.

p. 261   " 'The open and emotional . . .' " Bernstein and Kane, p. 601.

p. 261   "Interestingly, nonexpressive . . ." Bernstein and Kane, pp. 600, 606.

p. 261   ". . . twice as likely . . ." R. Cooperstock, "Psychotropic Drug Use Among
            Women," *CMA Journal* 115 (1976): 760.

p. 262   "In conversations . . ." Mary C. Howell, Sounding Board, "What Medical Schools
            Teach About Women," *New England Journal of Medicine* 291.6 (1974): 305.

p. 262   "A decade later . . ." Wendy D. Savage and Pat Tate, "Medical Students' Attitudes
            Towards Women: A Sex-Linked Variable?" *Medical Education*, 17 (1983): 159, 161.

p. 262   "One study found . . ." Jonathan N. Tobin, et al., "Sex Bias in Considering Cor-
            onary Bypass Surgery," *Annals of Internal Medicine* 107.1 (1987): 19.

p. 262   "Concerned about this . . ." Council on Ethical and Judicial Affairs, American
            Medical Association, "Gender Disparities in Clinical Decision Making," *JAMA*
            266.4 (1991): 561.

p. 263   "Beth Meyerowitz . . ." Beth Meyerowitz, personal interview, 12 Aug. 1993.

p. 263   "As Bernstein . . ." Bernstein and Kane, p. 607.

11: WOMEN'S MENTAL HEALTH
A Cruel Double Standard

p. 264   "The reality is . . ." Myrna M. Weissman, et al., "Sex Differences in Rates of De-
            pression: Cross-National Perspectives," *Journal of Affective Disorders*, 1993: 77–84.
            See also Ellen McGrath, Gwendolyn Puryear Keita, Bonnie R. Strickland, Nancy
            Felipe Russo, eds., *Women and Depression: Risk Factors and Treatment Issues* (Wash-
            ington, D.C.: American Psychological Association, 1990), pp. 1–2.

p. 264   "Close to 25 percent . . ." Ronald C. Kessler, et al., "Sex and Depression in the National Comorbidity Survey I: Lifetime Prevalence, Chronicity and Recurrence," *Journal of Affective Disorders* 1993: 85–96.

p. 264   "Studies suggest that . . ." Uriel Halbreich and Lucille A. Lumley, "The Multiple Interactional Biological Processes That Might Lead to Depression and Gender Differences in Its Appearance," *Journal of Affective Disorders* 1993: 159–73.

p. 264   "Ultimately the truth . . ." McGrath, et al., pp. 7–33.

p. 264   "One study found . . ." Nancy Wartik, "Blue Moods: New Findings on Why Women Feel Down More Often Than Men," *Working Woman*, Dec. 1992, p. 92.

p. 265   " 'You don't have . . .' " Judy Mann, "Our Culture as a Cause of Depression," *Washington Post*, 7 Dec. 1990. Cited in Peter R. Breggin, *Toxic Psychiatry: Why Therapy, Empathy, and Love Must Replace the Drugs, Electroshock, and Biochemical Theories of the "New Psychiatry"* (New York: St. Martin's Press, 1991), p. 320.

p. 265   "For instance, recent . . ." Wanda Taylor, personal interview, 7 March 1994. See Kessler. Also Marti Loring and Brian Powell, "Gender, Race, and DSM-III: A Study of the Objectivity of Psychiatric Diagnostic Behavior," *Journal of Health and Social Behavior* 29 (1988): 5. Loring and Powell write, "One area of contention is whether the true prevalence of mental illness among females exceeds that among males. . . . A considerable amount of epidemiological evidence suggests that women are more likely than men to be treated for cases of what can be labeled as intropunitive problems, . . . namely disorders resulting from the internalization of conflict. Disorders such as depression would belong to this set of problems. . . . In contrast, males are more likely to be treated for extropunitive difficulties, in which they 'act out' the conflict (for example, antisocial and paranoid personality disorders)."

p. 265   "The newly published . . ." American Psychiatric Association, *Diagnostic and Statistical Manual of Mental Disorders*, 4th ed. (Washington, D.C.: American Psychiatric Association, 1994).

p. 265   "It has grown . . ." Daniel Goleman, "Revamping Psychiatrists' Bible," *New York Times*, 19 April 1994, p. C11.

p. 266   "The problem in including . . ." Carol Tavris, *The Mismeasure of Woman* (New York: Simon & Schuster, 1992), p. 179.

p. 266   "Even the results of . . ." Inge K. Broverman, et al., "Sex-Role Stereotypes and Clinical Judgments of Mental Health," *Journal of Consulting and Clinical Psychology* 34.1 (1970): 2, 5.

p. 266   "For a woman . . ." Broverman, pp. 3–6. See Broverman for remaining points in this paragraph.

p. 266   "For instance, because . . ." Jodie Waisberg and Stewart Page, "Gender Role Noncomformity and Perception of Mental Illness," *Women & Health* 14.1 (1988): 10–11.

p. 266   "Even so, women . . ." Marcie Kaplan, "A Woman's View of DSM-III," *American Psychologist*, July 1983. pp. 786–92.

p. 266   "As psychologist . . ." Kaplan, p. 788.

p. 266   "A case in point . . ." American Psychiatric Association, *Diagnostic and Statistical Manual of Mental Disorders*, 3rd ed., revised (Washington, D.C.: American Psychiatric Association, 1994): 348–49.

p. 266   "To be diagnosed . . ." DSM-III-R, p. 349.

p. 267   "Remember: 'more excitable . . .' " Broverman, pp. 3–5.

p. 267   "Not surprisingly . . ." Kaplan, p. 787.

p. 267   "Although the diagnostic . . ." DSM-IV, pp. 655–58.

p. 267   " 'Is it possible . . .' " Anita Eichler and Delores Parron, eds., *Women's Mental Health: Agenda for Research* (Rockville, MD: Alcohol, Drug Abuse, and Mental Health Administration, National Institute of Mental Health, 1986), p. 5.

p. 267   "After objections . . ." DSM-III-R, pp. 371–74.

p. 267   "Feminists had . . ." Paula Caplan, personal interview, 17 April 1993.

p. 268   "To point out . . ." Caplan.

p. 268   "Although SDPD's criteria . . ." DSM-III-R, p. 373–74.

p. 268   "Despite the . . ." Caplan.

p. 268   "In fact a study . . ." Paul Cotton, "Psychiatrists Set to Approve DSM-IV," *Journal of the American Medical Association* 270.1 (1993): 14. The study involved 100 applicants for inpatient care at the New York State Psychiatric Institute and 100 applicants for outpatient care at Columbia University's Center for Psychoanalytic Training and Research.

p. 268   "Psychiatrist Margaret Jensvold . . ." Margaret Jensvold, personal interview, 18 April 1993.

p. 269   "Despite contentious . . ." Judith Gold, personal interview, 19 April 1993. Also DSM-III-R, pp. 367–69.

p. 269   "It was also . . ." "Statement from the American Psychiatric Association Board of Trustees on Inclusion of Premenstrual Dysphoric Disorder in the Appendix of *DSM-IV*," press release, American Psychiatric Association, 10 July 1993, p. 2.

p. 269   "This gobbledygook . . ." DSM-III-R, pp. 367–69.

p. 269   "In 1931 gynecologist . . ." Tavris, p. 138. See also Judith H. Gold and Sally K. Severino, eds., *Premenstrual Dysphorias: Myths and Realities* (Washington, D.C.: American Psychiatric Press, 1994), p. 173.

p. 269   "At about the same . . ." Tavris, p. 140.

p. 269   "In 1953 she coined . . ." Judith Gold, "Historical Perspective of Premenstrual Syndrome," in Gold and Severino, p. 173.

p. 269   "In the preface . . ." Katherina Dalton, *The Menstrual Cycle* (New York: Pantheon, 1969), p. vii.

p. 269   " 'The old cliché . . .' " Dalton, p. vii.

p. 269   "One cannot even . . ." Nada L. Stotland and Bryna Harwood, "Social, Political, and Legal Considerations," in Gold and Severino, p. 189.

p. 270   "It's telling that . . ." Gold.

p. 270   "Work-group member . . ." Jean Endicott, personal interviews, 23 April 1993 and 15 Jan. 1994.

p. 270   "Endicott has studied . . ." Endicott.

p. 270   "Research by LLPDD . . ." DSM-IV Literature Review, "Late Luteal Phase Dysphoric Disorder," unpublished, undated, p. 31.

p. 270   "The literature . . ." DSM-IV Literature Review, p. 13.

p. 270   "If this is ∴ . ." Caplan.

p. 270   "Then, too, 'why . . .' " Nada Stotland, personal interview, 17 Feb. 1994.

p. 271   "Studies going . . ." D. E. Stewart, "Positive Changes in the Premenstrual Period," *Acta Psychiatr Scand* 79 (1989): 400, 404.

p. 271   "In 1980 . . ." Stewart, pp. 400, 404.

p. 271   "Intrigued with . . ." Stewart, pp. 400–405.

p. 271   " 'I've heard . . .' " Stewart, personal interview, 26 Feb. 1994.

p. 271   "As Margaret Jensvold . . ." Jensvold.

p. 271   "There's plenty . . ." Stotland and Harwood, in Gold and Severino, p. 187.

p. 271   " 'There's clear . . .' " Stotland.

p. 272   "In order to get . . ." Gold, in Gold and Severino, p. 175.

p. 272   "Jensvold disagrees . . ." Jensvold.

p. 272   "Stotland is convinced . . ." Stotland and Harwood, in Gold and Severino, p. 187.

p. 272   "Paula Caplan . . ." Caplan.

p. 272   "While the use . . ." Margaret F. Jensvold, "Psychiatric Aspects of the Menstrual Cycle," *Obstetrics and Gynecology in the Practice of Psychiatry* (Washington, D.C.: American Psychiatric Press, Inc., in press.)

p. 273   " 'It's clear it's . . .' " Caplan, quoted in Tori DeAngelis, "Controversial Diagnosis Is Voted into Latest DSM," *The APA Monitor*, Sept. 1993, p. 33.

p. 273   "PMDD proponent . . ." Robert Spitzer, personal interview, 19 April 1993.

p. 273   "To which Caplan . . ." Caplan.

p. 273   "Not only was . . ." DSM-IV Literature Review, p. 75.

p. 273   " 'Changing the name . . .' " Sally Severino, personal interview, 23 April 1993.

p. 273   "Ultimately the American . . ." "Statement from the American Psychiatric Association Board of Trustees on Inclusion of Premenstrual Dysphoric Disorder in the Appendix of *DSM-IV*," press release, American Psychiatric Association, 10 July 1993, pp. 1–2.

p. 273   "The American Psychological . . ." Raymond Fowler, personal correspondence to Judith Gold, 20 April 1993.

p. 273   "Raymond Fowler . . ." Fowler.

p. 273   "Gail Erlick . . ." Gail Erlick Robinson, personal correspondence to Allen Frances, 28 April 1993.

p. 274   "As the psychiatric . . ." Cotton, p. 14.

p. 274   "Said Deborah Glenn . . ." Cotton, p. 14.

p. 274   " 'The DSM-IV . . .' " Peter Breggin, personal interview, 16 Feb. 1994.

p. 274   "Consider the case . . ." James Goldberg, personal interview, 2 May 1994. Also J. Hamilton, clinical pharmacology panel report. In S. J. Blumenthal, P. Barry, J. Hamilton, B. Sherwin, eds., *Forging a Women's Health Research Agenda* Conference Proceedings, National Women's Health Resource Center, Washington, D.C., Oct. 1991, p. 4. Unless otherwise noted, all subsequent details about Wellbutrin are from these two sources.

p. 275   "Amazingly, the company . . ." Transcript, Psychopharmacologic Drugs Advisory Committee, 25 April 1986, pp. 83–84, 109.

p. 275   "However, in a reanalysis . . ." James P. Goldberg, "Buproprion Dose, Seizures, Women, and Age," Letters to the Editor, *Journal of Clinical Psychiatry* 51.9 (1990): 388. Also from personal interview with Dr. Goldberg. See also Jonathan Davidson, "Seizures and Buproprion: A Review," *Journal of Clinical Psychiatry* 50.7 (1989): 258.

p. 275   "Wellbutrin had stimulant . . ." Psychopharmacologic Drugs Advisory Committee, p. 15.

pp. 275–276 "Although women make . . ." Nancy Felipe Russo, ed., *A Woman's Mental Health Agenda* (Washington, D.C.: American Psychological Association, 1985), p. 20.

p. 276   "Women receive up to . . ." Russo, p. 21.

p. 276   "Overall, women have . . ." Jean Hamilton, Advanced Curriculum on Women's Health, Part I—Midlife and Mature Years, American Medical Women's Association, New York, 29 Oct. 1993.

p. 276   "A 1992 article . . ." Psychotropic Drugs and Myocardial Infarction: Cause for or Caused by Panic?" *Lancet* 340 (31 Oct. 1992): 1069.

p. 276   "Seventy percent more . . ." Eichler and Parron, p. 8.

p. 276   "While working at . . ." Jean A. Hamilton, "Biases in Women's Health Research," *Women & Therapy*, 12.4 (1992): 96–98. Also personal interview, 27 March 1993. Unless otherwise noted, subsequent information attributed to Hamilton came from this interview or the above-mentioned paper.

p. 277   "In 1983 Hamilton . . ." Jean A. Hamilton and Barbara Parry, "Sex-Related Differences in Clinical Drug Response: Implications for Women's Health," *Journal of the American Medical Women's Association* 38.5 (1983): 126–31.

p. 277   ". . . not one study . . ." Confirmed by Sophia Glezos of the Office of Scientific Information, NIMH, 27 June 1994.

p. 277   "The studies . . ." Hamilton.

p. 277   "At a November . . ." Jean A. Hamilton, "Sex Differences in Metabolism and Pharmacokinetics," Effects on Agent Choice and Dosing," Somatic Treatments of Mood Disorders in Women, Toward a New Psychobiology of Depression in Women: Treatment and Gender, National Institute of Mental Health, Bethesda, MD, 4 Nov. 1993.

p. 277   "Some twenty years . . ." Hamilton.

p. 277   "For instance it's . . ." Jean A. Hamilton and Margaret F. Jensvold, "Pharmacotherapy for Complicated Depressions in Women," *The Psychiatric Times* VIII.5 (1991): 50.

p. 277   "In women over sixty-five . . ." Hamilton, "Sex Differences in Metabolism . . ."

p. 278   "Some women . . ." Hamilton. Also Jensvold.

p. 278   "Margaret Jensvold . . ." Jensvold, personal interview, 22 Sept. 1991.

p. 278   " 'The moral is . . .' " Jensvold.

p. 278   "Judi Chamberlin knows . . ." Judi Chamberlin, personal interview, 25 Feb. 1994.

p. 279   "Like Chamberlin . . ." Jeanne Dumont, personal interview, 25 Feb. 1994.

p. 279   ". . . psychiatrist Peter Breggin . . ." Breggin.

p. 279   "It's particularly . . ." Breggin, *Toxic Psychiatry*, p. 322.

pp. 279–280 "Hospitalized women . . ." Breggin, p. 322.

p. 280   ". . . what psychologist Phyllis . . ." Phyllis Chesler, *Women and Madness*, cited in Breggin, p. 324.

p. 280   "Institutionalization is . . ." Peggy Thoits, position paper, in Eichler and Parron, p. 82.

p. 280   "Once hospitalized . . ." Breggin.

p. 280   "At the top . . ." Breggin.

p. 280   "As Chamberlin . . ." Chamberlin.

p. 280   "A psychiatric nurse . . ." A nurse who asked to remain anonymous, personal interview, 3 March 1993.

p. 280   "In a widely cited . . ." Sarah Rosenfield, "Sex Roles and Societal Reactions to Mental Illness: The Labeling of 'Deviant' Deviance," *Journal of Health and Social Behavior* 23 (1982): 19, 20, 22.

p. 281   "Women are more . . ." Angela Barron McBride, position paper, in Eichler and Parron, p. 30.

p. 281   "Vanessa Savage . . ." Vanessa Savage (a pseudonym), personal interview, 2 March 1994. All subsequent quotes attributed to Savage are from this interview.

p. 282   "Writes Breggin . . ." Breggin, p. 324.

p. 282   "Ultimately, writes . . ." Breggin, pp. 325–26.

p. 282   "Shock therapy . . ." Breggin, p. 185.

p. 282   "Although the . . ." *The Practice of Electroconvulsive Therapy: Recommendations for Treatment, Training, and Privileging*. A Task Force Report of the American Psychiatric Association (Washington, D.C.: American Psychiatric Association, 1990), pp. 51–55. See also "Neurological Devices: Proposed Rule to Reclassify the Electroconvulsive Therapy Device Intended for Use in Treating Severe Depression," Food and Drug Administration, *Federal Register* 55.172 (1990): 36580. In its proposed rule the FDA noted that 90 percent of patients treated with ECT improved, versus 74 percent treated with adequate drug therapy.

            A 1985 NIH Consensus Development Conference Statement (vol. 5, no. 11) noted ECT's "significant side effects, especially acute confusional states and persistent memory deficits for events during the months surrounding the ECT treatment."

p. 282   "Susan Witte . . ." Susan Witte, personal interview, 26 Feb. 1994.

p. 283   "No one told . . ." Harold Sackeim, et al., "Effects of Stimulus Intensity and Electrode Placement on the Efficacy and Cognitive Effects of Electroconvulsive Therapy," *New England Journal of Medicine* 328.12 (1993): 839–46. Forty-one (or 59 percent) of the seventy patients who responded to ECT in this study relapsed. For a discussion of continuation and maintenance ECT, see *The Practice of Electroconvulsive Therapy*, p. 112.

p. 283   "Lee Coleman . . ." Lee Coleman, personal interview, 7 March 1994.

p. 283   "Especially vulnerable . . ." Breggin.

p. 283   "In December 1993 . . ." Brief and Argument, Re estate of Lucille Austwick, Appellate Court of Illinois, First Judicial District, Fourth Division, pp. 13–20. Unless otherwise noted, all facts about Austwick come from this brief.

p. 284   " 'I've explained . . .' " "Woman, 80, Fights Forced Shock Therapy," *New York Times*, 31 Dec. 1993, A-18.

p. 284   " 'Back in the early . . ." Sharon Wilsnack, personal interview, 5 Jan. 1994.

p. 284   " . . . a book titled . . ." McClelland, D. C., et al., eds., *The Drinking Man* (New York: Free Press, 1972).

p. 284   "In one such study . . ." W. H. George, et al., "Male Perceptions of the Drinking Woman: Is Liquor Quicker?" Presented at the Eastern Psychological Association, New York, 1986. Cited in Sheila B. Blume, "Sexuality and Stigma: The Alcoholic Woman," *Alcohol Health & Research World* 15.2 (1991): 141.

p. 285   "Research shows . . ." Blume, p. 143.

p. 285   "In a survey . . ." Wilsnack.

p. 285   " 'Thus, the stereotype . . .' " Sheila B. Blume, "Women, Alcohol, and Drugs," *Comprehensive Handbook of Drug and Alcohol Addiction*, ed. Norman S. Miller (New York: Marcel Dekker, Inc., 1991), p. 149.

p. 285   "Concerned that women . . ." Sheila B. Blume, "Clinical Research on Alcohol and
               Women: Gaps and Opportunities," *Assessing Future Research Needs, Mental and Ad-
               dictive Disorders in Women,* Summary of an Institute of Medicine Conference, Oct.
               1991, pp. 79–80.

p. 285   "Investigators found . . ." Blume, pp. 79–80.

p. 285   "A second look . . ." Marsha Vannicelli, "Women and Alcohol: Health-Related Is-
               sues," Proceedings of a Conference, National Institute on Alcohol Abuse and Alco-
               holism, 23–25 May 1984, pp. 133–34.

pp. 284–285 "Likewise a review . . ." Constance Weisner, *Assessing Future Research Needs,* p. 85.

p. 286   " 'If one is . . .' " Beth Glover Reed, *Assessing Future Research Needs,* p. 98.

p. 286   "Thirty percent . . ." Thomas Murphy, "The Need for Women Specific Program-
               ming in Treatment for Drug and Alcohol Dependence," paper presented at the
               18th International Institute on the Prevention and Treatment of Drug Dependence,
               West Berlin, 1990. See also B. F. Grant, T. C. Harford, et al., "Prevalence of DSM-
               III-R Alcohol Abuse and Dependence: United States, 1988," *Alcohol Health & Re-
               search World* 15.1 (1991): 91–96. The authors reported that approximately 4.36
               percent of women met DSM-III-R criteria for alcohol abuse and dependence. An
               Institute of Medicine report, *Broadening the Base of Treatment for Alcohol Problems*
               (1990, p. 356) noted that "the male-to-female ratio in national prevalence rates for
               alcohol problems and dependence appears to be about 2 to 1."

p. 286   "When appropriate . . ." Anne Geller, Advanced Curriculum on Women's Health,
               Part I—Midlife and Mature Years, American Medical Women's Association, New
               York, 1 Nov. 1993.

pp. 286–287 " 'Women are misdiagnosed . . .' " Sheila Blume, personal interview, 26 Feb. 1994.

p. 287   "A number of simple . . ." The questions in the TWEAK test are:
               How many drinks does it take to make you feel high?
               Have close friends or relatives worried or complained about your drinking
               in the past year?
               Do you sometimes take a drink in the morning when you first get up?
               Has a friend or family member ever told you about things you said or did
               while you were drinking that you could not remember?
               Do you sometimes feel the need to cut down on your drinking?

p. 287   "Of more than . . ." Substance Abuse and Mental Health Services Administration,
               National Drug and Alcoholism Treatment Unit Survey (NDATUS), Main Findings
               Report (1991), pp. 21–22.

p. 287   "No one consciously . . ." Blume.

p. 287   "In the mid-seventies . . ." Dean R. Gerstein and Henrick J. Harwood, eds., Insti-
               tute of Medicine, *Treating Drug Problems* (Washington, D.C.: National Academy
               Press, 1990), p. 11.

p. 287   "Women alcoholics start . . ." *Broadening the Base of Treatment for Alcohol Problems*
               (Washington, D.C.: National Academy Press, 1990), p. 357.

p. 287   "Not only are female . . ." *Broadening the Base . . . ,* p. 357. Blume, in Miller,
               p. 159. Also Sharon Wilsnack, "Childhood Sexual Abuse and Women's Substance
               Abuse: National Survey Findings," paper presented at the American Psychological
               Association Conference, "Psychosocial and Behavioral Factors in Women's Health:
               Creating an Agenda for the 21st Century," Washington, D.C., 13 May 1994.
               Wilsnack found a significant association between a history of childhood sexual
               abuse and use of alcohol and drugs as an adult among a national sample of 1,100
               women age twenty-one and older.

p. 287   "In one survey . . ." Sharon Wilsnack, *Assessing Future Research Needs,* p. 16.

p. 287   "Another study found . . . ." Eichler and Parron, p. 35.

p. 288   "Women become physically . . ." Blume.

p. 288   "The phases of . . ." Blume.

p. 288   "Women reach higher . . ." Blume.

p. 288   "Blood alcohol . . ." Blume.

p. 288   "Women alcoholics tend . . ." Constance Weisner, "Treatment Services Research
               and Alcohol Problems: Treatment Entry, Access, and Effectiveness," *Assessing Future
               Research Needs,* p. 88.

p. 288   "Men abandon . . ." Geller.
p. 288   "Women develop . . ." Geller.
p. 288   "As few as . . ." W. C. Willett, et al., "Moderate Alcohol Consumption and the Risk
             of Breast Cancer," *New England Journal of Medicine* 316.19 (1987): 1174–80.
p. 288   "Women alcoholics are at . . ." Geller.
p. 288   "Women alcoholics are more . . ." Geller.
p. 288   "Back then . . ." Reed, p. 93.
p. 288   "Programs have traditionally . . ." Reed, p. 94.
p. 289   "Jean Kirkpatrick . . ." Jean Kirkpatrick, personal interview, 17 Jan. 1994.
p. 289   " 'There are a . . .' " LeClair Bissell, personal interview, 4 Jan. 1994.
p. 290   "Only 10 percent . . ." *NDATUS*, p. 64.
p. 290   "An evaluation of . . ." Wilsnack.
p. 290   "Eighteen studies . . ." Wilsnack.
p. 290   "Muses Sharon Wilsnack . . ." Wilsnack.
p. 290   "In an attempt . . ." Frances Del Boca, personal interview, 19 Jan. 1994.
p. 290   "Between 1985 and . . ." American Civil Liberties Union, *Criminal Prosecutions
             Against Pregnant Women: National Update and Overview* (New York: ACLU, 1992).
p. 290   "In a recent case . . ." Sheila B. Blume, "Women and Alcohol: Issues in Social Pol-
             icy," in Richard W. Wilsnack and Sharon C. Wilsnack, *Gender and Alcohol*, in
             press, p. 19.
p. 291   "Until recently . . ." Blume.
p. 291   "One woman, Ana R. . . ." Blume, pp. 19–20.
p. 291   " 'There was a tremendous . . .' " Paula Roth, personal interview, 19 Jan. 1994.
p. 291   "Fetal rights . . ." Wilsnack.
p. 291   "A 1990 General . . ." *Drug-Exposed Infants: A Generation at Risk*, General Account-
             ing Office, June 1990, p. 36.
pp. 291–292 "When Wendy Chavkin . . ." Wendy Chavkin, personal interview, 25 Feb. 1994.
p. 292   "Historically, psychiatry . . ." Karen Johnson, "The Making of a Woman's Psychi-
             atrist: Residency Training and Clinical Practice from a Feminist Biopsychosocial
             Perspective," *Psychiatric Annals* 23.8 (1993): 463.

12: DRUG MARKETING
Selling Women Out

p. 295   "They also pitch advertising . . ." The statistic that women make up 70 percent of
             drugstore shoppers comes from Dianne Tharp, "Editor's Note: Remember When
             We Only Whispered About Female Problems?," *Drugstore News for the Pharmacist*,
             16 Aug. 1993.
p. 295   "Studies show . . ." Jerry Avorn, et al., "Scientific versus Commercial Sources of In-
             fluence on the Prescribing Behavior of Physicians," *American Journal of Medicine*,
             73 (1982): 7. Also Russell R. Miller, "Prescribing Habits of Physicians," *Drug In-
             telligence and Clinical Pharmacy*, 8 (1974): 81–91. And Lawrence S. Linn and
             Milton S. Davis, "Physicians' Orientation Toward the Legitimacy of Drug Use and
             Their Preferred Source of New Drug Information," *Social Science & Medicine* 6
             (1972): 199–203.
p. 296   "Pharmaceutical drug-promotion . . ." Michael S. Wilkes, et al., "Pharmaceutical
             Advertisements in Leading Medical Journals: Experts' Assessments," *Annals of Inter-
             nal Medicine*, 116.11 (1992): 917.
p. 296   "One study found . . ." Wilkes, *Annals of Internal Medicine*, p. 914.
p. 296   " 'Clearly because of the number . . .' " Joellen Hawkins, personal interview, 7 Feb.
             1994.
p. 296   "Studies show that even when doctors . . ." Jerry Avorn, et al., "Scientific versus
             Commercial Sources of Influence on the Prescribing Behavior of Physicians," *Amer-
             ican Journal of Medicine* 73 (1982): 4–8.
p. 296   " 'Drug advertisements are simply more . . .' " Avorn, *American Journal of Medicine*,
             p. 8.
p. 296   "Three-quarters of physicians . . ." M. Gershenson, "Pharmaceutical Detailman
             Survey," *The Internist*, Feb. 1971, pp. 4–5.

p. 296   "An article in the professional journal . . ." Wilkes, *Annals of Internal Medicine*, p. 916.

p. 296   "The study also found . . ." Wilkes, *Annals of Internal Medicine*, p. 912.

p. 297   "Joellen Hawkins and colleague . . ." Joellen W. Hawkins and Cynthia S. Aber, "Women in Advertisements in Medical Journals," *Sex Roles*, 28.3-4 (1993): 233–42. Hawkins and Aber, "The Content of Advertisements in Medical Journals: Distorting the Image of Women," *Women & Health* 14.2 (1988): 43–59.

p. 297   " 'Interestingly, we did not find . . .' " Joellen Hawkins, personal interview, 7 Feb. 1994. All subsequent quotes from Ms. Hawkins, unless attributed to her published studies, are from this interview.

p. 297   "She found that the advertisers . . ." Ronda Macchello, personal interview, 15 Feb. 1994. All subsequent quotes from Dr. Macchello are from this interview.

p. 297   "Women in drug ads . . ." Hawkins and Aber, 1988, p. 52.

p. 297   " 'Not one ad portrays . . .' " Hawkins and Aber, 1988, p. 52.

p. 298   "Write Hawkins and Aber . . ." Hawkins and Aber, 1988, p. 53.

p. 298   "One popular ad . . ." This ad, by Mead Johnson Pharmaceuticals, a Bristol-Myers Squibb Company, was copyrighted 1991, and appeared, for example, on the back cover of the *New England Journal of Medicine*, 24 June 1993.

p. 298   "Women make up 80 percent . . ." Ronda Macchello, "Gender Issues in Medical Advertising." Dr. Macchello presented this paper at a conference titled, "Controversies in Women's Health" sponsored by the University of California, San Francisco, and held in San Francisco on December 2–3, 1993.

p. 298   " 'There's a real abuse of women . . .' " Ann Turkel, personal interview, 21 Jan. 1994.

p. 299   "Eva Lynn Thompson, who published . . ." Eva Lynn Thompson, "Sexual Bias in Drug Advertisements," *Social Science & Medicine*, 13A (1979): 187–91.

p. 300   "He wrote, 'The burden . . .' " Robert Seidenberg, "Drug Advertising and Perception of Mental Illness," *Mental Hygiene* 55.1 (1971): 22, 26.

p. 300   " 'That is, women may display . . .' " Jane Prather and Linda S. Fidell, "Sex Differences in the Content and Style of Medical Advertisements," *Social Science & Medicine* 9 (1975): 24.

p. 300   "Some of the comments were . . ." Christine McRee, et al., "Psychiatrists' Responses to Sexual Bias in Pharmaceutical Advertising," *American Journal of Psychiatry* 131.11 (1974): 1274.

pp. 300–301 "One early study listed . . ." E. H. Mosher, "Portrayal of Women in Drug Advertising: A Medical Betrayal," *Journal of Drug Issues* 6 (1976): 73.

p. 301   " 'It takes a certain amount of confidence . . .' " Joan Lemler, personal interview, 4 March 1994. All subsequent quotes from Ms. Lemler are from this interview.

p. 302   " 'Advertisers of over-the-counter drugs . . .' " R. Stephen Craig, personal interview, 16 Feb. 1994. All subsequent quotes from Mr. Craig, unless specified from his published study, come from this interview.

p. 302   "He writes, 'This supports . . .' " R. Stephen Craig, "Women as Home Caregivers: Gender Portrayal in OTC Drug Commercials," *Journal of Drug Education* 22.4 (1992): 303.

p. 302   "Unlike the men in prescription drug ads . . ." Craig, *Journal of Drug Education*, p. 310.

p. 303   "According to Craig's study . . ." Craig, *Journal of Drug Education*, p. 311.

p. 303   " 'I never understood the concept . . .' " Dr. Mitchell spoke at the conference, "Meeting the Health Care Needs of Women: Developing a Funders' Agenda" (sponsored by Grantmakers in Health, and Women and Foundations/Corporate Philanthropy), held in New York, 22 Jan. 1992.

p. 304   "One brochure for a birth control pill . . ." Brochures for Ovcon 35 and Ovcon 50, both from Mead Johnson Laboratories, a Bristol-Myers Squibb Company, ran this slogan. The brochures were dated Jan. 1993 and handed out to physicians at medical conferences throughout the year.

p. 304   "Another ad has a woman saying . . ." This ad, for Triphasil (Wyeth-Ayerst Laboratories), appeared in medical journals, including the back cover of *Obstetrics & Gynecology* 82.2 (1993).

p. 304   "In an ad for estrogen ..." This ad, for Premarin (Wyeth-Ayerst Laboratories), appeared in many women's magazines, and in *Health*, Sept./Oct. 1993.

p. 305   "In general, drugs are more expensive ..." Philip J. Hilts, "Canada Is Found to Lead U.S. in Holding Drug Prices Down," *New York Times*, 22 Feb. 1993, p. A11. Gina Kolata, "U.S. Is Asked to Control Prices of Drugs It Develops," *New York Times*, 25 April 1993, p. 36. Robert Pear, "Report Finds Pills Cost More in U.S. than Britain," *New York Times*, 3 Feb. 1994, p. A16. Greg Borzo, "Study: Rx Drugs Cost More in U.S. Than U.K.," *American Medical News*, 21 Feb. 1994, pp. 5–6.

p. 305   "A General Accounting Office study ..." Pear, *New York Times*, 3 Feb. 1994. Borzo, *American Medical News*, 21 Feb. 1994.

p. 305   "Premarin (estrogen), for example ..." Pear, *New York Times*, 3 Feb. 1994.

p. 305   "Norplant, the recently approved ..." This section, on Norplant's cost, was complied from a variety of sources, including Philip J. Hilts, "Contraceptive Maker to Charge Clinics Less," *New York Times*, 11 Nov. 1993, p. B12. "Drug Manufacturer Accused of Profiteering on Norplant," *American Medical News*, 6 Dec. 1993, p. 34. Warren E. Leary, "Long-Term Contraceptives' Cost Called Excessive," *New York Times*, 19 March 1994, p. 10.

pp. 305–306   "When Upjohn began marketing ..." Harvey F. Wachsman, "Regulate the Drug Monopolies," *New York Times*, 16 Jan. 1993, p. 21. And "Sticker Shock," *Time*, 25 Jan. 1993, p. 24.

p. 306   "For instance, when Levamisole ..." Wachsman, *New York Times*, 16 Jan. 1993.

p. 306   "Analysts predicted first-year sales ..." Terence Poltrack, "Blondes, Brunettes, Redheads, and Rogaine," *American Druggist*, June 1992, p. 39.

p. 306   " 'That nod of approval ...' " Poltrack, *American Druggist*, p. 39.

p. 307   "The average cost of treatment ..." Poltrack, *American Druggist*, p. 40.

p. 307   "U.S. sales of the drug are now ..." Jeff Palmer, Upjohn Company.

p. 307   "The *American Druggist* article ..." Poltrack, p. 40.

p. 307   "While K-Y jelly, the old standard ..." Diane Debrovner, "The New VD," *American Druggist*, Feb. 1993, p. 40.

p. 307   "An estimated forty million baby boomers ..." Andrew A. Skolnick, "At Third Meeting, Menopause Experts Make the Most of Insufficient Data," *Journal of the American Medical Association* 268.18 (1992): 2483.

p. 307   "Another article in *American Druggist* ..." Diane Debrovner, "The New VD," *American Druggist*, Feb. 1993, pp. 38–43.

p. 307   "According to the article ..." Debrovner, p. 39.

p. 307   "Says Georgia Witkin ..." Debrovner, p. 40.

p. 308   "The market is estimated at between ..." Debrovner, p. 40.

p. 308   "In one study ..." Debrovner, p. 42.

p. 308   " 'Traditionally, vaginal dryness has not ...' " Joseph Robinson of Columbia Laboratories, which developed Replens, quoted in Debrovner, p. 43.

p. 308   "One pharmacy industry newspaper ..." "Self Diagnosis Rockets Fem Hygiene Sales," *Drugstore News for the Pharmacist*, 16 Aug. 1993.

p. 309   "One pharmacy journal ..." Eliot Glazer, "Medical Marketing Case History: How Gyne-Lotrimin Cleared the Hurdles in Entering the OTC Market," *Medical Marketing & Media*, Feb. 1992, p. 60.

pp. 309–310   "In 1993 the FDA's Fertility ..." "FDA Committee Urges OC Labeling Change," *The Female Patient*, Aug. 1993, pp. 57–58.

p. 310   "Some of these health advocates ..." David A. Grimes, "Editorial: Over-the-Counter Oral Contraceptives—An Immodest Proposal?" *American Journal of Public Health* 83.8 (1993): 1092.

p. 310   "The National Women's Health Network ..." "Oral Contraceptive Availability Without a Prescription," press release, National Women's Health Network, Washington, D.C.

p. 310   "The poll, of 997 women ..." "Poll Shows Women Still Skeptical of Contraceptive Safety," press release, American College of Obstetricians and Gynecologists, 20 Jan. 1994.

p. 310   "In January 1993 the FDA ..." Elyse Tanouye and Rose Gutfeld, "Talks Canceled on Making 'Pill' Nonprescription," *Wall Street Journal*, 28 Jan. 1993, pp. B1, B6.

p. 311   "In 1993, jumping on the new women's . . ." "New Medicines in Development for
           Women," Pharmaceutical Manufacturers Association, Washington, D.C., June 1993.

                              13: WOMEN AND THE LAW
                                  Unhealthy Judgments

           In addition to the citations below, valuable background information was obtained
           from the following articles:

           On pregnant women's autonomy and maternal-fetal conflict:
           Andrews, Lori B. "A Delicate Condition," *Student Lawyer*, May 1985, pp. 30–36.
           Chavkin, Wendy, "Women and Fetus: The Social Construction of Conflict," *The
           Criminalization of a Woman's Body*, ed. Clarice Feinman (New York: The Haworth
           Press, 1992), pp. 193–202.
           Goldberg, Susan. "Medical Choices During Pregnancy: Whose Decision Is It Any-
           way?" *Rutgers Law Review* 41.2 (1989): 591–623.
           Hubbard, Ruth. *The Politics of Women's Biology* (New Brunswick: Rutgers Univer-
           sity Press, 1990). See chapter 12, "Medical, Legal, and Social Implications of Pre-
           natal Technologies," pp. 147–78.
           Johnsen, Dawn. "Shared Interests: Promoting Healthy Births Without Sacrificing
           Women's Liberty," *Hastings Law Journal* 43 (1992): 569–614.
           Mattingly, Susan S. "The Maternal-Fetal Dyad: Exploring the Two-Patient Obstet-
           ric Model," *Hastings Center Report*, Jan–Feb. 1992, pp. 13–18.

           On court-ordered cesarean sections:
           Curran, William J. "Court-Ordered Cesarean Sections Receive Judicial Defeat,"
           New England Journal of Medicine 323.7 (1990): 489–92.
           Daniels, Janean Acevedo. "Court-Ordered Cesareans: A Growing Concern for In-
           digent Women," *Clearinghouse Review: National Clearinghouse for Legal Services, Inc.*
           21.9 (1988): 1064–70.
           Gallagher, Janet. "Prenatal Invasions & Interventions: What's Wrong with Fetal
           Rights?" *Harvard Woman's Law Journal* 10 (1987): 9–58.
           Goetze, Andrea. "Court-Ordered Cesarean Sections: Probing the Wound," *Texas
           Journal of Women and the Law* 1 (1992): 59–94.
           Hewson, Barbara. "Mother Knows Best," *New Law Journal* 142.6575 (1992):
           1538–46.
           Nelson, Lawrence J. "The Mother and Fetus Union: What God Has Put Together,
           Let No Law Put Asunder?" in F. K. Beller and R. F. Weir (eds.), *The Beginning of
           Human Life* (The Netherlands: Kluwer Academic Publishers, 1994), pp. 301–17.
           Nelson, Lawrence J., Brian Buggy, and Carol J. Weil. "Forced Medical Treatment
           of Pregnant Women: 'Compelling Each to Live as Seems Good to the Rest,' " *Hast-
           ings Law Journal* 37 (1986): 703–63.
           Nelson, Lawrence J., and Nancy Milliken. "Compelled Medical Treatment of Preg-
           nant Women," *Journal of the American Medical Association* 259.7 (1988): 1060–66.
           Noble-Alligire, Alice. "Court-Ordered Cesarean Sections," *Journal of Legal Medicine*
           10.1 (1989): 211–49.
           Rhoden, Nancy K. "The Judge in the Delivery Room: The Emergence of Court-
           Ordered Cesareans," *California Law Review* 74.6 (1986): 1951–2030.
           Williams, Annette. "*In re A. C.*: Foreshadowing the Unfortunate Expansion of
           Court-Ordered Cesarean Sections," *Iowa Law Review* 74 (1988): 287–302.

           On prosecutions of pregnant women for substance abuse:
           Barrett, Kristen. "Prosecuting Pregnant Addicts for Dealing to the Unborn," *Ari-
           zona Law Review* 33 (1991): 221–37.
           Becker, Barrie L. "Order in the Court: Challenging Judges Who Incarcerate Preg-
           nant, Substance-Dependent Defendants to Protect Fetal Health," *Hastings Constitu-
           tional Law Quarterly* 19.1 (1991): 235–59.
           Callahan, Joan C. and James W. Knight, "Prenatal Harm as Child Abuse?" *The*

Criminalization of a Woman's Body, ed. Clarice Feinman (New York: The Haworth Press, 1992), pp. 127–55.

Capron, Alexander Morgan. "Fetal Alcohol and Felony," *Hastings Center Report* May–June 1992, pp. 28–30.

Dobson, Tracy, and Kimberly K. Eby. "Criminal Liability for Substance Abuse During Pregnancy: The Controversy of Maternal v. Fetal Rights," *Saint Louis University Law Journal* 36 (1992): 655–94.

Field, Martha A. "Controlling the Woman to Protect the Fetus," *Law, Medicine & Health Care* 17.2 (1989): 114–29.

Lowry, Susan Steinhorn. "The Growing Trend to Criminalize Gestational Substance Abuse," *Journal of Juvenile Law* 13 (1992): 133–43.

Merrick, Janna C. "Maternal Substance Abuse During Pregnancy," *Journal of Legal Medicine* 14.1 (1993): 57–71.

Rubenstein, Laurie. "Prosecuting Maternal Substance Abusers: An Unjustified and Ineffective Policy," *Yale Law & Policy Review* 9 (1991): 130–60.

Schiff, Nancy K. "Legislation Punishing Drug Use During Pregnancy: Attack on Women's Rights in the Name of Fetal Protection," *Hastings Constitutional Law Quarterly* 19.1 (1991): 197–234.

On so-called fetal-protection employment policies and discrimination:

Dayton, Kim. "Patriarchy, Paternalism, and the Masks of 'Fetal Protection,' " *Kansas Journal of Law & Public Policy* 2.1 (1992): 25–32.

Evans-Stanton, Sherri. "Gender Specific Regulations in the Chemical Workplace," *Santa Clara Law Review* 27 (1987): 353–72.

Hamlet, Pendleton Elizabeth. "Fetal Protection Policies: A Statutory Proposal in the Wake of *International Union, UAW* v. *Johnson Controls, Inc.*, *Cornell Law Review* 75.5 (1990): 1110–50.

Longi, Maria A. "*International Union, UAW* v. *Johnson Controls, Inc.*: Can Science Ever Justify Gender Discrimination?" *Northern Kentucky Law Review* 19.2 (1992): 425–48.

p. 314   " 'Sometimes the unfairness . . .' " Marcia Greenberger, personal interview, 7 March 1994. All subsequent quotes from Ms. Greenberger are taken from this interview.

p. 314   "Obstetrical suits are the most common . . ." "Suits Over Breast Cancer Exams Up," *Medical Tribune*, 9 July 1992. "Failure-to-Diagnose Suits Continue," *The Female Patient* 18 (1993): 47.

p. 314   "Along with articles . . ." Examples of these articles include: "Avoiding Suit Over Failure to Diagnose Breast Cancer," *Internal Medicine News*, 1–14 Aug. 1991, p. 8. Marvin A. Dewar and Neil Love, "Legal Issues in Managing Breast Disease," *Postgraduate Medicine* 92.5 (1992): 137.

p. 315   "The study found . . ." LaRae I. Huycke and Mark M. Huycke, "Characteristics of Potential Plaintiffs in Malpractice Litigation," *Annals of Internal Medicine* 120.9 (1994): 792–98.

p. 315   " 'Women were being destroyed . . .' " Harvey Wachsman, personal interview, 2 March 1994.

p. 315   " 'If a woman who has been . . .' " Karen Rothenberg, personal interview, 7 March 1994. All subsequent quotes from Ms. Rothenberg are from this interview.

p. 316   " 'The real conflict . . .' " Lawrence Nelson, personal interview, 9 March 1994. All subsequent quotes from Mr. Nelson are taken from this interview.

p. 317   " 'What would fetal rights be?' " Lynn Paltrow, personal interview, 8 March 1994. All subsequent quotes from Ms. Paltrow are from this interview.

p. 317   "According to Lori B. Andrews . . ." Lori Andrews spoke at a March of Dimes editorial luncheon, "Maternal-Fetal Conflict: The Ultimate Dilemma," New York, 28 May 1992.

p. 318   "In 1987 Angela Carder . . ." *In re A. C. Appellant*, 573 A.2d 1235 (D.C. App. 1990). Angela Carder's case was widely reported in the legal and popular press, and the details have been compiled from a variety of sources, including some of those listed in the chapter bibliography.

p. 318   "In 1987 the *New England Journal of Medicine* . . ." Veronika E. B. Kolder, et al., "Court-Ordered Obstetrical Interventions," *New England Journal of Medicine* 316.19 (1987): 1192.

p. 319   " 'In 99.9 percent of cases . . .' " Ann Allen, personal interview, 8 March 1994. All subsequent quotes from Ms. Allen are from this interview. ACOG's policy on maternal-fetal conflict is set out in a brief paper entitled, "Patient Choice: Maternal-Fetal Conflict," ACOG Committee Opinion No. 55, Oct. 1987.

p. 319   "Hundreds of thousands . . ." For more information on the exceptionally high rate of cesarean sections, see Chapter 7 on surgery.

p. 320   "Andrews says she knows . . ." Lori Andrews spoke at a March of Dimes editorial luncheon, "Maternal-Fetal Conflict: The Ultimate Dilemma," New York, 28 May 1992.

p. 320   " 'Going to court . . .' " Richard H. Schwarz spoke at the March of Dimes editorial luncheon, above.

p. 320   "In 1981 Jessie Mae Jefferson . . ." *Jessie Mae Jefferson* v. *Griffin Spalding County Hospital Authority et al.,* Ga., 274 S.E. 2d 457 (Supreme Court of Georgia, 3 Feb. 1981). Additional information on this case compiled from a wide variety of sources, including some of those listed in the chapter bibliography.

p. 321   "The decision . . ." *McFall* v. *Shimp*, 10 D&C 3d 90 (1978).

p. 321   "In mid-1993 . . ." Illinois case described in: Don Terry, "Illinois Is Seeking to Force Woman to Have Caesarean," *New York Times,* 14 Dec. 1993, p. A11. "Court Rebuffs Move to Force Woman to Have Caesarean," *New York Times,* 17 Dec. 1993, p. A33.

p. 322   "Consider the case of . . ." Lori Andrews, at March of Dimes editorial lunch, 28 May 1992. Also described in "Who Decides for Women?" by Andrea Boroft Eagan, *American Health,* Sept. 1990, p. 42.

p. 322   "Yet in 1986 . . ." "Mother Charged with Abuse for Drinking in Pregnancy," *American Medical News* 27 July 1992, p. 11. Also in Marilyn French, *The War Against Women* (New York: Summit Books, 1992), p. 144.

p. 323   "In 1993 there were fifty-one bills . . ." Terry Sollom, "State Legislation on Reproductive Health in 1992: What was Proposed and Enacted," *Family Planning Perspectives* 25.2 (1993): 90. Updated for 1993 by phone with the Alan Guttmacher Institute, April 1994.

p. 323   "For example, a new law . . ." Terry Sollom, *Family Planning Perspectives* 25.2 (1993): 90.

p. 323   "Minnesota, however . . ." The Alan Guttmacher Institute, April 1994.

p. 323   "In 1991 two Washington state waiters . . ." "Pregnancy Police Miss the Mark," *The Los Angeles Daily Journal* (reprinted from *The Progressive*), 11 June 1991, p. 6.

p. 324   "In mid-1994 . . ." Philip J. Hilts, "Hospital Is Accused of Illegal Experiments," *New York Times* 21 Jan. 1994, p. A7. Also Philip J. Hilts, "Hospital Is Object of Rights Inquiry," *New York Times,* 6 Feb. 1994, p. 29. And John Roberts, "Hospital Accused of Experiments on Pregnant Women," *Lancet* 308 (1994): 291–92. Additional information from Lynn Paltrow, personal interview, 8 March 1994.

p. 324   "All fifty states . . ." David A. Smith, "Ruling Undercuts Pregnancy Restrictions," *Choice in Dying News* 1.3 (1992): 4.

p. 324   "But in thirty-four states . . ." "Pregnancy Restrictions in Living Will Statutes," *Choice in Dying,* Sept. 1993.

p. 324   "According to David A. Smith . . ." *Choice in Dying News* 1.3 (1992): 4.

p. 325   "One disturbing survey . . ." Steven H. Miles and Allison August, "Courts, Gender, and the 'Right to Die,' " *Law, Medicine and Health Care* 18.1–2 (1990): 85–95.

p. 325   "Says study author Steven Miles . . ." "Courts, Wills and Women," *New York Times,* 23 July 1990, p. A13.

p. 326   "In 1993 a study reported . . ." "AZT May Block in Utero Transmission of HIV," *Medical World News* 35.1 (1994): 11.

p. 326   "Now that medical advances . . ." Information on male reproductive risks from alcohol, drugs, and other toxins compiled from a variety of sources, including: Jane Brody, "Personal Health," *New York Times,* 25 Dec. 1991, p. 64; Donna Alvarado, "Fathers' Health and Fetal Harm," *Washington Post Health,* 20 Aug. 1991, p. 6;

Beth Weinhouse, "Dangerous Dads," *Redbook*, Dec. 1991, p. 150; and a March of Dimes editorial luncheon, "Real Men Do Get Pregnant: The Father's Role in Creating a Healthy Baby," *New York*, 10 Dec. 1991.

p. 326   "In 1991 the *Journal of the American Medical Association* . . ." Ricardo A. Yazigi, et al., "Demonstration of Specific Binding of Cocaine to Human Spermatozoa," *JAMA* 266.14 (1991): 1956–59.

pp. 326–327 "Commenting on the study . . ." "Paternal-Fetal Conflict," *Hastings Center Report*, March–April 1992, p. 3.

p. 327   "According to the ACLU's Joan Bertin . . ." Peter Jaret, "How Fathers Affect Their Babies," *Glamour*, Aug. 1991, p. 232.

p. 328   "Not long after . . ." "A Sterile Market," *Hastings Center Report*, July–Aug. 1992, p. 45.

14: WOMEN AND DOCTORS
A Troubled Relationship

p. 329   " 'The usual experience . . .' " John M. Smith, *Women and Doctors* (New York: Atlantic Monthly Press, 1992), p. 13.

p. 329   " 'The general mood is anger . . .' " Marianne J. Legato, "Reaching Across the Gender Gap," *The Female Patient* 18 (1992): 11.

p. 329   "Because women's health care . . ." Legato, *The Female Patient*.

p. 329   " 'Women, the old . . .' " Marianne Legato, personal interview, 23 May 1993.

p. 330   " 'If she's premenopausal . . .' " Isadore Rosenfeld, "Health Care for Women: Taking Affirmative Action," *Vogue*, Feb. 1993, p. 134.

p. 330   "In this century . . ." Barbara Ehrenreich and Deirdre English, *For Her Own Good: 150 Years of the Experts' Advice to Women* (Garden City, N.Y.: Anchor Press/ Doubleday, 1978), pp. 248–49.

p. 330   "One 1947 obstetrics textbook . . ." Joseph B. DeLee, and J. Greenhill, *Principles and Practice of Obstetrics* (Philadelphia: W. B. Saunders and Co., 9th ed., 1947), p. 112. (Dr. DeLee was the obstetrician responsible for the routine use of episiotomies—the incision between vagina and rectum supposedly performed to hasten a birth and prevent tearing, but which studies have found to be virtually useless and perhaps even harmful.)

p. 330   " 'Women are consistently described . . .' " Diana Scully and Pauline Bart, "A Funny Thing Happened on the Way to the Orifice: Women in Gynecology Textbooks," *American Journal of Sociology* 78.4 (1973): 1045.

p. 330   "A popular 1971 ob-gyn textbook . . ." J. R. Wilson, et al., *Obstetrics and Gynecology*, 4th ed. (St. Louis, MO: C. V. Mosby Co, 1971), cited in Kay Weiss, "What Medical Students Learn About Women," *Seizing Our Bodies*, ed. Claudia Dreifus (New York: Vintage Books, 1977), pp. 213–14.

p. 330   "When *JAMA* . . ." Ernest H. Friedman, letter, *Journal of the American Medical Association* 266.21 (1991): 2984.

p. 331   "In a 1993 Commonwealth Fund survey . . ." *The Commonwealth Fund Women's Health Survey* (New York: Louis Harris and Associates, Inc., 1993), p. 3.

p. 331   "A study of one thousand complaints . . ." Daniel Goleman, "All Too Often, the Doctor Isn't Listening, Studies Show," *New York Times*, 13 Nov. 1991, p. C15.

p. 331   " 'The most common complaints . . .' " Goleman, *New York Times*.

p. 331   "As an example, Frankel describes . . ." Goleman, *New York Times*.

p. 331   "Frankel has found . . ." Howard B. Beckman, and Richard M. Frankel, "The Effect of Physician Behavior on the Collection of Data," *Annals of Internal Medicine* 101.5 (1984): 694.

p. 332   " 'Physicians often experience . . .' " Richard Frankel, personal interview, 21 Jan. 1994.

p. 332   " 'Women are patronized . . .' " Ann Turkel, personal interview, 21 Jan. 1994.

p. 333   " 'I think women are kept waiting longer . . .' " Turkel, 21 Jan. 1994.

p. 333   "Advice columnist Ann Landers . . ." Dennis L. Breo, "A Few Words of Advice from a Woman of Letters—Ann Landers," *Journal of the American Medical Association* 268.14 (1992): 1930–31.

p. 333   "Women tend to ask more questions . . ." Debra L. Roter and Judith A. Hall, "Examining Gender-Specific Issues in Patient-Physician Communications," presented at the Women's Health and Primary Care Conference: Building a Research and Policy Agenda. Landsdowne Conference Resort, Leesburg, VA, June 1993.

p. 333   "Women also show more emotion ..." Roter and Hall, "Examining Gender-Specific Issues ..."

p. 333   "Men, on the other hand ..." Roter and Hall, "Examining Gender-Specific Issues ..."

p. 333   "During a typical ..." Sherrie Kaplan, speaking at the Annual Meeting of the Association for Health Services Research, Washington, D.C., July 1993. Reported in "Male Patients Suffer for Being Taciturn," *Wall Street Journal,* 9 July 1993, p. B7.

p. 333   " 'Practice makes perfect ...' " Sherrie Kaplan, personal interview, 26 Jan. 1994. All subsequent quotes attributed to Ms. Kaplan are from this interview.

p. 334   "Researchers have actually found ..." J. A. Hall, et al., "Physicians' Liking for Their Patients: More Evidence for the Role of Affect in Medical Care," *Health Psychology* 12 (1993): 140–46.

p. 334   "One study reported ..." Jacqueline Wallen, et al., "Physician Stereotypes About Female Health and Illness: A Study of Patients' Sex and the Informative Process During Medical Interviews," *Women & Health* 4.2 (1979): 145.

p. 334   " 'Medical textbooks from around ...' " Richard Frankel, personal interview, 27 Nov. 1991.

p. 335   " 'Physician folklore says ...' " Karen Carlson, in a talk entitled, "What Do Women Want in a Physician?" presented at the Annual Meeting of the American Medical Women's Association, New York, 30 Oct. 1993.

p. 335   "A 1979 study compared ..." Karen J. Armitage, et al., "Response of Physicians to Medical Complaints in Men and Women," *Journal of the American Medical Association* 241.20 (1979): 2186.

p. 335   "Another study found ..." Charlotte F. Muller, *Health Care and Gender* (New York: Russell Sage Foundation, 1990), p. 13. Muller's information comes from 1985 data provided by the U.S. Department of Health and Human Services.

p. 335   " 'The myth is that women complain more ...' " Karen Carlson, AMWA annual meeting, 30 Oct. 1993.

p. 336   "At a recent workshop ..." Susan E. Skochelak and Frederic W. Platt, "Patient/Physician Partner Workshop," presented at the Annual Meeting of the American Medical Women's Association, New York, 30 Oct. 1993.

p. 336   "When men without a ..." Muller, *Health Care and Gender,* p. 6.

p. 336   "In the Commonwealth Fund poll ..." *The Commonwealth Fund Women's Health Survey,* 1993, p. 33.

pp. 336–337 " 'If you brought your car ...' " Richard Frankel, personal interview, 27 Nov. 1991.

p. 337   "One 1993 article ..." Neil Baum, "How to Market Your Medical Practice to Women," *American Medical News,* 5 July 1993, p. 25.

p. 337   "Ob-gyn John Smith ..." *Women and Doctors,* p. 2.

p. 337   "A study of nearly 100,000 women ..." Nicole Lurie, et al., "Preventive Care for Women—Does the Sex of the Physician Matter?," *New England Journal of Medicine* 329.7 (1993): 478.

p. 338   "Male physicians are more likely ..." Edith B. Gross, "Gender Differences in Physician Stress," *Journal of the American Medical Women's Association* 48.4 (1992): 109.

p. 338   "Male doctors tend to interrupt ..." Candace West, "When the Doctor Is a 'Lady': Power, Status and Gender in Physician-Patient Encounters," *Symbolic Interaction* 7.1 (1984): 87.

p. 338   "Women physicians are more inclined ..." "When the Going Gets Tough," *Hastings Center Report,* July–Aug. 1993, p. 2.

p. 338   " 'Gender isn't something ...' " Candace West, personal interview, 29 Jan. 1994.

p. 338   " 'From the patient's point of view ...' " Deborah Allen, personal interview, 2 Feb. 1994. See also Deborah Allen, et al., "Caring for Women: Is It Different?" *Patient Care,* 15 Nov. 1993, pp. 183–99.

p. 339   "Julie was twenty-three ..." Anna Quindlen, "Mother and Child: The Legacy and Lesson of DES," *New York Times,* 9 May 1993, Sect. 4, p. 15.

p. 339   "When women patients are paired . . ." Debra Roter, et al., "Sex Differences in Patients' and Physicians' Communication During Primary Care Medical Visits," *Medical Care* 29.11 (1991): 1083–93.

p. 339   "Male and female physicians . . ." Candace West, personal interview, 28 Jan. 1994. Also see her article, "Not Just 'Doctors' Orders': Directive-Response Speech Sequences in Patients' Visits to Women and Men Physicians," *Discourse and Society* 1 (1990): 85–112.

p. 339   "The relationship between a woman physician . . ." Candace West, personal interview, 28 Jan. 1994. Also see her article, "Reconceptualizing Gender in Physician-Patient Relationships," *Social Science & Medicine*, Jan. 1993, pp. 57–66.

p. 339   "Candace West, whose work . . ." Personal interview, 28 Jan. 1994, plus "Not Just 'Doctors' Orders,' " *Discourse and Society* 1 (1990).

p. 339   "John Smith believes . . ." *Women and Doctors*, p. 29.

p. 339   "The caseload of female doctors . . ." Muller, *Health Care and Gender*, p. 10.

p. 339   " 'Women doctors spend more time . . .' " Steven Cohen-Cole, personal interview, 21 Jan. 1994.

p. 340   " 'The studies on how male and female . . .' " Debra Roter, personal interview, 31 Jan. 1994.

p. 340   "Recognizing that those skills . . ." Dennis H. Novack, et al., "Medical Interviewing and Interpersonal Skills Teaching in U.S. Medical Schools," *Journal of the American Medical Association* 269.16 (1993): 2101.

p. 340   "In 1993 the American College . . ." "Physicians Urged to Go 'Back to Basics,' " press release, American College of Obstetricians and Gynecologists, 5 May 1993. Report of ACOG's 41st Annual Clinical Meeting, Washington, D.C.

p. 340   "Said Richard S. Hollis, M.D. . . ." ACOG press release, 5 May 1993.

p. 341   " 'From one perspective women physicians . . .' " Richard Frankel, personal interview, 21 Jan. 1994.

p. 342   " 'Continuity of care is . . .' " Deborah Allen, personal interview, 2 Feb. 1994.

p. 342   " 'From my viewpoint . . .' " Dr. Lillian Gonzalez-Pardo, quoted in Judith Mandelbaum-Schmid, "An Unequal Past, A Common Future," *MD*, May 1992, p. 100.

15: THE FUTURE OF WOMEN'S HEALTH

p. 343   " 'It isn't enough . . .' " Karen Johnson, personal interview, 13 Sept. 1993.

p. 344   "One study found . . ." B. A. Bartman and K. B. Weiss, "Women's Health Care in the Ambulatory Care Setting," *Clinical Research* 39 (1991): 595A. Cited in Carolyn M. Clancy and Charlea T. Massion, "American Women's Health Care: A Patchwork Quilt with Gaps," *JAMA* 268.14 (1992): 1918–19.

p. 344   "Carolyn Clancy . . ." Clancy, *JAMA*.

p. 344   "In one telling . . ." Patricia A. Carney, et al., "The Periodic Health Examination Provided to Asymptomatic Older Women: An Assessment Using Standardized Patients," *Annals of Internal Medicine* 119.2 (1993): 129, 130, 132, 133.

p. 344   "In another study . . ." Survey of Women's Health, Commonwealth Fund, 14 July 1993, 6.

p. 344   "There's even evidence . . ." Nicole Lurie, et al., "Preventive Care for Women: Does the Sex of the Physician Matter?" *New England Journal of Medicine* 329.7 (1993): 478.

p. 344   " 'Medicine responded . . .' " Johnson.

p. 345   "In terms of services . . ." A Gallup Study of Women's Attitudes Toward the Use of Ob/Gyn for Primary Care, Oct. 1993, pp. 18, 20. Ob-gyns were much more likely to perform Pap smears (94 percent versus 53 percent for other types of doctors) and pelvic exams (91 percent versus 50 percent).

p. 345   "Now gynecologists . . ." Eileen Hoffman, personal interview, 13 March 1994.

p. 345   "The demographics . . ." Andrew A Skolnick, *Journal of the American Medical Association* 268.18 (1992): 2483.

p. 345   " 'By focusing on . . .' " Hoffman.

p. 345   "In 1993 the college . . ." *The Obstetrician-Gynecologist and Primary-Preventive Health Care*, American College of Obstetricians and Gynecologists, vol. V, 1993, 12–15.

p. 345   "These guidelines were . . ." *Primary Care Update for Ob/Gyns* 1.1 (1993): 1.

p. 346   "Although two-thirds . . ." Clancy.

p. 346   " 'The intestines . . .' " Hoffman, presentation, The New School, New York 10 March 1994.

p. 346   "An internist . . ." Hoffman, New School.

p. 346   " 'Medicine had divvied . . .' " Hoffman, New School.

p. 346   " 'I knew next to . . .' " Vivian Terkel, personal interview, 14 March 1994.

p. 346   "As Carolyn Clancy . . ." Clancy.

p. 347   " 'Nowhere does . . .' " Hoffman, New School.

p. 347   " 'If medicine was . . .' " Hoffman, New School.

p. 347   " 'My antenna . . .' " Hoffman, New School.

pp. 347–348 " 'There's nothing more . . .' " Marcia Greenberger, personal interview, 7 March 1994.

p. 348   "Right now . . ." Joan Kuriansky, Press Conference, Campaign for Women's Health, a project of the Older Women's League, Washington D.C., 24 Sept. 1993.

p. 348   " 'When women are . . .' " Greenberger.

p. 348   "As Leslie Wolfe . . ." Leslie Wolfe, personal interview, 18 June 1993.

p. 349   "At the new clinical . . ." Janet Henrich, personal interview, 22 Dec. 1992.

p. 349   "In late 1993 . . ." Terkel.

p. 349   " 'Women are starving . . .' " Terkel.

p. 349   "As Hoffman says . . ." Hoffman.

p. 350   "Yale is planning . . ." Henrich.

p. 350   "A study is currently . . ." Mary Lou Russell, Commonwealth Fund, personal conversation, 23 March 1994. The Commonwealth Fund is funding the Johns Hopkins study.

p. 350   "At a time when . . ." "Nursing Facts," the American Nurses Association (undated).

p. 350   "Studies show . . ." "A Meta-Analysis of Process of Care, Clinical Outcomes, and Cost Effectiveness of Nurses in Primary Care Roles: Nurse-Practitioners and Nurse-Midwives," American Nurses Association, rev. 7 Jan. 1993, p. 4.

p. 350   "To meet women's . . ." "Women's Primary Care Nursing" and "Women's Health Nurse-Practitioner," School of Nursing, University of California San Francisco (undated), pp. 2–7.

p. 350   " 'The public has . . .' ' Muriel Shore, personal interview, 13 May 1993.

p. 350   ". . . while nurse-practitioners . . ." Shore.

p. 350   "Women who are . . ." Deborah Morrill, N.P., personal interview, 16 May 1993.

p. 350   "The AMA strongly . . ." Randolph Smoak, Jr., AMA, personal interview, 18 May 1993.

p. 351   "Asks Janet Henrich . . ." Henrich.

p. 351   " 'As medical curricula . . .' " Karen Johnson, Plenary Session II, "Women's Health: A Medical Specialty?" 1st Annual Congress on Women's Health, Washington, D.C., 3 June 1993. See also Karen Johnson, "Women's Health: Developing a New Interdisciplinary Specialty," *Journal of Women's Health* 1.2 (1992): 95–99.

p. 351   "Physicians do not . . ." Johnson, 13 Sept. 1993.

p. 351   "Sue Rosser . . ." Sue V. Rosser, "A Model for a Specialty in Women's Health," *Journal of Women's Health* 2.2 (1993): 99–103.

p. 352   "When Carolyn Clancy . . ." Clancy.

p. 352   "Psychiatrist Michelle Harrison . . ." Michelle Harrison, Plenary Session II, "Women's Health: A Medical Specialty?" 1st Annual Congress on Women's Health, Washington, D.C., 3 June 1993. See also Michelle Harrison, "Women's Health as a Specialty: A Deceptive Solution," *Journal of Women's Health* 1.2 (1992): 101–106.

p. 352   "Currently fewer . . ." Karen Johnson, transcript of testimony before the Senate Committee on Insurance, Claims and Corporations, "Women's Health Insurance: Policy Options," San Francisco, 14 Dec. 1993, p. 3.

p. 352   " 'I shared my . . .' " Henrich.

p. 352   "Albert Einstein . . ." Program announcement, the Department of Medicine, Albert Einstein College of Medicine, 1993.

p. 352   "Women's health programs . . ." Rosser, p. 102.

p. 352   " 'I refer to this . . .' " Henrich.

p. 352   "To that end ..." News release, Medical College of Pennsylvania, 13 May 1994.
             Also Henrich.

p. 353   "On a larger scale ..." Lila Wallis, Course Announcements, Advanced Curriculum
             on Women's Health, American Medical Women's Association, New York, 29 Oct.
             1993.

p. 353   "By the year 2010 ..." *Women in Medicine in America* (Chicago: American Medical
             Association, 1991), p. 33.

p. 353   " 'Feminism is about ...' " Laura Helfman, "Feminism in Medicine," Women Pro-
             moting Women's Health, American Medical Women's Association, 78th Annual
             Meeting, New York, 7 Nov. 1993.

p. 353   "At the Breast Service ..." Alison Estabrook and Freya Schnabel, personal inter-
             views, 18 Aug. 1993.

INDEX

ABOUT THE AUTHORS

LESLIE LAURENCE is a medical journalist and author of a syndicated column, "Her Health," that appears in more than seventy-five newspapers nationwide. Her writing also appears in *Glamour, Town & Country,* and *Ladies' Home Journal.* She is a former reporter at *Money,* and a former senior writer at *Self* and *Condé Nast Traveler,* where she shared in a National Magazine Award.

BETH WEINHOUSE is a medical journalist who writes for *Glamour, Redbook,* and many other magazines. She has been a regular medical columnist for *Ladies' Home Journal, Self, Redbook,* and *Travel & Leisure,* and currently writes a column for *Remedy.* A former senior editor at *Ladies' Home Journal* and contributing editor at *Self,* she is the author of *The Healthy Traveler.*